Ethical Approaches to the Practice of Anesthesiology - Part 1: Overview of Ethics in Clinical Care: History and Evolution

Editors

NEAL H. COHEN
GAIL A. VAN NORMAN

ANESTHESIOLOGY CLINICS

www.anesthesiology.theclinics.com

Consulting Editor
LEE A. FLEISHER

September 2024 • Volume 42 • Number 3

ELSEVIER

1600 John F. Kennedy Boulevard • Suite 1800 • Philadelphia, Pennsylvania, 19103-2899

http://www.theclinics.com

ANESTHESIOLOGY CLINICS Volume 42, Number 3
September 2024 ISSN 1932-2275, ISBN-13: 978-0-443-24678-4

Editor: Joanna Gascoine
Developmental Editor: Anita Chamoli

Anesthesiology Clinics (ISSN 1932-2275) is published quarterly by Elsevier Inc., 360 Park Avenue South, New York, NY 10010-1710. Months of issue are March, June, September, and December. Periodicals postage paid at New York, NY and at additional mailing offices. Subscription prices are $100.00 per year (US student/resident), $398.00 per year (US individuals), $492.00 per year (Canadian individuals), $100.00 per year (Canadian student/resident), $225.00 per year (foreign student/resident), $528.00 per year (foreign individuals). For institutional access pricing please contact Customer Service via the contact information below. To receive student and resident rate, orders must be accompanied by name of affiliated institution, date of term, and the *signature* of program/residency coordinator on institutions letterhead. Orders will be billed at individual rate until proof of status is received. Foreign air speed delivery is included in all *Clinics'* subscription prices. All prices are subject to change without notice. Orders, claims, and journal inquiries: Please visit our Support Hub page https://service.elsevier.com for assistance.

Reprints. For copies of 100 or more of articles in this publication, please contact the Commercial Reprints Department, Elsevier Inc., 360 Park Avenue South, New York, NY 10010-1710. Tel.: 212-633-3874; Fax: 212-633-3820; E-mail: reprints@elsevier.com.

Anesthesiology Clinics, is also published in Spanish by McGraw-Hill Inter-americana Editores S. A., P.O. Box 5-237, 06500 Mexico D. F., Mexico.

Anesthesiology Clinics, is covered in *MEDLINE/PubMed (Index Medicus), Current Contents/Clinical Medicine, Excerpta Medica, ISI/BIOMED*, and *Chemical Abstracts*.

Contributors

CONSULTING EDITOR

LEE A. FLEISHER, MD
Emeritus Professor and Former Chair of Anesthesiology and Critical Care, Perelman School of Medicine at University of Pennsylvania, Philadelphia, Pennsylvania, USA

EDITORS

NEAL H. COHEN, MD, MPH, MS
Distinguished Professor Emeritus, Anesthesia and Perioperative Care and Medicine, Vice Dean, UCSF School of Medicine, San Francisco, California, USA

GAIL A. VAN NORMAN, MD
Professor Emeritus, Department of Anesthesiology and Pain Medicine, Past Adjunct Professor Bioethics, University of Washington, Seattle, Washington, USA

AUTHORS

AGNESE ACCOGLI, MD
Critical Care Resident, Department of Surgical Science, University of Turin, Torino, Italy

DENISE BATTAGLINI, MD, PhD
Consultant, Department of Anesthesia and Intensive Care, IRCCS Ospedale Policlinico San Martino, Genoa, Italy

ANDREA CORTEGIANI, MD
Professor, Department of Precision Medicine in Medical, Surgical and Critical Care Area (Me.Pre.C.C.), University of Palermo, Department of Anesthesia Analgesia Intensive Care and Emergency, University Hospital Policlinico 'Paolo Giaccone', Palermo, Italy

TERA CUSHMAN, MD, MPH
Assistant Professor, Department of Anesthesiology and Perioperative Medicine, Oregon Health & Science University, Portland, Oregon, USA

JO DAVIES, MB BS, FRCA
Professor, Department of Anesthesiology and Pain Medicine, University of Washington, Associate Medical Director for Professional Affairs, University of Washington Medical Center, Seattle, Washington, USA

CARLOS DELGADO, MD
Associate Professor, Department of Anesthesiology and Pain Medicine, University of Washington, Associate Director, Division of Obstetric Anesthesia, Residency Education Site Director, University of Washington Medical Center, Seattle, Washington, USA

MICHAEL J. DEVINNEY, MD, PhD
Assistant Professor, Department of Anesthesiology, Duke University School of Medicine, Durham, North Carolina, USA

ELIZABETH HAYS, MD
Assistant Professor, Department of Anesthesiology and Perioperative Medicine, Oregon Health & Science University, Portland, Oregon, USA

KATHERINE O. HELLER, MD
Assistant Professor, Department of Anesthesiology and Pain Medicine, University of Washington Medical Center, Seattle, Washington, USA

JAMES HUNTER, MD
Associate Professor, Department of Anesthesiology and Perioperative Medicine, University of Alabama at Birmingham, Birmingham, Alabama, USA

MARIACHIARA IPPOLITO, MD
Department of Precision Medicine in Medical, Surgical and Critical Care Area (Me.Pre.C.C.), University of Palermo, Medical Director of Anesthesia and Resuscitation, Department of Anesthesia Analgesia Intensive Care and Emergency, University Hospital Policlinico 'Paolo Giaccone', Palermo, Italy

STEPHEN H. JACKSON, MD
Chair, Department of Anesthesiology, Bioethics Committee, Good Samaritan Hospital, San Jose, California, USA

GRACE LIM, MD, MSc
Associate Professor, Department of Anesthesiology and Perioperative Medicine, University of Pittsburgh School of Medicine, UPMC Magee Women's Hospital, Pittsburgh, Pennsylvania, USA

LESLIE MATTHEWS, MD, PharmD
Assistant Professor, Department of Anesthesiology and Pain Medicine, Nationwide Children's Hospital, Columbus, Ohio, USA

SEBASTIANO MERCADANTE, MD
Medical Director of Anesthesia and Resuscitation, Main Regional Center of Pain Relief and Supportive/Palliative Care, Nutrition (S.M.), La Maddalena Cancer Center, Palermo, Italy

ANDREA K. NAGENGAST, MD
Clinical Assistant Professor, Portland VA Medical Center, Portland, Oregon, USA

ANDREW P. NOTARIANNI, MD, FASE, FASA
Assistant Professor, Department of Anesthesiology, Yale University School of Medicine, New Haven, Connecticut, USA

MATTHEW W. PENNINGTON, MD, PhD
Assistant Professor, Department of Anesthesiology and Pain Medicine, University of Washington, University of Washington Medical Center, Seattle, Washington, USA

MARCUS J. SCHULTZ, MD, PhD
Full Professor, Department of Intensive Care, Amsterdam University Medical Centers, Location 'AMC', Amsterdam, Netherlands; Mahidol Oxford Tropical Medicine Research Unit (MORU), Mahidol University, Bangkok, Thailand; Nuffield Department of Medicine, University of Oxford, Oxford, United Kingdom; Division of Cardiothoracic and Vascular

Anesthesia and Critical Care Medicine, Department of Anesthesia, General Intensive Care and Pain Management, Medical University of Vienna, Vienna, Austria

SEBASTIAN M. SEIFERT, MD
Instructor, Department of Anesthesiology, Perioperative and Pain Medicine, Harvard Medical School, Brigham and Women's Hospital, Boston, Massachusetts, USA

GENTLE S. SHRESTHA, MD, FACC, EDIC, FCPS, FRCP (Edin), FSNCC (Hon), FNCS
Associate Professor, Department of Critical Care Medicine, Tribhuvan University Teaching Hospital, Maharajgunj, Kathmandu, Nepal

KANWALPREET SODHI, DA, DNB, IDCCM, EDIC, FICCM
Director and Head of Critical Care, Department of Critical Care, Deep Hospital, Ludhiana, India

KAREN J. SOUTER, MB, BS, FRCA, MACM, PCC
Full Professor, Department of Anesthesiology and Pain Medicine, University of Washington Medical Center, Seattle, Washington, USA

MICHAEL J. SOUTER, MB, CHB, FRCA, FNCS
Professor, Department of Anesthesiology and Pain Medicine, University of Washington, Adjunct Professor, Department of Neurological Surgery, University of Washington, Seattle, Washington, USA

LINDSAY K. SWEEN, MD, MPH
Northside Anesthesiology Clinicians, Northside Hospital, Atlanta, Georgia, USA

MIRIAM M. TREGGIARI, MD, PhD, MPH
Paul G. Barash Professor, Department of Anesthesiology, Duke University School of Medicine, Durham, North Carolina, USA

LAWRENCE C. TSEN, MD
Associate Professor, Department of Anesthesiology, Perioperative and Pain Medicine, Harvard Medical School, Brigham and Women's Hospital, Boston, Massachusetts, USA

GAIL A. VAN NORMAN, MD
Professor Emeritus, Department of Anesthesiology and Pain Medicine, Past Adjunct Professor Bioethics, University of Washington, Seattle, Washington, USA

MARCO VERGANO, MD
Consultant, Department of Anesthesia and Intensive Care, San Giovanni Bosco Hospital, Torino, Italy

DAVID WAISEL, MD
Chief, Division of Pediatric Anesthesiology, Department of Anesthesiology, Yale School of Medicine, New Haven, Connecticut, USA

JAMES M. WEST, MD, MA
Director of Transplant Anesthesia, Emeritus, Methodist Transplant Institute, Medical Anesthesia Group, Ret., Memphis, Tennessee, USA

JOEL B. ZIVOT, MD, FRCP(C), MA, JM
Associate Professor of Anesthesiology and Surgery, Emory University School of Medicine, Senior Fellow, Emory Center for Ethics, Emory University, Atlanta, Georgia, USA

Contents

Foreword: Do no Harm: What Are the Ethical Tenets of Modern Perioperative Practice

xiii

Lee A. Fleisher

Preface

xv

Neal H. Cohen and Gail A. Van Norman

Managing the Labyrinth of Complex Ethical Issues in Anesthesia Practice: The Anesthesiologist's Ariadne's Thread 357

Agnese Accogli and Marco Vergano

> Facing ethical dilemmas is challenging and sometimes becomes a real burden for anesthesiologists, particularly because they rarely have previous or long-standing patient relationships that help inform clinical decision-making. Although there is no ideal algorithm that can fit all clinical situations, some basic moral and ethical principles, which should be part of every clinician's armamentarium, can guide the decision-making process. Dealing with conflicting views among providers and/or patients can be distressing but can lead to meaningful professional and personal growth for each clinician.

The Evolution of the Ethical Guidelines of the American Society of Anesthesiologists 367

Stephen H. Jackson and David Waisel

> In 1992, the American Society of Anesthesiologists Committee on Ethics was formed primarily to address the rights of patients with existing Do-Not-Resuscitate orders presenting for anesthesia. Guidelines written for the ethical management of these patients stated that such orders should be reconsidered—not rescinded—thus respecting patient self-determination. The Committee also rewrote the reigning Guidelines for the Ethical Practice of Anesthesiology by expanding its ethical foundations to reflect the evolving climate of ethical opinions. These Guidelines described ethically appropriate conduct and behavior, including anesthesiologists' ethical responsibilities to patients, themselves, colleagues, health-care institutions, and community and society.

The role of Advance Directives and Living Wills in Anesthesia Practice 377

Michael J. Devinney and Miriam M. Treggiari

> Preoperative review of existing advance directives and a discussion of patient goals should be routinely done to address any potential limitations on resuscitative therapies during perioperative care. Both surgeons and anesthesiologists should be collaboratively involved in these discussions, and all perioperative physicians should receive training in shared decision making and goals of care discussions. These discussions should center around patient preferences for limitations on life-sustaining medical

therapy, which should be accurately documented and adhered to during the perioperative period. Patients should be informed that limitations of life-sustaining medical therapy may increase their risk of postoperative mortality.

Perioperative Care of the Patient with Directives Limiting Life-Sustaining Treatments   393

Tera Cushman, Elizabeth Hays, and Andrea K. Nagengast

Like most complex aspects of procedural care, sound perioperative management of limits to life-sustaining medical therapy requires a multidisciplinary team-based approach bolstered by appropriate care management strategies. This article discusses the implications of care for the patient for whom limitations of life-sustaining care are in place and the roles and responsibilities of each provider in supporting quality procedural care compatible with patients' right to self-determination. The authors focus on the roles of the surgeon, preoperative clinic provider, anesthesiologist, and postoperative care consultants and discuss how the health care system and care pathways can support and improve adherence to best practices.

End-of-life Care in the Intensive Care Unit and Ethics of Withholding/Withdrawal of Life-sustaining Treatments   407

Andrea Cortegiani, Mariachiara Ippolito, and Sebastiano Mercadante

The medical progress has produced improvements in critically ill patients' survival to early phases of life-threatening diseases, thus producing long intensive care stays and persisting disability, with uncertain long-term survival rates and quality of life. Thus, compassionate end-of-life care and the provision of palliative care, even overlapping with the most aggressive of curative intensive care unit (ICU) care has become crucial. Moreover, withdrawal or withholding of life-sustaining treatment may be adopted, allowing unavoidable deaths to occur, without prolonging agony or ICU stay. Our aim was to summarize the key element of end-of-life care in the ICU and the ethics of withholding/withdrawal life-sustaining treatments.

Brain Death: Medical, Ethical, Cultural, and Legal Aspects   421

Matthew W. Pennington and Michael J. Souter

The development of critical care stimulated brain death criteria formulation in response to concerns on treatment resources and unregulated organ procurement. The diagnosis centered on irreversible loss of brain function and subsequent systemic physiologic collapse and was subsequently codified into law. With improved critical care, physiologic collapse (while predominant) is not inevitable—provoking criticisms of the ethical and legal foundation for brain death. Other criteria have been unsuccessfully proposed, but irreversibility remains the conceptual foundation. Conflicts can arise when families reject the diagnosis—resulting in ethical, cultural, and communication challenges and implications for diversity, equity, and inclusion.

Ethics Consultation in Anesthesia Practice   **433**

Andrew P. Notarianni

Because modern surgical and medical care have advanced, patients increasingly present for procedural and surgical intervention with life-limiting diagnoses and/or advanced care goals such as "do not resuscitate." Anesthesiologists now care for these patients across the complete perioperative setting and frequently find themselves at the crossroads of these mounting pressures. As the boundaries and capabilities of anesthetic care and critical care anesthesiology expand so too do the specialty's needs for support in ethical decision-making. Herein, we review the role of the ethics consultation in anesthesia practice and special ethic issues encountered by the anesthesiologist.

Public Good versus Private "Goods": Ethical Implications of Drug Shortages on Anesthesiology Practice   **445**

Joel B. Zivot

Drug shortages remain a serious and widespread problem affecting all health systems and patients. Anesthesiology practice is strongly impacted by shortages of sterile injectable drugs, resulting in a negative impact on the quality of care. Understanding the root causes of drug shortages guides the anesthesiologist toward an ethical response. While rationing is a common consideration in secular ethics, and indeed rationing strategies are utilized, the use of rationing alone risks normalizing and perpetuating the drug shortage problem. Drug shortages are the direct result of a market failure brought on by lack of oversight of drug production standards in some cases as well as by the impact of intermediary purchasing groups on costs and availability of drugs. Legislation needs to reestablish a responsible, competitive, and robust manufacturing drug market.

Medical Triage: Ethical Implications and Management Strategies   **457**

Gentle S. Shrestha, Denise Battaglini, Kanwalpreet Sodhi, and Marcus J. Schultz

Natural or man-made medical disasters have repeatedly affected human communities. The impact on health care resources may vary depending on the magnitude of each crisis, catastrophe or pandemic, and the resources available. Medical triage protocols serve as invaluable tools to address clinical needs, particularly when resources, including supplies, equipment, and personnel, are limited. Although resources should be allocated to maximize the benefit, resource allocations need to be ethically sound. Existing triage protocols have inherent limitations.

Ethics of Preanesthesia Mandatory Laboratory Testing   **473**

James Hunter, Stephen H. Jackson, and Gail A. Van Norman

Some practices require mandatory preoperative laboratory testing for select patients presenting for anesthesia and surgery. Such mandatory preanesthesia laboratory testing has significant ethical implications related to informed consent and patient autonomy. Assumptions that a patient provides "presumed consent" by merely presenting for a test are flawed because such consents are often not informed and do not acknowledge patient autonomy. By placing a condition on access to a medical treatment, mandatory preanesthesia testing may not be ethically justifiable. Not all laboratory tests are "ethically equal"; several raise specific questions regarding informed consent, related to their potential to cause significant harm.

Maternal–Fetal Conflicts in Anesthesia Practice
491

Sebastian M. Seifert, Leslie Matthews, Lawrence C. Tsen, and Grace Lim

Anesthesia clinicians often navigate a delicate balance between maternal and fetal safety. Interventions for at fetal well-being may introduce risks of harm to the mother and raise ethical dilemmas. Emergency procedures often focus on direct fetal safety, sidelining maternal physical and mental well-being. The clash between ethical principles, particularly nonmaleficence and beneficence, often arises, with maternal autonomy guiding decisions. Fetal surgery exemplifies risking maternal health for fetal benefit, whereas emergent cesarean deliveries pose physical and psychological challenges for both the mother and child.

Ethical Care of Pregnant Patients During Labor, Delivery, and Nonobstetric Surgery
503

Carlos Delgado and Jo Davies

The 4 basic principles of ethics (beneficence, nonmaleficence, autonomy, and justice) can guide clinical decision-making for the pregnant patient during labor and delivery, as well as when undergoing nonobstetric surgery. An evidence-based decision-making conversation with the patient facilitates obtaining informed consent. When maternal-fetal conflict arises, both during labor and delivery and nonobstetric surgery, beneficence-based obligations to both parties should be considered, with discussions and decisions well documented. Labor is not an impediment to women providing consent for care. A careful balance between evidence-based clinical judgment and patient autonomy is necessary when addressing cesarean delivery.

Ethical Issues in the Care of Patients Whose Personal, Religious, or Cultural Beliefs Impact Clinical Management Strategies
515

Lindsay K. Sween and James M. West

Ethical principles regarding respect for patient autonomy in medical decision-making and the impact of religion, culture, and other issues on clinical care have been extensively reviewed in the medical literature. At the same time, despite physicians having an understanding of the underlying ethical principles in clinical decision-making, challenges arise when managing complicated clinical problems for which medical treatment is available, but not acceptable to the patient. For example, many anesthesiologists are challenged when caring for one of Jehohah's Witnesses who refuses to receive blood or blood products despite the potential consequences of doing so.

Disclosure of Adverse Events and Medical Errors: A Framework for Anesthesiologists 529

Katherine O. Heller and Karen J. Souter

Ethical disclosure of adverse events (AE) presents opportunities and challenges for physicians and has unique ramifications for anesthesiologists. AE disclosure is supported by patients, regulatory organizations, and physicians. Disclosure is part of a physician's ethical duty toward patients, supports fully informed patient decision making, and is a critical component of root cause analysis. Barriers to AE disclosure include disruption of the doctor–patient relationship, fear of litigation, and inadequate training. Apology laws intended to support disclosure and mitigate concern for adverse legal consequences have not fulfilled that initial promise. Training and institutional communication programs support physicians in providing competent, ethical AE disclosure.

Conscientious Objection 539

Gail A. Van Norman

Physicians may under some circumstances decline to provide a clinical service that is within accepted medical standards due to a deeply held moral belief that to do so would be wrong. Conscience objection in medicine is legally protected, but ethically limited by physician obligations to put patient interests first. Accommodation to conscientious objections, when possible, recognizes the diverse moral perspectives and benefits for both the objectors and the profession as a whole. When these situations arise, physicians have obligations to respectfully resolve the distress of conscientious objectors while still honoring the primacy of patient care needs.

ANESTHESIOLOGY CLINICS

FORTHCOMING ISSUES

December 2024
Ethical Approaches to the Practice of Anesthesiology - Part 2: Ethical Constructs that Impact Health Policy, Research and Professional Integrity
Neal H. Cohen and Gail A. Van Norman
Editors

March 2025
Gender, Racial and Socioeconomic Issues in Perioperative Medicine
Katherine Forkin, Lauren Dunn, and Edward Nemergut, *Editors*

September 2025
Artificial Intelligence in Anesthesiology
Ali Dabbagh and A. Sassan Sabouri, *Editors*

RECENT ISSUES

June 2024
Sports Anesthesia
Ashley M. Shilling, *Editor*

March 2024
Preoperative Patient Evaluation
Zdravka Zafirova and Richard Urman, *Editors*

December 2023
Perioperative Safety Culture
Matthew D. McEvoy and James H. Abernathy, *Editors*

SERIES OF RELATED INTEREST

Critical Care Clinics

THE CLINICS ARE AVAILABLE ONLINE!
Access your subscription at:
www.theclinics.com

Foreword

Do no Harm: What Are the Ethical Tenets of Modern Perioperative Practice

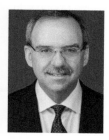

Lee A. Fleisher, MD
Consulting Editor

Practicing medicine has changed dramatically since the time of Hippocrates with new advances only accelerating during recent years. With these advances, including the ability to prolong life through mechanical means, come more complex ethical dilemmas. In the first of a two-part series on the Ethical Approaches to the Practice of Anesthesiology, an international group of authors have written on multiple aspects of perioperative care and the application of clinical ethics.

In order to commission two issues on ethics tenets of care, two leaders in anesthesiology clearly were the obvious choice. Neal H. Cohen, MD, MPH, MS is Distinguished Professor Emeritus of Anesthesia and Perioperative Care and Medicine and Vice Dean at the UCSF School of Medicine. He received his MD from UCSF School of Medicine, an MPH in Epidemiology from the University of California, Berkeley, and an MS in Management from the Stanford University Graduate School of Business Sloan Program. He served in leadership roles in the Accreditation Council for Graduate Medical Education, the American Board of Anesthesiology Critical Care Examination Committee, and the National Board of Respiratory Care. Gail A. Van Norman, MD is Professor Emeritus of Anesthesiology and Pain Medicine and Adjunct Professor of Bioethics at the University of Washington. Dr Van Norman is a clinical ethicist who served as a member of the Committee on Ethics for the American Society of Anesthesiologists for 19 years and chaired the Committee. She was also a resident scholar of the Brocher

Anesthesiology Clin 42 (2024) xiii–xiv
https://doi.org/10.1016/j.anclin.2024.05.003
1932-2275/24/© 2024 Published by Elsevier Inc.

anesthesiology.theclinics.com

Foundation in Geneva, Switzerland. Together they have created an outstanding two-part series.

Lee A. Fleisher, MD
Perelman School of Medicine at
University of Pennsylvania
3400 Spruce Street, Dulles 680
Philadelphia, PA 19104, USA

E-mail address:
Lee.Fleisher@pennmedicine.upenn.edu

Preface

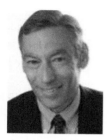 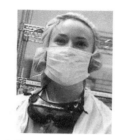

Neal H. Cohen, MD, MPH, MS   Gail A. Van Norman, MD
Editors

From the time of Hippocrates, the medical profession has been distinguished by common moral values and principles, and by special obligations to patients, colleagues, and society. The specialty of anesthesiology is built upon these fundamental principles and played a rich role in defining twentieth century bioethical principles. In 1957, for example, the World Congress of Anesthesiologists sought and received advice from Pope Pius XII that administration of opioids to relieve pain at end of life was acceptable, even if the use of opioids hastened death. In addition, the Pope declared that women should receive labor analgesia (previously opposed on biblical grounds), and that refusal of invasive, life-sustaining medical care, such as mechanical ventilation, was neither suicide nor a sin. Henry Beecher, the first chair of the Department of Anesthesiology at the Harvard Medical School, chaired the committee that first proposed brain death as a medicolegal concept. He also exposed medical research practices in the United States that violated the Nuremburg Code and thereby hastened the development of institutional research boards to protect human subjects from exploitation and harm. In addition to these advances in bioethical practices, the expansion in the scope of anesthesiology practice and research also creates both opportunities and challenges for anesthesiologists to address complex ethical issues. Anesthesia practice now touches nearly every aspect of medicine—reaching far beyond the operating room to include perioperative and pain medicine, critical care, emergency medicine, palliative care, and more—providing care across the continuum of clinical needs from reproductive medicine and perioperative care to end-of-life care. Anesthesiologists have demonstrated their commitment to advancing medical care, promoting patient quality and safety, and ensuring equitable access to care. As a result, it is hardly a surprise that the specialty plays a leading role in addressing many of the most challenging ethical issues in medicine.

We dedicate two issues of *Anesthesiology Clinics* to exploring a variety of ethical issues confronted by anesthesiologists during the course of their careers as physicians, researchers, and administrators. Part 1 explores ethical issues primarily facing

Anesthesiology Clin 42 (2024) xv–xvi
https://doi.org/10.1016/j.anclin.2024.05.002
1932-2275/24/© 2024 Published by Elsevier Inc.
anesthesiology.theclinics.com

anesthesiologists in clinical practice, while Part 2 addresses ethical issues in research, publication, and societal issues.

In Part 1, we are delighted to welcome esteemed authors from Italy, Austria, India, Nepal, the Netherlands, and the United States to present basic principles in biomedical ethics, ethics consultation, the history of the American Society of Anesthesiologists Committee on Ethics statements and guidelines in ethical practice, and ethical aspects of clinical practice. Clinical topics range from end-of-life care, medical triage in emergencies, ethical concerns in laboratory testing, to care of pregnant patients. The issue concludes with ethical aspects of medical error, and conscientious objection in anesthesia practice.

Neal H. Cohen, MD, MPH, MS
Anesthesia and Perioperative Care and Medicine
UCSF School of Medicine
513 Parnassus Street, S-224
San Francisco, CA, 94143-0410, USA

Gail A. Van Norman, MD
University of Washington Medical Center
1959 NE Pacific Street
Seattle, WA 98195, USA

E-mail addresses:
cohenn@ucsf.edu (N.H. Cohen)
gvn@uw.edu (G.A. Van Norman)

Managing the Labyrinth of Complex Ethical Issues in Anesthesia Practice

The Anesthesiologist's Ariadne's Thread

Agnese Accogli, MD[a], Marco Vergano, MD[b],*

KEYWORDS

- Bioethics • Clinical ethics • Clinical decision-making • Anesthesiology • Critical care
- Palliative care

KEY POINTS

- Awareness and understanding of the ethical component in every clinical decision is paramount. Basic ethics teaching should be part of routine medical training to optimize decision-making and foster trust.
- Bioethics is multidimensional, encompassing juridical, sociopolitical, cultural, and medical issues while preserving basic human rights.
- Any medical intervention should always be both clinically appropriate and ethically proportionate.
- Prognostic uncertainty should not lead to "prognostic paralysis."
- There is no one-size-fits-all solution in medical decision-making, rather a tailored and shared decision process should be applied to every individual situation. Professionals have different views: reasoned discussion is essential to identify and address areas of disagreement.

The technical and moral aspects of medicine are inseparable
—Albert R Jonsen

The following day, no one died.

This fact, being absolutely contrary to life's rules,

ª Department of Surgical Sciences, University of Turin, Corso Dogliotti 14, Turin, Italy;
ᵇ Department of Anesthesia and Intensive Care, San Giovanni Bosco Hospital, Torino, Italy
* Corresponding author. Department of Anesthesia and Intensive Care, San Giovanni Bosco Hospital, Piazza del Donatore di Sangue 3, Turin 10154, Italy.
E-mail address: marco.vergano@aslcittaditorino.it

Anesthesiology Clin 42 (2024) 357–366
https://doi.org/10.1016/j.anclin.2023.12.006
1932-2275/24/© 2024 Elsevier Inc. All rights reserved.

anesthesiology.theclinics.com

provoked enormous and, in the circumstances,

perfectly justifiable anxiety in people's minds…

Death with Interruptions

—Jose Saramago

LOST IN ETHICAL DILEMMAS

When addressing ethical dilemmas, the already tortuous clinical pathway of a critically ill patient can become a real labyrinth, whether in the operating room, intensive care unit, emergency department, or other environments, leaving the anesthesiologist lost in anguished wondering. Religious factors or maternal–fetal critical cases, for example, present additional complexities. Unlike maze brain games, there is often no single right solution. Yet, the player must not be left alone: teamwork—and the input of colleagues, patients, and their families—is needed. Some general ethical principles can guide clinicians, such as an Ariadne's thread out of the labyrinth.

MANDATORY TRAINING, NOT PERSONAL CHARACTER

It is a misleading, though common perception that ethical thinking, as well as communication skills, is grounded in personal character and sensibility. Although some clinicians' aptitude for critical and philosophic thinking may be innate, as with any other medical skill most will require training to achieve basic expertise. Every physician should be able to handle a set of basic tools: from accessing the right vocabulary to defend a position in ethical discussions, to knowledge of the basic principles of bioethics. Knowledge in ethics should be an integral part of medical education and residency programs and not left to a single physician's personal interests. Professionals who are often involved in ethically challenging situations should build personal awareness about which ethical approach suits them best and evolve their own view based on impartiality and consistency. A debate argued on solid consolidated theories provides clear conclusions, and not surprisingly, the same deliberations can be reached through different ethical approaches.

COMMON MORALITY AND THE *GEORGETOWN MANTRA*

Tom Beauchamp and James Childress, two of the "founding fathers" of biomedical ethics, embraced different ethical theories and it was with wonder that they found themselves in agreement on several relevant and complex issues, thus leading them to elaborate a theory for bioethical reasoning (**Tables 1** and **2**). They had different backgrounds: Beauchamp was a rule-utilitarian, whereas Childress was a deontologist.[1] According to the authors, their outlined principles correspond to an analytical framework of general rules derived from *common morality* and constitute a starting point for discussion about bioethical dilemmas. They defined *common morality* not as a particular, specific, morality, but rather as a set of universally standard rules that remain valid regardless of geographic, social, religious, or cultural identity.[2]

The "label" principlism was at first used as a negative by some philosophers who considered the theory to be reductive and simplistic. On the contrary, this approach has the credit of bringing together medical ethics tradition and contemporary society moral consideration, a valuable and broad scope ethical merging. Two of four ethical principles from Beauchamp and Childress, *beneficence* and *non-maleficence,* directly derive from the Hippocratic heritage, whereas the remaining two, *autonomy* and *justice*, come from the modern juridical and sociopolitical thinking.[1]

Table 1 Based on data from "Ethics in Intensive Care Medicine"[3] and "Una introduzione alle teorie morali"						
Summary of the Principle Bioethical Theories						
	Utilitarianism	Liberalism	Virtue Ethics	Ethics of Care	Deontology	Narrative Ethics
Subject evaluated	Consequences	Actions	Acting agent	Relationships	Actions	Stories
General rule	Maximizing benefits	Autonomy/ rights	Virtues	Care	Duties	Patients' values
Reference philosopher	J Bentham	J B Rawls	Plato and Aristotle	C Gilligan	I Kant	P Ricoeur

From Mordacci, R. Una introduzione alle teorie morali - Confronto con la bioetica. (Feltrinelli, 2003).

The strength of this approach lies on the one hand in shaping a basic shared vocabulary and common landmarks and on the other hand in encompassing all of the issues that arise in clinical practice for patients, health care professionals and society.[1]

However, the four basic principles can frequently conflict. One of the challenges in using these principles is determining the relative weight or priority each applies in any decision-making process, because no fixed hierarchy exists among the four basic principles.[2,4] To better understand the inherent conflicts that arise when applying each principle, it is worth summarizing the main features of each of them.

- *Autonomy* is a double-shaped principle: it considers both positive and negative actions, for example, to support patients in their choices versus to not interfere unfairly in patients' choices. They highlight that autonomy can also result in a patient's desire *not* to be informed, and also result in proxy designation and that we must think in terms of a new concept of *relational autonomy*, progressively abandoning the traditional individualistic view.[2]
- *Beneficence* involves a concept of moral obligation in terms of benefit not only to the single patient but also to society, in a wider view of mutual duty of health care professionals and patients, for a shared commitment to let medicine thrive.[2]
- *Non maleficence* is intended by the authors as a comprehensive principle: excessive protection can harm patients no less than insufficient protection, an interesting consideration to keep in mind when weighing the burdens of every intervention. They also focus on some specific issues regarding end-of-life care and palliative care, interpreting and discussing them in light of a deep analysis of the *primum non nocere* principle. They confute three traditional distinctions: the one between withholding and withdrawing life-sustaining treatment; the one between medically administered nutrition/hydration and treatments; and the fine line between foreseen but unintended harmful effects (*doctrine of double effect*).[2]
- *Justice* is perhaps the most complex and debated of the four principles. It comes into play every time we have to deal with allotment of scarce resources, from equipment to organ transplants, when we manage uninsured patients, and when we face triage choices. Although it was a bit neglected for decades, *distributive justice* took central stage in the recent past, in the darkest moments of COVID-19 emergency, showing how much reflection is still needed to find a shared approach to such events.[5,6]

Table 2 The four principles approach	
Principle Definition	**Specific Rules**
Autonomy Respect patients' free and informed choices and support patients in the exercise of self-determination	• Tell the truth • Respect privacy • Protect confidential information • Obtain consent for interventions • Support autonomous decisions
Beneficence Act for patients' benefit and remove the potential harm, balancing risks and advantages	• Protect and defend the rights of others • Prevent harm from occurring to others • Remove conditions that will cause harm • Help persons with disabilities • Rescue persons in danger
Nonmaleficence Not to harm patients	• Do not kill • Do not cause pain or suffering • Do not incapacitate • Do not cause offense • Do not deprive others of the goods of life
Justice Distribute fairly advantages, risks, and costs	Fair, equitable, and appropriate distribution of benefits and burdens according to six different theories: • Utilitarianism • Libertarianism • Communitarianism • Egalitarianism • Capabilities theory • Welfare theory

From Beauchamp, T. L. & Childress, J. F. Principles of Biomedical Ethics. (Oxford University Press, 2019).

CROSS-CULTURAL BIOETHICS

In a world where medicine should know no borders and where multiethnicity is a matter of fact, another complex challenge of bioethics stands out: how to deal with cultural diversity. The principlist approach considers *common morality* as a universally valid set of general moral judgments. This mindset describes the so-called *moral objectivism*. To be thorough, we must clarify that there is another predominant ethical theory that attempts to answer this matter: *moral relativism*. Moral relativists recognize two different points of view: descriptive moral relativism and metaethical moral relativism. The former claims that there is broad divergence in moral values between different cultures, both currently and across time. The metaethical relativists identify only views about right and wrong, arguing that even our tolerance of the customs of others can lead, in some circumstances, to unavoidable contradictions.[3]

By and large we can say that on the one hand we have Western societies with "self-determination"-oriented medical ethics versus developing countries with family-oriented or community-oriented decision-making where traditions and relationships are valued the most. Apart from this rough distinction, we must keep in mind the wide religious and cultural diversity of modern societies, especially in large urban areas in Western countries.

From the unquestionable starting point of respect for others and for other points of view, a pathway of knowledge, empathy, acceptance, and comprehension must be followed. If imposing an individualistic mindset is not always feasible nor correct, legitimizing individual rights violations through the dominance of extremely conservative communities must certainly be avoided.[7] We should pursue an interculturally sensitive bioethics approach, capable of embracing cultural diversity while preserving fundamental human rights.

"To ACT OR NOT TO ACT"

The mere application—even when perfect—of clinical guidelines, is not sufficient to perform excellent medical care. What is *adequate* for a patient's biology may not be the *right choice* for their biology. We often limit our "duty to care" to an automatic chain of actions: this behavior is driven by distorted interpretations on three different levels.

- From a *philosophic point of view*, we believe that only decisions to limit treatments require justification. Nevertheless, if we consider the patient as a person with their biography, goals, and values and not just as a broken machine that we have to fix at all costs, we realize that every medical intervention we perform needs serious consideration and justification, according to the "first do no harm" paradigm.
- From a *deontological point of view*, the doctrine with which we have been raised as physicians is driven by the goal to "save lives." However, the equation "to cure = to care" is not always valid. A fully invasive treatment strategy is not always the best choice for every patient and if we do not want to be mere executors of medical automatisms, we must conduct a continuous reevaluation of the goals of care, ensuring a patient-centered approach to care and decision-making.
- From a *legal point of view*, the rise of defensive medicine is leading to a "must do" mindset. Physicians deem doing more is more defensible, not realizing that iatrogenic harm, especially when derived from an inappropriate intervention, has the same weight as not performing the intervention.[8]

INFORMED CONSENT: NOT MERELY A SIGNED FORM

From a legal perspective, informed consent is often perceived as a "security blanket" for physicians and health systems. In our hectic daily routine, we collect thousands of patients' signatures in paternalistic fashion, which have little or no legal or ethical value. In so doing, we unconsciously approach patients with a paternalistic method. Confident that we are offering the best treatment option and overwhelmed by the workload, we believe that the patients' nodding in response to our quick and technical explanation really corresponds to true understanding and agreement. This common scenario does not demonstrate therapeutic alliance. The gap in knowledge between the two parties of the agreement puts the patient in a disadvantaged position where the patient entrusts to the physician the management of his health, like a child totally relies on his parents.

These are just a few of the requirements of a legitimate informed consent process: time, communication skills, continuous assessment of the patient's or surrogate's understanding, acknowledgment of the patients' goals, and bias-free explanations. Presuming to know what is best for our patients, even with the best of intentions, nourishes incomprehension, mistrust, and lawsuits.

With respect to communication, Ezekiel and Linda Emanuel[9] proposed a description of four possible doctor–patient relationship models. The first two approaches are asymmetrical: the *paternalistic model* puts information and decision control entirely in the physician's hands, whereas the *informative model* leaves all the choice responsibility to the patient and the physician role is limited to a "purveyor" of thorough but aseptic technical information. The third kind of relationship corresponds to the *interpretative model,* where the physician, while keeping his informative role, also acts as a counselor or moderator in the process of reconstructing and interpreting the patient's values and priorities. Fourth and last, the *deliberative model* is based on the critical discussion of alternative health-related values where both subjects are engaged in a mutual understanding of reasons and preferences, like in a dialogue between two friends.[9]

APPROPRIATENESS AND PROPORTIONALITY

To optimize clinical decision-making and management, an intervention must be both clinically appropriate and ethically proportionate (**Fig. 1**).

- Clinical appropriateness is achieved when the proposed medical intervention is reasonably expected to attain a beneficial effect in the pertaining case and represents the best suitable current therapeutic chance.
- Ethical proportionality means that the proposed intervention is in line with the patient's life project and their personal idea of dignity and acceptable quality of life.

These two criteria perfectly sum up the above discussion about the ideal therapeutic alliance: on the one hand, the knowledge and expertise of the physician who is able to present the best current evidence-based treatment options for the specific case and, on the other hand, alignment of the decision-making process with the patient's goals and values. This approach ensures a process of bilateral comprehension that leads to the best possible matching of means and goals.

NOT EVERYTHING THAT IS PERMITTED IS HONORABLE

Ethics and law intersect, but are not equivalent. The legal system aims at regulating broader spheres of human activity, affecting society as a whole. Even if addressed

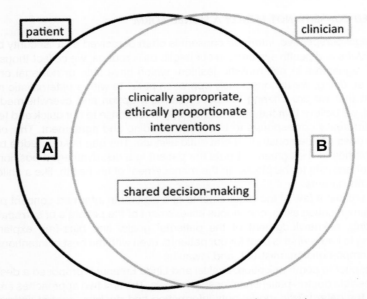

Fig. 1. A: Requests for inappropriate or futile treatments, for example, extracorporeal life support for a patient with terminal cancer; B: Clinically appropriate treatments refused or deemed not acceptable by the patient, for example, transfusion of blood products for a Jehovah's Witness with capacity. (*From* Vergano M et al, Clinical Ethics: what the Anesthesiologist and the Intensivist need to know. Minerva Anestesiol 2018;84(4):515-22.)

to similar issues and concerns, the underlying rationales and the approaches taken "may fail to mirror or indeed consciously sacrifice ethical principles on utilitarian and/or pragmatic grounds."[10] Laws direct and judge cases and phenomena on standard general bases. Bioethics attempts to identify the ethical issues that arise and to propose solutions to address specific ethical dilemmas.[11] Thus, beyond the overlapping perspectives, there are large areas where ethics and law can be profoundly divergent and where what is legal could be unethical and vice versa. This fact can have a great impact on health care professionals' choices and potentially lead to moral distress.[12]

JOIN FORCES, SHARE THE BURDEN!

Another piece of our Ariadne's thread is *shared decision-making*. Depending on the scenario we face, shared decision-making can be interprofessional and/or between team and patients/families. We have already fully examined the options for engaging the competent patient in shared decision-making with competent patients, but frequently the time for decisions comes in worse conditions.

Different countries have different legislation regarding surrogates' and proxies' rights to make decisions on behalf of their loved ones. Depending on the status of surrogate decision-makers, their role may or may not have legal authority. However, it is always desirable and crucial to involve families continuously in the process of assessment of the patient's condition and reevaluation of the goals of therapy. This is extremely relevant to make relatives feel involved, understood, and supported and gains even more value when there are no advanced directives because families and friends become a source of information that helps physicians clarify the patient's wishes, values, and beliefs.[13,14]

In one of the worst-case scenarios, when unconscious, pharmacologically sedated or delirious patients have no advanced directives, previously expressed wishes or available proxies, interprofessional decision-making aimed at what is judged to be the patient's best interest comes into play. Shared discussions and decision-making can reduce the emotional burden of choices that may be distressing, allow consideration of all the treatment options and the available evidence, minimize the amount of uncertainty, and avoid decisions based on the individual health care professionals' personal views and values.[15]

This approach to case discussion is also important for the staff, to avoid moral distress and to increase cohesion of the team. Good communication skills, adequate training and planned shared methods/tools can help deal with disagreements. Intra-team conflicting views can be distressing but should be considered a chance for professional enrichment.

In cases of unsurmountable controversy, another opportunity is *ethics consultation*. Hospital ethics committees or clinical ethics committees (CECs) provide nonbinding counseling that has been proved to lead to significant changes in patient treatment and a decrease of moral distress in health personnel.[16] Besides health care professionals' satisfaction and the resolution of single cases, CECs contribute to the intra-hospital dissemination of critical thinking and to the shaping of an active and accessible space for moral reflection.[17]

MEDICINE, NOT MATHEMATICS

We are living in the era of evidence-based medicine, often shaped by a "technological imperative." In view of the well-settled metaphor of fighting illnesses, death is too often regarded as a defeat, especially in critical care. Medicine, though properly considered part of the realm of science, is an imperfect one. Physicians deal on a daily basis with clinical decisions based on limited and imperfect data. Interindividual variability leads to unpredictable treatment responses.[18] Facing real cases often makes the strength of statistics wreck into pieces, generating a deep sense of uncertainty at a time when decision-making is most critical. Nevertheless, prognostic uncertainty should never lead to "prognostic paralysis."[8] Although time-limited intensive care trials or the wait-and-see approach can both be valuable strategies if used consciously, they must not be used extensively and routinely as an escape path. Keeping patients in a state of limbo when there is no reasonable recovery probability or maintaining life-sustaining interventions that are of no value is detrimental in many ways: it feeds un-realistic relatives' expectations, it leads to unequal resources allocation, it triggers staff moral distress, and it is often an egoistic defense, due to our inability to accept death, both as physicians and human beings. Tolerance for uncertainty is thus another essential tool of the physicians' armamentarium.[18] It takes courage, honesty, and hu-mility to take the step through decisions and not hide behind the alibi of uncertainty. This is a lesson that must be taught and learned.[19]

THE DUAL-ROLE EXPERIENCE OF CLINICIAN-RESEARCHERS AND RESEARCH ETHICS

Because advancing medical progress has become a moral obligation to society, almost every physician finds themselves in the dual role of clinician and researcher. This results in both ethical and methodological implications. Competing expectations and obligations lead clinician-researchers to experience situations of conflict between their sense of clinical duty and methodological requirements. This dual role must be clarified to both patients and ourselves, and the concurrence of ethical norms of both clinical practice and research must be deeply considered. The role of the physi-cian as clinician-researcher has advantages in the research setting, providing clinical expertise and judgment, as well as patient trust due to a preexisting clinical relation-ship. At the same time, physician-researchers must maintain a rigorous research method, which could be particularly challenging.[20]

With this background, we cannot overlook the importance of providing training in issues related to research methodology and ethics in addition to providing training related to clinical ethics.[21] The four Georgetown principles perfectly apply to research: the new paradigm of *beneficence* as a mutual commitment to medical development discussed above and *distributive justice* are clearly implicated in research in terms of obligation to research participation and results diffusion, access, and application. Looking back in research history we can better understand the concept of avoiding excessive protection cited about the nonmaleficence principle: the "stop protecting us to death!" of the early 80s AIDS patients to whom the experimental treatments were denied in the name of vulnerable patients' protection is a meaningful example.[17]

SUMMARY

Clinical ethics is a multifaceted and complex subject. It implies a pathway of both inner and outer knowledge. Bioethics education and training can improve clinical practice and work environment as well as optimize the experience and well-being of providers, patients, and their families. As tangled as the bioethics labyrinth can appear, the "thread" of bioethics will trace, case after case, an increasingly easier path to follow as one's training, experience, and exposure to diverse perspectives expands. For most anesthesiologists who do not confront major ethical challenges regularly, it may take time to begin to feel confident in dealing with ethically complex situations, and sometimes that time never comes: it is nevertheless our duty to take on this challenge. After all, as Hippocrates of Kos taught us,

Ὁ βίος βραχύς, ἡ δὲ τέχνη μακρή, ὁ δὲ καιρὸς ὀξύς, ἡ δὲ πεῖρα σφαλερή, ἡ δὲ κρίσις χαλεπή» *(Vita brevis, ars longa, occasio praeceps, experimentum periculosum, iudicium difficile). Life is short and art long; opportunity is fleeting, experimentations perilous and judgment difficult.*

—Hippocrates

DISCLOSURE

The authors have nothing to disclose.

REFERENCES

1. Furlan, E. Il principialismo di Beauchamp e Childress. Una ricostruzione storiofilosofica. (2020).
2. Beauchamp TL, Childress JF. Principles of biomedical ethics. New York, NY: Oxford University Press; 2019.
3. Michalsen A, Sadovnikoff N, Kesecioglu J. Ethics in intensive care medicine. Berlin, Germany: Springer International Publishing; 2023. https://doi.org/10.1007/978-3-031-29390-0.
4. Shea M. Forty years of the four principles: Enduring themes from Beauchamp and Childress. J Med Philos 2020;45:387–95.
5. Craxì L, Vergano M, Savulescu J, et al. Rationing in a Pandemic: Lessons from Italy. Asian Bioeth Rev 2020;12:325–30.
6. Varkey B. Principles of Clinical Ethics and Their Application to Practice. Med Princ Pract 2021;30:17–28.
7. Ekmekci,' PE, Arda B. Interculturalism and Informed Consent: Respecting Cultural Differences without Breaching Human Rights.
8. Vergano M, Magavern E, Zamperetti N. Clinical ethics: What the anesthesiologist and the intensivist need to know. Minerva Anestesiol 2018;84:515–22.
9. Emanuel EJ. Four models of the physician-patient relationship. JAMA, J Am Med Assoc 1992;267:2221–6.
10. Charlesworth A, Tonkin EL. If You find Yourself in a Hole, stop Digging. In working with Text: tools, Techniques and approaches for Text mining. Elsevier; 2016. p. 61–88. https://doi.org/10.1016/B978-1-84334-749-1.00003-2.
11. Stoeklé HC, Deleuze JF, Vogt G Society. law, morality and bioethics: A systemic point of view. Ethics, Medicine and Public Health 2019;10:22–6.
12. Dzeng E, Bein T, Curtis JR. The role of policy and law in shaping the ethics and quality of end-of-life care in intensive care. Intensive Care Med 2022;48:352–4.
13. Lind R. Sense of responsibility in ICU end-of-life decision-making: Relatives' experiences. Nurs Ethics 2019;26:270–9.
14. McAndrew NS, Leske JS. A Balancing Act: Experiences of Nurses and Physicians When Making End-of-Life Decisions in Intensive Care Units. Clin Nurs Res 2015;24:357–74.
15. Michalsen A, Long AC, DeKeyser Ganz F, et al. Interprofessional Shared Decision-Making in the ICU: A Systematic Review and Recommendations From an Expert Panel. Crit Care Med 2019;47(9):1258–66.
16. Crico C, Sanchini V, Casali PG, et al. Evaluating the effectiveness of clinical ethics committees: a systematic review. Med Healthc Philos 2021;24:135–51.

17. Tusino S, Viafora C, Furlan E. Questioni di vita. Un'introduzione alla bioetica. (2019).
18. Simpkin AL, Schwartzstein RM. Tolerating Uncertainty — The Next Medical Revolution? N Engl J Med 2016;375:1713–5.
19. Hillman KM, Cardona-Morrell M. The ten barriers to appropriate management of patients at the end of their life. Intensive Care Med 2015;41:1700–2.
20. Hay-Smith EJC, Brown M, Anderson L, et al. Once a clinician, always a clinician: a systematic review to develop a typology of clinician-researcher dual-role experiences in health research with patient-participants. BMC Med Res Methodol 2016;16:1–17.
21. Accogli A, Vergano M. Be an ethicist not a stranger. Journal of Anesthesia, Analgesia and Critical Care 2023;3:26.

The Evolution of the Ethical Guidelines of the American Society of Anesthesiologists

Stephen H. Jackson, MD[a],*, David Waisel, MD[b]

KEYWORDS

- ASA ethical guidelines • Patients with DNR orders
- Anesthesiologists' ethical responsibilities • Medical ethics

KEY POINTS

- The history and evolution of the ethical guidelines for the American Society of Anesthesiologists is detailed.
- The self-determination of patients with existing Do-Not-Resuscitate (DNR) orders undergoing anesthesia and surgery/procedure is to be honored.
- Existing DNR orders should be reconsidered (not automatically rescinded) with the patient before anesthesia and surgery/procedure.
- Ethical behavior of anesthesiologists to patients, themselves, colleagues, nurses, hospitals, and society is binding for American Society of Anesthesiologists membership.

INTRODUCTION

For the most part, philosophers have been content to ignore the practical problems of real-time decision-making, regarding the brute fact that we are all finite and forgetful, and have to rush to judgment, as a real but irrelevant element of friction in the machinery whose blueprint they are describing. It is as if there might be two disciplines ethics proper, which undertakes the task of calculating the principles determining what the ideal agent ought to do under the circumstances – and then the less interesting "merely practical" discipline of Moral First Aid, or What to Do Until the Doctor of Philosophy Arrives, which tell, in rough and ready terms, how to make "online" decisions under time pressure.[1]

—Daniel Dennett

[a] Department of Anesthesiology, Bioethics Committee, Good Samaritan Hospital, 2425 Samaritan Drive, San Jose, CA 95124, USA; [b] Division of Pediatric Anesthesiology, Department of Anesthesiology, Yale Medical School, Yale School of Medicine, 333 Cedar Street, New Haven, CT 06510, USA
* Corresponding author.
E-mail address: hojacks@gmail.com

Anesthesiology Clin 42 (2024) 367–376
https://doi.org/10.1016/j.anclin.2023.12.004
1932-2275/24/© 2023 Elsevier Inc. All rights reserved.

anesthesiology.theclinics.com

Ethics is the study and analysis of morals and addresses concerns with other people's welfare and our responsibility to them, whereas moral precepts and codes refer to actions that may either harm or benefit others. Medical ethics tasks physicians to conduct their behavior as both a doctor and an ethicist, and therefore, studies the intentional actions that physicians carry out with sufficient knowledge and choice with respect to their being right or wrong. Every clinical anesthetic has ethical implications. Historically, anesthesiologists have played pivotal roles in the development of the field of medical ethics by responding to prominent ethical questions and proposing new ones.[2]

The Hippocratic Oath required a new physician to uphold ethical standards of conduct. With the passage of time, this Oath has been rewritten to conform to the values of different cultures. One popular version was created in 1964 by Louis Lasagna MD[a],[3] emphasizing a wholistic and compassionate approach to medicine: "*I shall remember that there is art to medicine as well as science, and that warmth, sympathy and understanding may outweigh the surgeon's knife or the chemist's drug.*"[4]

Throughout the history of Western culture, the work of human healing has intertwined with ethics and morals. Recurring themes brought to bear on the practice of healing include the character of the healer, the obligations of the healer to others, and their social responsibilities that engender public trust and authority.[5]

In 1847, 1 year after its founding, the American Medical Association (AMA) wrote its initial *Code of Medical Ethics*,[6] a document firmly rooted in the 1803 *Code of Ethics* written by British physician and moral philosopher/deontologist Thomas Percival that defined the responsibilities and relationships among physicians, surgeons, and apothecaries in hospitals.[7],[8] In 1927, a modernized version of Percival's *Code* was edited by Chauncey Leake PhD[b], who emphasized that Percival's *Code* was one of "etiquettes" rather than "ethics."[8–11] Nonetheless, he claimed that Percival did his best to promote the spirit of idealism and dignity of the medical profession. Leake advocated for basing professional ethics on a foundation of moral ethics concerned with the conduct of physicians toward their patients and society. The AMA's frequent revisions of its *Code* later were retitled *Principles of Medical Ethics*[6] and reflected the moral maturation of contemporary society that recognizes the value of the patient in the physician–patient relationship. These AMA *Principles* represent the fundamental ethical precepts of medical practice across all specialties and circumstances.[12,13]

To our knowledge, the earliest so-called Code of Ethics for an anesthesia society was proposed in 1949 by anesthesiologist William Neff MD.[c] Neff's Code focused on the interactions and interface of anesthesiologists with hospitals,[14] and a portion of this document's intent was reflected in the initial 1967 American Society of Anesthesiologists (ASA) *Guidelines to the Ethical Practice of Anesthesiology*.[15]

These 1967 *Guidelines* offered detailed legal and administrative definitions and descriptions of the rights and duties of anesthesiologists, addressing the behavior of

---

[a] Renowned physician and clinical pharmacologist and Dean of the Tufts University School of Graduate Medical Sciences who, early in his career, was a coinvestigator with Harvard Professor of Anesthesia, Henry Beecher.

[b] Renowned Professor of Pharmacology, discoverer of divinyl ether, popular author and lecturer on anesthesia.

[c] Coauthor of seminal articles on the clinical use of cyclopropane with Ralph Waters, MD and Emery Rovenstine, MD, and who established the first formal anesthesia training program in California (at Stanford).

anesthesiologists' interactions with their patients, colleagues and nurse anesthetists, and the hospitals in which they practiced. In 1977, however, the section of the *Guidelines* on "Financial Aspects of Anesthesia Practice"—in particular, the mandate that ASA members practice on a fee-for-service basis and not as an employee of an entity such as a hospital—instigated the Federal Trade Commission (with support of the Department of Justice) to claim the *Guidelines* thwarted competition and violated federal antitrust laws.[16] This forced a negotiated consent decree in 1979 in which the ASA agreed to revise their *Guidelines* by removing this federally offending portion.[17] This 1979 version also "recognized" the AMA *Principles of Medical Ethics* as *"the basic guide to the ethical conduct of its members,"* while concomitantly acknowledging that *"the practice of anesthesiology involves special problems relating to the quality and standards of patient care."*[17]

Because the ASA had not previously appointed a committee on ethics, its ethical guidelines had never received input from anesthesiologist-ethicists. Nonetheless, the 1979 *Guidelines* were ethically credible in that they addressed the anesthesiologist's relationship to patients, other physicians, nurse anesthetists and other nonphysician personnel; and their duties, responsibilities and relationship to the hospital. They spoke against unfair exclusion of qualified anesthesiologists from obtaining medical staff appointments; exploitation of patients and other anesthesiologists; unreasonable billings; and charging for anesthesia care that was not provided personally.

In 1992, the ASA appointed its first ever Committee on Ethics, prompted primarily by medical ethicists' concerns with the routine practice of automatically suspending existing Do-Not-Resuscitate (DNR) orders for patients entering the operating room, an act clearly failing to honor a patient's informed refusal for resuscitation. The Committee soon created 2 landmark documents: *Guidelines for Anesthesia Care of Patients with Do-Not-Resuscitate Orders or Other Directives Limiting Care* and *Guidelines for the Ethical Practice of Anesthesiology*. These constitute the primary focus of the remainder of this article.

AMERICAN SOCIETY OF ANESTHESIOLOGISTS GUIDELINES FOR THE ETHICAL PRACTICE OF ANESTHESIOLOGY

In 1993, the Committee on Ethics incorporated the *actual text* of the AMA's *Principles* into the "Preamble" portion of the existing (1979) *Guidelines for the Ethical Practice of Anesthesiology*. The Committee also determined that the still-in-force 1979 *Guidelines* were ethical only in the broadest sense, and that there was a need to expand its ethical foundations to assure longevity while concomitantly establishing a vehicle to facilitate modifications reflecting the evolving climate of ethical opinions. Consequently, in 1995 the "Body" of the *Guidelines* underwent extensive revision, reformation, and expansion.

These revised ASA *Guidelines* featured a description of acceptable physician conduct and behavior and were adopted in 1995.[18] The construct of these *Guidelines* focused on ethical values and behaviors and adhered to the 4 foundational principles of Western bioethics: patient autonomy (self-determination), physician beneficence (to confer benefit to the patient), physician nonmaleficence (to avoid inflicting harm), and social/distributive justice.[19] Today, social justice, often the least emphasized of these principles, holds a prominent footing in modern day population ethics and societal function. It refers to a just or fair distribution/allocation in society of our limited health-care resources so that benefits and risks are borne fairly by different groups, and it underscores physicians' responsibilities not only to the individual patient but also to society.

At its core, the practice of medicine is based on a covenant of trust among patients, physicians, and society,[20] one in which the ethics of medicine must seek to balance physicians' responsibility to each patient and the collective professional obligation to all who need medical care. Indeed, *"medicine, at its center, is a moral enterprise grounded in a covenant of trust,"*[20] morally obliging physicians to deploy their intellectual competence in the patient's best interests, continually renewing their covenant with patients and society. With only a few but important additions, the 1995 *Guidelines* have served well as a standard of physician behavior for almost 3 decades.

The first section of the *Guidelines*[18] addresses anesthesiologists' ethical responsibilities to their patients. Because the uniquely encompassing characteristic of the covenantal relationship between anesthesiologists and their patients is the vulnerability of the patient, emphasis is placed on administering "competent medical care with compassion and respect for human dignity and rights." In the process of obtaining informed consent, constituting the practical application of respect for the right of patients to self-determination, persuasion is ethically permissible but coercion and manipulation are forbidden. Respecting the right of every patient's autonomous moral agency, the *Guidelines* have added that minors should be included (assent) in medical decision-making that is appropriate to their developmental capacity and the medical issues involved.[21]

Prominently, the patient's interests are to be paramount because the anesthesiologist faithfully cares for the patient, is obligated to maintain patient confidentiality, and is honest and truthful. There should be commitment to lifelong learning and advancement of the science. Financial exploitation of patients and colleagues are forbidden. Moreover, anesthesiologists are to be forthcoming regarding their degree of participation in the patient's care, and to be continuously available to directly participate in the most demanding aspects of perioperative care. All of these obligations apply to *all* patients, irrespective of the ability of patients to pay for their care.

The second section introduces anesthesiologists' ethical responsibilities to respect their physician and nonphysician colleagues and to participate in enhancing the quality, effectiveness and efficiency of medical care. First among the medical specialties to incorporate maintaining physician physical and mental well-being into their ethical guidelines, anesthesiologists are obligated to observe, identify, and advise colleagues whose ability to practice has become impaired, and, when feasible, to assist them to rehabilitate for the purpose of returning to practice.

The third section, anesthesiologists' ethical responsibilities to the health-care facilities in which they work, advises them to be good citizens within their institutions, including to observe and report the potential of anyone whose negligent practice or behavior could inflict harm to patients, and to be vigilant for both the security and abuse of anesthetic drugs.

The fourth section requires anesthesiologists to have ethical responsibilities to themselves. With the prescient awareness of the epidemic of physician burnout, the *Guidelines* exhorted anesthesiologist to maintain their mental as well as physical health. Moreover, their primary professional duty is to achieve and maintain competence and skills through the vehicle of lifelong learning.

Although the first 4 sections have remained largely the same since their inception, the fifth Section, calling on anesthesiologists to have ethical responsibilities to their community and to society, had a decidedly rockier start within the ASA. The Committee's initial proposal for this section contained several statements of which the first essentially repeated a statement in Section 1 and was deleted. Another, addressing diversity, inclusion, and equity, was politically 30 years ahead of its time and also deleted. Finally, a statement that encouraged thoughtful use of local and planetary resources was mocked as a product of "West Coast tree huggers" and "moon-bea-mers"[2,d] and rejected. This notwithstanding, the ensuing years witnessed an expansion of this section's ethical horizons with additions involving expert witness testimony, misconduct in research and publication,[22] and, most recently, environmental sustainability because it relates to clinical anesthesia management.[23,24]

Because the first declaration in these *Guidelines* is that *"membership in the ASA is a privilege of physicians who are dedicated to the ethical provision of health care,"* they are actually *binding* for ASA membership. Initially this sentence was displayed for signature on the front of members' annual membership cards:

> *As a member of good Standing of the American Society of Anesthesiologists, I agree to adhere to the ASA "Guidelines for the Ethical Practice of Anesthesiology."*

Currently, while membership cards no longer are mailed to members, one can be accessed on the ASA website and printed out. Reassuringly, membership applications do require "click agreement" for *"I agree to the Guidelines for the Ethical Practice of Anesthesia."*

AMERICAN SOCIETY OF ANESTHESIOLOGISTS GUIDELINES FOR ANESTHESIA CARE OF PATIENTS WITH DO-NOT-RESUSCITATE ORDERS OR OTHER DIRECTIVES LIMITING CARE

A series of articles, most notably one published in 1991,[25] catalyzed the Committee on Ethics to create the *Guidelines for the Anesthesia Care of Patients with Do-Not-Resuscitate Orders or Other Directives Limiting Care*. These *Guidelines* codified that limitations on potentially life-sustaining treatment should be reviewed and reconsidered for the perioperative period rather than automatically revoked. It proposed procedure-directed limitations similar to those used on ward medicine. On request, the America College of Surgeons[26] and the Association of Operating Room Nurses[27] followed with similar statements.

In the procedure-directed approach, physicians are guided by a checklist of permissible interventions, such as mask ventilation, tracheal intubation, chest compressions, vasoactive drugs, and cardiac electric shock. A procedure-directed approach made sense for ward medicine where various physicians present in the hospital at the time of an arrest—often without knowledge of the patient or the etiology of the event initiating the code—had to respond to an arrest without the privilege of a personal discussion with the patient to ascertain their code status and how they wanted it managed.

These ASA *Guidelines* spawned objections, including the overlap of most procedure-directed limitations with standard anesthesia practice (such as intubation). Moreover, limitations on potentially life-sustaining treatment might lead an anesthesiologist to change an anesthetic technique to one that may be less likely to require resuscitation despite it being less optimal overall. Furthermore, concerns relating to the ethical and legal culpability of the anesthesiologist for not administering potentially life-sustaining treatment could be misapplied.

Perhaps, the most legitimate concern with the 1993 *Guidelines* was the fundamental incoherency between the vicissitudes of anesthetics requiring patient-tailored interventions and the absolute prohibitions of certain techniques of the procedure-

---

[d] Alluding to then California governor Jerry Brown.

directed approach. Anesthesiologists were uneasy with having limited flexibility to do what likely was consistent with the patient's overall goals, as for example, with sedation for a procedure that required temporary airway management, or pharmacologic reversal of bradycardia or hypotension.

This inflexibility exposed a persistent ambiguity and ambivalence among anesthesiologists regarding the care of patients who possess a moral right with respect to their existing orders expressing a desire to limit their resuscitation. This unease impeded a widespread acceptance and implementation of patient-desired limitations on perioperative potentially life-sustaining treatment. However, it paved the way to a landmark proposal for a goal-directed approach that presented an opportunity to honor patient's wishes without creating a moral hazard for the anesthesiologist.[28] This goal-directed approach presented the unique situation for anesthesiologists to manage events consistent with the patient's overall goals and values. It untied anesthesiologists' hands, letting them address conditions, typically temporary and reversible, that were consistent with the patient's goals. The resultant operating room scenario has the advantage of a patient having an anesthesiologist who would be able to discuss options and goals with the patient preanesthetically, and then implement them during the procedure. As compared with the procedure-directed approach, where the reversibility of the crisis would be unknown, the same anesthesiologist would be immediately present to assess the etiology and the likelihood of successful treatment leading to outcomes consistent with the patient's goals.

As a result, in 2001, a goal-directed approach to perioperative/periprocedural limitations of potentially life-sustaining treatment was incorporated into the existing *Guidelines* and remains in place through the present day. Reaffirmed in 2023,[29] these *Guidelines* offer 3 approaches to potentially life-sustaining treatment: (1) full attempt at resuscitation; (2) limited attempt at resuscitation defined by procedures; and (3) limited attempt at resuscitation defined by a patient's goals and values. The *Guidelines* also offer recommendations on documentation, including that for postsurgical/procedural care, such as when presurgery/procedure limitations on potentially life-sustaining treatment should be reinstituted, including whether to use a time-limited or event-limited trial of therapy to more closely achieve the patient's goals. This invaluable and ethical approach offers anesthesiologists opportunities while also creating demands with respect to the process of informed consent.[30]

In addition, these *Guidelines* propose a practical pathway to resolve any conflict of the anesthesiologist's moral beliefs about this ethical standard of care with those of the patient or the surgeon/proceduralist.

Despite these seeming enhancements, there has been only a slow adoption of this *Guideline* into routine clinical practice. It is our opinion that this ethically frustrating pace will continue until there is a sufficient number of anesthesiologists and surgeons/proceduralists who are trained to incorporate these limitations into routine practice.

A preview of the next iteration of patient-determined limitations on perioperative resuscitation may be represented by a 2021 article that proposes using an understanding of the variables affecting the outcomes of perioperative resuscitation, the increased recognition of approaches to goal-concordant care in geriatrics, and a promotion of shared decision-making that includes offering perioperative limitations on potentially life-sustaining treatment in those patients *without* current limitations.[31] Identifying patients at high risk for conventionally undesirable outcomes of perioperative resuscitation and tailoring the resuscitation efforts to their goals and likelihoods of the range of outcomes may further enhance the fulfillment of the basic ethical principle of patient self-determination.

THE AMERICAN SOCIETY OF ANESTHESIOLOGISTS COMMITTEE ON ETHICS RESPONDS TO CLINICAL EVENTS

Over time, ongoing events in clinical practice have influenced the work of the Committee on Ethics. Emblematic of this was the response to the question of physician nonparticipation in legally authorized executions. The AMA had a longstanding statement prohibiting physician participation in lethal injection.[32] In 2005, concerns about whether inmates are sufficiently anesthetized during lethal injection led some states to suggesting the involvement of an anesthesiologist in lethal injection to ensure that the inmate was properly anesthetized. In response to these concerns, ASA President Orin Guidry wrote a *Message from the President* emphasizing that the AMA guidelines prohibit physician participation, and that the ASA endorses these guidelines.[33] At the next ASA Annual Meeting in October 2006, the ASA produced a formal statement developed by the Committee on Ethics stating:

Capital punishment in any form is not the practice of Medicine.[34]

The current statement on *Physician Nonparticipation in Legally Authorized Executions*, last amended in 2021, does not differ significantly from the original 2006 statement.

The question then arose as to whether the ASA should enforce professional standards through various mechanisms, such as forfeiture of ASA membership. The American Board of Anesthesiology had declared that participation in lethal injection, a violation of AMA guidelines, could result in revocation of diplomate status.[35] In fact, the contemporaneous chair and a previous chair of the ASA Committee on Ethics distinguished between the roles of the American Board of Anesthesiology and ASA, and they emphasized that the ASA itself had "no regulatory authority" or ability to affect an anesthesiologist's practice, making enforcement ineffectual.[36]

On another front, a stunning increase in drug shortages required anesthesiologists to make difficult decisions regarding use of scarce resources and presented challenges as to how to communicate to patients about the use of alternative drugs or techniques. In 2013, the Committee published a comprehensive *Statement* guiding anesthesiologists through these difficult issues.[37] In part, the *Statement* suggests that anesthesiologists disclose to patients if the increased risk of an alternative technique was "significant." It indirectly reminded anesthesiologists of the professionalism associated with contributing to national databases to help determine the risk of alternative approaches, and it also warned against hoarding of drugs. The most important part of the statement, however, may have been the admonition that anesthesiologists have an "ethical obligation to examine and manage shortage of drugs that are essential to safe practice,"[37] prompting anesthesiologists to consider ethical obligations beyond direct patient care.

The Committee also expanded its domains for consideration with a Statement on Fatigue that identified not only the ethical aspects of patient safety and physician well-being but also defined requirements for education and mitigation of fatigue.[38] The Committee additionally has contributed to ASA's development of comprehensive policies on conflicts of interest, as well as statements regarding organ donation after circulatory death[39] and pregnancy testing before anesthesia and surgery.[40]

SUMMARY

The ASA Committee on Ethics has helped anesthesiologists navigate complexities in professionalism, clinical care and science, and even with nonclinical participation in events, both preemptively when a need was recognized and in response to a wide range of issues. Furthermore, the work of the Committee, along with perhaps generational and societal change, has increased the number and productivity of anesthesiologists involved in academic and clinical medical ethics, promoting recognition and concern with the broad spectrum of ethical issues facing the anesthesiologist. Indeed, the Committee has been central to the development of the specialty of anesthesiology.

CLINICS CARE POINTS

- DNR orders of patients presenting for anesthesia should be reconsidered and not automatically rescinded, thus honoring patient autonomy.
- Anesthesiologists have ethical obligations to their patients (including minors), physician and nonphysician colleagues, themselves, health-care institutions, and their community and society.

ACKNOWLEDGMENTS

The authors wish to gratefully acknowledge the help of Gabrielle Jackson, PhD, from the Department of Philosophy, Stanford University, for her kind review of an early draft and recommended inserting the quote from the eminent philosopher Daniel Dennett (recently passed) that introduces the article, and in so doing, set the "focus and thrust" for the entire article. She has also served as a co-member of the Bioethics Committee of Boston Children's Hospital.

DISCLOSURE

The authors have nothing to disclose.

REFERENCES

1. Dennett D. Darwin's dangerous idea – evolution and the meaning of life. New York, N.Y: Touchtone/Simon and Schuster; 1995.
2. Jackson S, Van Norman G. Anesthesia, anesthesiologists and modern medical ethics. In: Eger E, Saidman L, Westhorpe R, editors. The wondrous story of anesthesia. New York, NY: Springer; 2014. p. 205–18.
3. Mashour G. From LSD to the IRB: Henry Beecher's Psychedelic research and the foundation for clinical ethics. In: Lowenstein E, McPeek B, editors. Enduring contributions of Henry K. Beecher to medicine, science, and society. Hagerstown, MD: International Anesthesiology Clinics. (Wolters Kluweer); 2007. p. 105–11.
4. Lasagna L. The Hippocratic Oath: Modern Version. Available at: https// www.pbs.org/wgbh/nova/oath_medicine. Accessed 09-18-2023.
5. Jonsen A. The birth of bioethics. New York: Oxford University Press; 1998.
6. Riddick F Jr. The Code of Medical Ethics of the American Medical Association. Ochsner J 2003;5:6–10.
7. Percival P. Medical ethics: or, a code of institutes and precepts, adapted to the professional conduct of physicians and surgeons. Birmingham, Alabama: The Classics of Medicine Library; 1985.
8. Leake C, editor. Percival's medical ethics. Baltimore: Williams and Wilkins; 1927.
9. Pelligrino E, Thomas Percival's Ethics. The Ethics Beneath the Etiquette. In: Percival P., Medical ethics. Birmingham, AL: The Classics of Medicine Library; 1985. p. 1–52.

10. Leake C. Percival's medical ethics: promise and problems. West J Med 1971;114: 68–70.
11. Leake C. Percival's Medical Ethics. NEJM (Boston Medical and Surgical Journal) 1927;197(#9):357–61.
12. American Medical Association. Principles of medical ethics. https://code-medical-ethics.ama-assn.org/principles. Last Accessed date 23 September 2023.
13. Patuzzo S, Goracci G, Ciliberti R, et al. Discussing the foundations of medical ethics. Acta Biomed 2018;89:343–8.
14. Jackson, S. A scrapbook collation of the history of organized California anesthesia societies predating the California Society of Anesthesiologists.
15. American Society of Anesthesiologists. Guidelines to the Ethical Practice of Anesthesiology. Member Directory, 1967.
16. Scott M. 1979 adventures in antitrust: some justice here, some FTC there. ASA Newsl 2004;68:18–9.
17. American Society of Anesthesiologists. Guidelines for the Ethical Practice of Anesthesiology. Directory of Members, 1982.
18. American Society of Anesthesiologists. Guidelines for the Ethical Practice of Anesthesiology. Last amended October 13, 2020. www.asahq.org Last Accessed 29 September 2023.
19. Beauchamp T, Childress J. Principles of biomedical ethics. 4th edition. Oxford, UK: Oxford University Press; 1994. p. 12.
20. Crawshaw R, Rogers D, Pelligrino E, et al. Patient-physician covenant. JAMA 1995;273:1553.
21. Waisel D. Ethical issues in pediatric anesthesiology. In: Cote C, Lerman J, Anderson B, editors. A practice of anesthesia for infants and children. 6th edition. Amsterdam: Elsevier; 2019. p. 69–80.
22. Jackson S, Van Norman G. Ethics in research and publication. In: Jericho B, editor. Ethical issues in anesthesiology and surgery. Cham: Springer; 2015. p. p199–214.
23. Van Norman G, Jackson S. The anesthesiologist and global climate change: an ethical obligation to act. Cur Opin Anes 2020;33:577–83.
24. American Society of Anesthesiologists Task Force on Environmental Sustainability Committee on Equipment and Facilities. Greening the operating room and perioperative arena; environmental sustainability for anesthesia practice. American Society of Anesthesiologists. ASAhq.org. Last accessed 11/09/2023.
25. Truog RD. "Do-not-resuscitate" orders during anesthesia and surgery. Anesthesiology 1991;74(3):606–8.
26. American College of Surgeons. Statement of the American College of Surgeons on advance directives by patients: "Do not resuscitate" in the operating room. Bull Am Coll Surg 1994;79(9):29.
27. Association of peri-Operative Registered Nurses. Position Statement on Perioperative Care of Patients with Do-Not-Resuscitate or Allow-Natural-Death Orders. 1995 and reaffirmed by the Board of Directors, 2020. Available at: https://www.aorn.org/docs/default-source/guidelines-resources/position-statements/patient-care/posstat-dnr-w-0620.pdf?sfvrsn=b4a9796d_1. Last Accessed date November 8, 2023.
28. Truog RD, Burns JP, Waisel DB. DNR in the OR: A goal-directed approach. Anesthesiology 1999;90:289–95.
29. American Society of Anesthesiologists. Statement on Ethical Guidelines for the Anesthesia Care of Patients with Do-Not-Resuscitate Orders. Reaffirmed:

October 18, 2023. (original approval: October 17, 2001). https://www.asahq.org/standards-and-practice-parameters/statement-on-ethical-guidelines-for-the-anesthesia-care-of-patients-with-do-not-resuscitate-orders?&ct=6fd89a56f0c 16f42540bd59b6891d7cfe986683546c2fd70353bb3c2375a115f0fcd531b4193e 28886e374525f722c32d114f90efa7c9db7915792201e2c5b55 Accessed November 3, 2023.

30. Jackson S, Van Norman G. Goals- and values-directed approach to informed consent in the "DNR" patient presenting for surgery: More demanding of the anesthesiologist? (editorial). Anesthesiology 1999;90:3–6.

31. Allen MB, Bernacki R, Gewertz, et al. Beyond the do not resuscitate order: An Expanded Approach to Decision-making Regarding Cardiopulmonary Resuscitation in Older Surgical Patients. Anesthesiology 2021;135:781–7.

32. AMA Code of Medical Ethics. Opinion 9.7.3. Capital Punishment. Available at: https://code-medical-ethics.ama-assn.org/ethics-opinions/capital-punishment#:~:text=An%20individual's%20opinion%20on%20capital,in%20a%20legally%20authorized%20execution. Accessed November 3, 2023.

33. Guidry OF. Message from the President. Observations regarding lethal injection. American Society of Anesthesiologists Newsletter 2006;70(8):6–8.

34. American Society of Anesthesiology. Statement on Physician Nonparticipation in Legally Authorized Executions. Amended October 13, 2021. https://www.asahq.org/standards-and-practice-parameters/statement-on-physician-nonparticipation-in-legally-authorized-executions Last accessed November 9, 2023.

35. American Board of Anesthesiology. Policy Book. Policy 7.06, Professional standing. Raleigh, NC: American Board of Anesthesiology; 2023:68-69. https://www.theaba.org/wp-content/uploads/pdfs/Policy_Book.pdf Accessed November 3, 2023.

36. Van Norman GA, Jackson SH. The importance of enforcing professionalism at ASA. ASA Newsl 2011;75(5):10–2.

37. American Society of Anesthesiology. Statement on the Ethical Considerations with Drug Shortages. Approved October 16, 2013. https://www.asahq.org/standards-and-practice-parameters/statement-on-the-ethical-considerations-with-drug-shortages Accessed November 3, 2023.

38. American Society of Anesthesiology. Statement on Fatigue. Approved October 15, 2014; last amended October 13, 2021. https://www.asahq.org/standards-and-practice-parameters/statement-on-fatigue#:~:text=Anesthesia%20providers%20must%20receive%20training,to%20include%20potential%20staffing%20solutions Accessed November 3, 2023.

39. American Society of Anesthesiologists. Statement on Controlled Organ Donation After Circulatory Death. Committees on Critical Care, Ethics and Transplant Anesthesia. Last amended October 25, 2017. https://www.asahq.org/standards-and-practice-parameters/statemetn-on-controlled-organ-donation-after-circulatory-death.

40. ASA Committee on Quality Management and departmental Administration. Pregnancy testing prior to anesthesia and surgery. American Society of Anesthesiologists. October, 2021. Available at https://www.asahq.org/standards-and-guidelines/statement-on-pregnancy-testing-prior-to-anesthhesia-and-surgery. Last accessed June 9, 2023.

The role of Advance Directives and Living Wills in Anesthesia Practice

Michael J. Devinney, MD, PhD[a,b],
Miriam M. Treggiari, MD, PhD, MPH[a,c],*

KEYWORDS

- Advance care planning • End-of-life • Patient-centered care
- Shared decision-making

KEY POINTS

- A discussion of advance directives and any limitations on life-sustaining medical therapy should occur before procedures, to ensure that patient's wishes are being honored, to improve quality of care, and to minimize unnecessary medical care.
- Perioperative physicians, including anesthesiologists and surgeons, are best poised to lead these discussions and establish perioperative directives through shared decision-making with patients.
- Enhanced perioperative workflows and physician communication training have potential to improve the consistency for preoperative advance care planning and improve quality of perioperative care.

INTRODUCTION

Advance directives (ADs) refer to written instructions recognized under state laws that indicate the patient's or a surrogate's authorization to provide health care to the patient when the patient is incapacitated and unable to make decisions.[1–3]

This process is supported by the Patient Self-Determination Act that was passed by Congress and became effective in 1991.[4,5] The act requires that all health care institutions that receive Medicare or Medicaid funds provide written information to patients

[a] Department of Anesthesiology, Duke University School of Medicine, 2301 Erwin Road, Durham, NC 27710, USA; [b] Department of Anesthesiology, Duke University School of Medicine, 40 Medicine Circle, Room 4317, Orange Zone, Duke Hospital South, Durham, NC 27710, USA; [c] Department of Anesthesiology, Duke University School of Medicine, 3 Genome Court, MSRB-3, 6116, Durham, NC 27710, USA
* Corresponding author. Department of Anesthesiology, Duke University School of Medicine, 3 Genome Court, MSRB-3, 6116, Durham, NC 27710.
E-mail address: miriam.treggiari@duke.edu

Anesthesiology Clin 42 (2024) 377–392
https://doi.org/10.1016/j.anclin.2024.02.001
1932-2275/24/© 2024 Elsevier Inc. All rights reserved.
anesthesiology.theclinics.com

and/or their families concerning their state-recognized rights to establish ADs before any serious procedure.[5] Each health care institution must provide patients with information regarding ADs and their right to refuse medical treatment.[1,5]

The American Association of Nurse Anesthesiology recommends that, whenever possible, patients, family members, proceduralists, and the anesthesia team should meet at the time of obtaining informed consent for anesthesia, thoroughly review and discuss the patient's ADs, and develop a plan for care that completely aligns with the wishes of the patient.[6,7] Furthermore, since the mid-1970s, the American Medical Association recommends that decisions of "do-not-resuscitate" (DNR) should be formally documented in the medical records.[8]

On the other hand, the American Society of Anesthesiologists (ASA) published more extensive guidelines for the anesthesia care of patients with DNR orders.[9] These guidelines emphasize that it is very important that the parties involved practice proper and prompt communication and patients and their designated surrogates should have all the necessary information to make their decisions concerning ADs.[1,2] Every practitioner must provide clear and accurate information to patients, an essential element of preoperative preparation and perioperative care for patients with DNR orders or other directives directing treatment.[9]

In regard to the preoperative discussion of existing directives (including DNR orders) to guide the use of resuscitation efforts during perioperative care, the ASA guidelines present 3 possible resulting outcomes.[9]

(1) *Full attempt at resuscitation*: "The patient or a surrogate may request full suspension of the existing directives at the time of anesthesia and immediately following the postoperative (PO) procedures. In other words, there is implicit consent to perform resuscitation procedures if they can provide successful outcomes."

(2) *Limited attempt at resuscitation according to some specific procedures*: "A patient or a surrogate is free to refuse certain specific resuscitation procedures (for example, chest compressions, defibrillation or tracheal intubation). Because of this instruction, it is imperative that the anesthesiologists inform the patients or their surrogates which procedures are essential for the success of the anesthesia and the proposed procedure, and which ones are not essential; and therefore may be refused."

(3) *Limited attempt at resuscitation because of the goals and values of the patient*: In this case, "with the agreement of the patient or the designated surrogate, the anesthesiologist and the procedural team may use clinical judgment to determine those resuscitation procedures that are appropriate regarding the situation and the goals and values of the patient."

In summary, particularly in patients with advanced age or life-limiting illnesses,[10] it is of the outmost importance to discuss existing ADs and DNR orders to determine if there will be any perioperative resuscitation limitations. The outcome of the discussion should be documented clearly in the medical record. By doing so, perioperative care can be tailored according to the goals and values of the patient. These health care plans should be revisited periodically as well as prior to any future anesthesia and surgical services to ensure that they remain in agreement with what the patient has previously indicated. Most recommendations discourage automatic DNR orders during surgery and emphasize the importance of documenting patients' resuscitation decisions based on their personal values, although in some cases, a DNR order may be temporarily removed during the immediate perioperative period after discussion with all providers and the patient or family.[10,11]

Recommendations About Anesthesia Care for Patients with Do-not-Resuscitate Orders

Guidelines on anesthesia care for patients with DNR orders discourage automatic DNR suspension during the perioperative period because this practice could lead to perioperative interventions that are incongruent with the patient's wishes. For example, while some interventions that the patient would normally decline (such as intubation) may be temporarily necessary for the provision of anesthesia, these interventions may not be desired in other clinical scenarios, such as progressive organ failure or critical illness.[10,11] Thus, a perioperative physician must develop a plan for perioperative life-sustaining medical treatment (LSMT) centered on the patient's preferences.[12] This plan should be communicated to all perioperative team members, including prespecified criteria (such as time) guiding PO reinstitution of the DNR orders.

The Role of Patient Preferences in Perioperative Resuscitation Planning

According to the ASA guidelines, the wishes and goals of the patient must be prioritized in all health care decisions, including resuscitation.[9] If there is a need for suspension or modification of limitations on LSMT, the duration of this suspension should be determined preoperatively, well-documented, and communicated to all personnel involved. The patients and/or their surrogates must be informed about any potentially life-threatening problems and about any approaches that the physician may follow to deal with such problems.[13] In summary, understanding patients' values and wishes is essential in perioperative resuscitation care.

PREOPERATIVE PLANNING: THE ROLE OF THE PERIOPERATIVE PROVIDER IN ADVANCE DIRECTIVES

Perioperative discussions of advance care planning (ACP) should include the entire multidisciplinary perioperative care team including nurses, anesthesiologists, surgeons, and any other consultants (including a primary care provider) involved in perioperative care. In the context of perioperative and anesthetic risks, the preferences of the patient and their attitudes toward ACP should be personally reviewed by the health care provider administering anesthesia.[11,14–16] While anesthesiologists have a positive view of the importance of ACP, they may sometimes lack adequate training to address these conversations with the patients.[17] Yet, it is important that anesthesiologists initiate these discussions in part because of key differences in relationships of anesthesiologists and surgeons with surgical patients. Due to the discussion leading up to surgery, surgeons may expect that their patients accept aggressive forms of life support despite indications from patients and their surrogates that this is not consistent with their goals.[18,19] Thus, although surgeons tend to form durable personal relationships with their patients, anesthesiologists may be better poised to have critical conversations that will elicit important values to inform perioperative care ADs. Finally, it is paramount to recognize that there are legal and medical consequences of resuscitation against documented patient wishes, which in some circumstances have had significant implications that resulted in diminished public trust.[16]

Primary Goals of Advanced Care Planning

Advanced care planning's (ACP) primary goal is to engage the patients and/or their surrogate in a conversation about their goals, values, and preferences for end-of-life medical care.[20] This discussion should be directed at allowing the patient to manifest their wishes regarding medical treatments, in particular life-sustaining treatments such that health care providers know what is expected of them in order to satisfy the patient's decisions during the perioperative period.

Importance of the Advanced Care Planning in the Perioperative Period

In the perioperative period, ACP is important because it ensures that the resuscitation preferences of the patients are respected during all involved procedures.[21–23] These plans are particularly relevant when procedural outcomes do not meet best case scenario expectations or if there are perioperative complications. ACP engages patients in conversations to determine their goals and preferences for end-of-life medical care, including whether to limit or continue PO LSMTs. The attending anesthesiologist should re-evaluate the fundamental limitations of the potentially life-sustaining treatments before the anesthetic is administered in order to determine the perioperative resuscitation preferences of the patients.[10,24] Furthermore, ACP discussions facilitate accurate documentation of the end-of-life care preferences of the patients, including their wishes concerning resuscitation.

The attitudes, knowledge, and training of anesthesiologists regarding DNR orders have evolved since they were first published in the early 90s.[10] Currently, there are more anesthesiologists following professional directives that recommend against automatically suspending DNR orders in the perioperative period.[24] Per a recent study in 2013,[25] anesthesiologists are half as likely to automatically suspend DNR orders perioperatively compared to both internists and surgeons (18% vs 34%–38%). In general, anesthesiologists have a positive view concerning ACP, and compared with previous years, they are currently better trained to address ACP conversations with the patients and their families. In addition, recent survey data have shown that most surgical patients are interested in having ACP discussions, particularly surrounding their desire for life-saving treatments versus life-prolonging treatments.[26]

Because of the nuances of determining whether a treatment is likely to be life-saving versus simply life-prolonging,[26] perioperative physicians should be the primary leader engaging patients in ACP conversations to determine their wishes for end-of-life care preferences, documenting their decisions, and respecting their choices (such as code status) during the operation. Furthermore, physicians should conduct the patient-centered re-evaluation of fundamental limitations of potential LSMTs before administering anesthesia (including DNR directives).[21,27] Using specialized knowledge of perioperative LMST, physicians are well positioned to guide ACP discussions to determine when a patient would prefer to limit or continue LSMT that incorporates their end-of-life care preferences.[28] Thus, all perioperative physicians should be properly prepared to readily discuss ACP and LSMT with the patients during the perioperative period.[24] Finally, the patients' perioperative resuscitation preferences must be respected during surgical procedures, based on these sincere and open conversations regarding ACP between patients and physicians.

Perioperative physicians should collaboratively engage patients in ACP conversations before anesthesia, so that their desired end-of-life care preferences are documented, such as situations in which LSMTs should be withheld to ensure that these choices are respected perioperatively. Surgeons and anesthesiologists must work together to incorporate ACP conversations into their preoperative workflow. This collaboration will enable clinicians to have a holistic approach to patient care and ensure that the patient is actively involved in the process. Further, patients who participate in these conversations report higher satisfaction levels and feel more at ease knowing that their wishes are respected.[29]

Potential Consequence of Resuscitating a Patient Against Their Documented Wishes

Resuscitating a patient against their documented wishes may result in potential legal action from the patient or their families.[1,9] Providers and medical institutions have been held liable for legal charges such as assault, battery, or negligence, and for causing emotional distress. Additionally, resuscitation-related injuries may result in public health citations, institutional fines, medicolegal damages, and increased medical bills. Cases of resuscitation against documented patient wishes have also received high-profile coverage in the media, leading to a public distrust in the medical field.[10]

CLINICAL OUTCOMES: IMPLICATIONS OF LSMT ON POSTOPERATIVE MORBIDITY AND MORTALITY

Although surgical patients with preoperative limitations on LSMT are consistently associated with higher mortality compared to age-matched, procedure-matched, and comorbidity-matched patients without LSMT limitations,[30–37] these groups exhibit no significant differences in the rates of major PO complications. This finding potentially reflects an equivalent quality of care but less-aggressive PO resuscitation, consistent with the patient's goals or surrogate wishes. Patients with preoperative limitations on LSMT status also do not appear to have increased rates of common PO complications.[31] It is essential to note that these findings are limited to the rates of PO complications and do not apply to patients' survival or mortality.

The Study to Understand Prognoses and Preferences for Outcomes and Risks of Treatments (SUPPORT) trial, conducted between 1989 and 1994, was designed to study the effect of different intensities of medical care on seriously ill patients and their families.[38] This study was focused on potential improvements in communication, decision-making, and patients' outcomes. SUPPORT was designed to determine whether improving communication between patients, families, and health care providers about their expectations for medical treatments and their possible benefits and burdens would lead to better alignment of the treatments with the patients' goals, values, and preferences, thereby improving patients' outcomes. For the SUPPORT study, 2652 patients were enrolled in the intervention arm while 2152 were enrolled in the control arm.[39] Patients found that they had major issues with (1) understanding their situation, (2) communication and decision-making, (3) ACP, (4) DNR orders, and (5) general support, including support for loss and grieving. There is no evidence to suggest that patients with preoperative limitations on LSMT status receive poorer quality of care compared to those without such limitations.[10] In fact, it is suggested that the increased mortality but not morbidity among surgical patients with preoperative LSMT limitations may reflect an equivalent quality of care but less-aggressive PO resuscitation, consistent with the patient's goals or wishes.[33,34,36]

The Effects of DNR Instructions on Morbidity and Mortality

Patients with preoperative DNR instructions undergoing surgery have consistently shown higher PO mortality rates than those without DNR orders.[24,34] A surgical subgroup analysis of the SUPPORT trial phase 1 cohort found that of the patients with DNR orders, 57 proceeded to surgery, and only 31 survived to discharge. Additionally, 4 patients with preoperative DNR orders who underwent surgery experienced cardiopulmonary arrest either intraoperatively or postoperatively with attempted resuscitation, but none survived.[38] These findings suggest that preoperative DNR orders may be associated with increased mortality among patients undergoing surgery.[30–37] However, it is important to note that this conclusion is limited only to mortality and does not provide evidence of how DNR orders may affect morbidity. In contrast to mortality, there were similar rates of common PO complications in those with preoperative limitations on LSMT status (vs those without), suggesting that increased mortality seen in those with preoperative limitations on LMST are not due to higher complication rates.[33]

Evidence suggests that having pre-existing limitations on LSMT leads to higher PO mortality.[30–37] A significant proportion of patients aged over 65 years undergoing surgery have pre-existing limitations on LSMT, and this subgroup consistently has higher PO mortality than those without preexisting limitations.[10] It is not clear whether information about postsurgical survival for patients with preoperative limitations on LSMT is appropriately and clearly communicated to patients as part of their surgical and anesthesia consent process.[10] Therefore, there are potential concerns that patients with limitations on LSMT may not be fully informed about their PO survival rates during the surgical and anesthesia consent process.[29,40]

In summary, compared to those without limitations, patients aged older than 65 years undergoing surgery with pre-existing limitations on LSMT have higher PO mortality but do not appear to have increased rates of common PO complications. Thus, increased mortality but not morbidity may reflect equivalent quality of care but less-aggressive resuscitation following surgery, consistent with the patient's goals or wishes. Finally, information about lower PO survival rates in those with preoperative limitations on LSMT status is not consistently communicated to patients as part of their surgical and anesthesia consent process.

CURRENT PRACTICE AND ADHERENCE TO GUIDELINES

Despite increasing awareness of ADs and many guidelines recommending preoperative discussion of ADs, these discussions occur less often than they do when care is being provided by nonprocedural specialties.[10] The difference may be related to the extent of involvement in the care of the patient (ongoing primary care vs procedure-specific perioperative care) or the training and experience of the providers. To address the latter, there needs to be improvement in training perioperative physicians to have these important conversations that includes decision-making skills and implementation of documentation and communications strategies.[41–44] There also is a need for further research investigating the impact of discussing preoperative limitations of LSMT on PO patient-centered outcomes.

The Role of Cultural Tolerance

Procedural specialties may have lower cultural tolerance for uncertainty (ie, full consideration of worst-case scenario) and thus an aversion to limitations on aggressive care than internal medicine or primary care specialists. It has been suggested that even while some perioperative physicians are aware of the guidelines, they are not consistently working with patients to establish their treatment goals or do not deliver care according to those goals.[10,45] Further research documenting the positive impact of preoperative AD discussions on patient-centered outcomes could be helpful to convince perioperative physicians and procedural specialists about the importance of these discussions.

Research and Educational Programs Can Improve the Delivery of Patient-centered Perioperative Care

Additional studies are likely to demonstrate how delivery of patient-centered perioperative care can be improved by clearly addressing goals of care, particularly for patients at the end-of-life. By prioritizing research that addresses these outcomes, medical practitioners can better understand the needs of patients and tailor care plans to meet those needs. In addition, developing and evaluating educational programs could improve procedural physicians' shared decision-making skills, and encourage implementation of new care systems that emphasize documentation and communication of patient wishes, in order to improve the delivery of patient-centered perioperative care. The content of these programs should focus on improving physicians' skills to elicit patient goals for treatment limitation and deliver care consistent with those goals. By improving their shared decision-making skills, procedural physicians can better communicate with their patients and understand their end-of-life care wishes. Furthermore, new care systems could be implemented emphasizing documentation and communication of patient wishes in order to provide the best possible procedural care for patients near the end-of-life. Such care systems may include better and more easily accessible information about patients' advance care directives and documented wishes for limitations on life-sustaining therapy in the electronic health records.

FUTURE DIRECTIONS: PATIENT-CENTERED OUTCOME DATA

Better patient-centered outcome data, especially for patients with LSMT who tend to prefer quality over quantity of life, are needed. These data must include PO outcomes, including length of stay, mortality, morbidity, and other PO quality metrics such as functional and cognitive status, decision remorse, and perceptions of care of the caregiver or the survivor. Furthermore, better tools for assessing frailty, psychological status, and social support are also needed to help educate patients and providers about each patient's status and improve the patient-centered decision-making process. Annotated data can be used to improve communication practices among patients, providers, and/or surrogates regarding preoperative preparations and the potential outcomes of surgery, including PO care.[10,46–50]

Patient-centered Outcome Data

Patient-centered outcome data systems collect the information about the impact of health care interventions on each individual patient; these data are collected directly from the patient rather than relying on the evaluations of experts.[10] These data may include measures of functional status, symptoms, health-related quality of life, decision-making, satisfaction with care, and other patient-reported outcomes that indicate the experience of the patient as related to health care. The data can help patients and their providers make decisions about health care that are aligned with the patient's experiences, goals, values, and priorities.

The patient-centered outcome data can be used to improve health care in several ways. First, it can help patients make informed decisions about their care by providing them with information on how different health care interventions impact their symptoms, functional status, and quality of life. Second, it can help providers understand what matters most to their patients and how to tailor care accordingly. Third, it can help health care systems and policymakers measure the quality of care delivered to patients and identify areas for improvement. Finally, it can help researchers design better studies on health care interventions that account for the perspectives and priorities of patients. In summary, patient-centered outcome data are a valuable tool for improving health care quality and can be used to inform the decisions of patients, providers, health care systems, policymakers, and researchers.[10]

Differences Between Patient-centered Outcome Data in the Perioperative Setting Versus in the Intensive Care Unit

The perioperative setting is more appropriate for structured communication, shared decision-making, and patient optimization than the intensive care unit (ICU), where many clinical issues require emergency response, leaving little opportunity for discussion of ADs. On the other hand, for patients admitted to the ICU with pre-existing ADs or for patients able to communicate their wishes early in the ICU course, the discussions can provide similar guidance as is available during the less-emergent perioperative care environment. ICU literature has validated culturally tailored instruments for measuring the quality of intensive care for relatives and has defined key quality domains for end-of-life care in the ICU. In contrast, there are limited data on patient-centered and surrogate-centered PO outcomes in patients with limitations on LSMT, and many of the measured outcomes remain "hospital length of stay, 30 day mortality, and 30 day morbidity" rather than PO quality metrics such as the "impact of surgery on pain and symptoms, decision regret, and caregiver or survivor perceptions of care."[10,19,46–51]

Along these lines, robust preoperative screening tools to assess preprocedure cognitive and psychological status, activities of daily living, frailty, and social support have been partially developed and implemented. Some of the known screening tools for evaluating frailty include the Clinical Frailty Scale[52] and the Groningen Frailty Indicator.[53] For social support, the Lubben Social Network Scale[54] and the Medical Outcomes Study Social Support Survey[55] can be used. Additionally, standardized preoperative assessments such as anesthesia preoperative instructions and Patient-Reported Outcomes Measurement Information System[56,57] measures of function, depression, and anxiety can assist in evaluating patient baseline characteristics ahead of surgery, all of which can impact shared decision-making between providers and patients about goals of care.

The Process of Shared Decision-making in the Perioperative Setting

In shared decision-making, patients are questioned about their clinical goals, values, and priorities. This also allows providers to discuss what options of care are appropriate based on patients' goals and expectations, including potential outcomes associated with each option. For many patients, preoperative frailty can be an important consideration in the discussion about goals of care and potential limitations on PO life sustaining medical therapy. There are many other factors that should be considered since they also correlate with PO complications, including other measures of preoperative functional status. Identifying these factors can inform the strategy of care and improve outcomes.[10] Further research designed to identify these key factors will help improve the decision-making process. For example, artificial intelligence may be a useful tool for evaluating outcomes in diverse patient populations, which could impact advance decision-making by informing clinicians and patients about potential outcomes that impact advance decision-making.

Several instruments used to measure patient-centered outcomes are more focused palliation of symptoms, and the value of spiritual and emotional support.[58,59] While important, these outcomes are not as well studied and their impact on decision-making is less clear.[10]

Practical Applications for Improved Perioperative Outcome studies that Focus on Functional Status in the Context of LMST Limitations

Improved perioperative outcome data based on "functional status" and "predefined patient goals" should facilitate communications with the patients and their families, including potential outcomes of surgery and PO care.[10] Improved communications of patient-centered values should be informed by patient goals and wishes, and help make better decisions about whether or not to proceed to surgery, and finally should result in improved outcomes.[10]

Finally, shared decision-making models can be particularly effective. Steps that could help improve the measurement and use of patient-centered outcome data include (1) improve perioperative outcome data that focus on functional status and predefined patient goals, which can help patients and families make better-informed decisions about the benefits and risks of surgery; (2) increase the accuracy of information on the likelihood of PO outcomes that typically matter to patients with LMST limitations to inform a patient-centered shared decision-making process; (3) use preoperative tools to assess perioperative cognitive and psychological status, activities of daily living, instrumental activities of daily living, frailty, and social support to identify patients who are at an increased risk of PO complications; and (4) leverage the use of robust preoperative assessments to guide a patient-centered shared decision-making process.[10]

FUTURE DIRECTIONS: PERIOPERATIVE PHYSICIAN TRAINING

Structural perioperative physician training programs should include improving communication skills, specifically in having discussions with patients about serious illnesses and ACP and goals of care.[10] There is a general perception by anesthesiologists that care planning and discussions of goals of care are important; however, they feel less confident of being able to initiate these discussions. While primary care providers may have the advantages of longer access and well-established therapeutic relationships with the patients, they may not have the proper understanding of the risks and benefits of a procedure and possible courses of perioperative care. Novel information about procedural outcomes and the course of perioperative care during the preoperative discussion may lead to a change in patient's goals and wishes that will influence perioperative AD and decision-making. Although some perioperative physicians may feel that AD conversations should be conducted by other providers with long-term therapeutic relationships with the patient, it is imperative that perioperative physicians conduct these conversations. Therefore, perioperative physicians need to have adequate training in shared decision-making and goals of care discussions.

Training Programs Available to Improve Physicians' Communication Skills for Emotionally Charged Conversations

It is of the outmost importance to develop and implement training and educational programs designed to improve the skills of physicians and their comfort with perioperative discussions of treatment limitations and goals of care. There exist several communication training programs to improve the communication skills of physicians for stressful discussions about serious illness. These programs include the Center to Advance Palliative Care Continuing Medical Education modules,[60] VitalTalk,[61] the Serious Illness Care Program at Ariadne Labs,[62] Respecting Choices,[63] and the Education on Palliative and End-of-Life Care at Feinberg School of Medicine.[64]

Existing communication training programs related to perioperative care cover several issues, including[1] identification of patient goals and values,[2] how to request permission to offer a clinical perspective to help in the decision-making process,[3] proper language use,[4] how to anticipate strong emotions and to be ready to respond accordingly,[5] how to conduct a proper interpretation of the goals and values of the patients,[6] and how to recommend a proper treatment pathway.[10]

Several key indicators of the quality of code status discussions by medical residents include communication skills training and simulations of code status and goals of care discussions, including references to statements about nonabandonment and the importance of understanding and guiding care based on patient goals and values.[10,65,66] One study found significant variability with respect to anesthesiology residents' capability to demonstrate compassionate communication during simulated informed consent, with approximately 15% of residents failing to address the patient's specific concerns about anesthetic complications.[67] This is concerning because a study by Back and colleagues[68,69] showed that improved discrete communication skills among physicians about serious illnesses and goals of care are associated with better clinical outcomes.[10] In addition, there is evidence that engaging patients in early discussion of their goals and values can help avoid unwanted and ineffective treatments, reduce length of stay and cost of care, and improve patient and family satisfaction.[10] Overall, there is a clear positive correlation between better communication skills and better clinical outcomes. When considering goals of care discussions with patients or their families, anesthesiologists and surgeons must acknowledge their importance, and ensure that there is sufficient time allocated to the discussions without creating undue delays in surgical scheduling. Some of the discussion must take place prior to the day of the procedure, with appropriate review of goals of care on the day of surgery. When possible, coordination with the primary care provider, if available, can also help facilitate communication and foster shared decision-making related to perioperative management.

In summary, it is important that perioperative physicians receive proper training to improve their communication skills about serious illnesses, goals and wishes of the patients, and the surgical options available to them. Finally, it has been proposed that conversations about perioperative care are best conducted by physicians with an established therapeutic relationship with the patient. Health care professionals should be aware of those resources that can help them improve their communication skills with their patients.

FUTURE DIRECTIONS: IMPROVING QUALITY AND CONSISTENCY OF CARE

Organizational policies, workflow structure, and electronic medical record systems can be used to improve the quality and consistency of care, including improving communication strategies.[10] Patient-centered perioperative strategies and communication between providers and patients may be improved by workflows that emphasize advance care plans. Furthermore, advance care plans can prove valuable for improving care both in and out of the hospital according to the goals and wishes of the patients. These include Physician Orders for Life-Sustaining Treatment (POLST), which are portable medical orders that document treatment limitations for prehospital emergency care to help prevent undesirable treatments at the end-of-life.[70]

Strategies that Can Be Used by Health Care Organizations to Improve Quality and Consistency of Care in the Perioperative Period

- Implement system cues and decision support tools to prompt the discussion of goals of care and code status at the most important points during perioperative care.[10]

- Develop, evaluate, and implement workflows to improve the identification of patients with LSMT and increase the awareness of clinicians concerning advance care plans such as POLST.
- Improve multidisciplinary communication among providers by incorporating assessments of the advance care plans in the systematic workflow changes.
- Leverage the skill sets of the providers with formal communication training to better understand the patients' goals and wishes.

A particular example is represented by an automated, multidisciplinary workflow, which was developed at the Oregon Health & Science University (OHSU) emergency department to improve the clinician's awareness of active POLST among elderly or seriously ill patients. The OHSU POLST database is accessible to emergency medical personnel both in the field and in the acute care setting and has been shown to improve instances of goal-concordant care when accessed in a timely manner.[10]

Potential Role of Anesthesia Preoperative Evaluations in Facilitating Goals of Care Discussions

Preoperative evaluations before anesthesia can facilitate goals of care discussions by including targeted questions about perioperative code status.[71] By including this discussion in routine preoperative evaluation, patient goals of care can be documented often prior to the day of surgery; these discussions can leverage workflow structures and electronic medical record systems to improve the quality and consistency of care.[10]

Perioperative Workflows Should Include Assessments of Advance Care Plans

The demonstration that there is an association between clinician acknowledgment of an active POLST and fewer ICU days suggests that including assessments of advance care plans in systematic workflow changes and using the information generated effectively in the perioperative period can improve communication among providers and increase goal-concordant perioperative care for patients.[10]

Despite clear recommendations from expert groups about seeking the appropriate times to discuss goals of care, workflows often hinder effective communication of these goals. Furthermore, existing advance care plan data are rarely used effectively either in research about perioperative outcomes or in efforts to improve goal concordance in the perioperative settings. Finally, perioperative care should be patient-centered and more research should be conducted about effectively incorporating patients' goals and values during the decision-making process.[10]

SUMMARY

The perspectives of the patients are crucial for determining the quality of life; therefore, quality care must align with patient values and promote the achievement of patient goals. Patient goals, values, and wishes should be properly discussed, established, and formally recorded. While medical care tends to prioritize achieving optimal technical outcomes, the procedure planning should be placed in the context of the goals of care that have been discussed. Anesthesiologists need to receive proper training to discuss patient's goals and wishes, communicate these to the perioperative team, and then incorporate collaborative decision-making into care pathways that adhere to these goals. A partnership among anesthesiologists, proceduralists, and primary care physicians to develop care pathways that incorporate collaborative decision-making should become standard practice. Collaboration among clinical teams may enable more effective perioperative shared decision-making with patients about their goals of care and will allow for better incorporation of patient values and their diverse cultural backgrounds. Goal-concordant care plans are plans that are developed by health care providers that take into account the goals, values, and preferences of the patients during the perioperative stages of surgery. These plans are designed to increase the chances of achieving the patient's anticipated outcomes. This practice can improve patient satisfaction and quality of care and reduce unnecessary care.

CLINICS CARE POINTS

- Before surgery, shared decision-making with an interdisciplinary perioperative team should be done to elicit the patient's values and wishes.
- The patient's goals of care should be discussed and documented prior to surgery, including any limitations on life-sustaining medical therapy.
- Perioperative care plans concordant with the patient's goals improve patient satisfaction and quality of care.

DISCLOSURE

The authors have nothing to disclose. No funding supported this work. MJD acknowledges additional support from a Foundation for Anesthesia and Education Research GEMSSTAR grant, Merck Investigator Studies Program grant, and a National Alzheimer's Coordinating Center New Investigator Award. MMT acknowledges additional support from the NIH/NHLBI, NIH/NIGMS, and Edwards Lifesciences.

REFERENCES

1. NIH. Advance Care Planning: Advance Directives for Health Care. Available at: https://www.nia.nih.gov/health/advance-care-planning-advance-directives-health-care. [Accessed 26 September 2023].
2. Clinic M. Living wills and advance directives for medical decisions: Plan ahead and get the medical care you want at the end of life. Available at: https://www.mayoclinic.org/healthy-lifestyle/consumer-health/in-depth/living-wills/art-20046303. [Accessed 26 September 2023].
3. mndh. Federal Law Regarding Advance Directives, Information BUlletin 98-4. Available at: https://www.health.state.mn.us/facilities/regulation/infobulletins/ib98_4.html. [Accessed 26 September 2023].
4. Kelley K. The Patient Self-Determination Act. A matter of life and death. Physician Assist 1995;19(3):49, 53-46, 59-60.
5. Teoli D, Ghassemzadeh S. Patient Self-Determination act. Treasure Island (FL): StatPearls; 2023.
6. AANA. Reconsideration of Advance Directives: Practive guidelines and policy considerations. 2023. Available at: https://issuu.com/aanapublishing/docs/10_-_reconsideration_of_advance_directives. [Accessed 26 September 2023].
7. Mannino MJ. The AANA code of ethics. AANA J (Am Assoc Nurse Anesth) 1986; 54:473-5.
8. Yuen JK, Reid MC, Fetters MD. Hospital do-not-resuscitate orders: why they have failed and how to fix them. J Gen Intern Med 2011;26:791-7.
9. Anesthesiologists ASo. Statement on Ethical Guidelines for the Anesthesia Care of Patients with Do-Not-Resuscitate Orders. 2018. Available at: https://www.asahq.org/standards-and-practice-parameters/statement-on-ethical-guidelines-for-the-anesthesia-care-of-patients-with-do-not-resuscitate-orders.

10. Cushman T, Waisel DB, Treggiari MM. The Role of Anesthesiologists in Perioperative Limitation of Potentially Life-Sustaining Medical Treatments: A Narrative Review and Perspective. Anesth Analg 2021;133:663–75.

11. Sumrall WD, Mahanna E, Sabharwal V, et al. Do Not Resuscitate, Anesthesia, and Perioperative Care: A Not So Clear Order. Ochsner J 2016;16:176–9.

12. Wang XS, Gottumukkala V. Patient-reported outcomes: Is this the missing link in patient-centered perioperative care? Best Pract Res Clin Anaesthesiol 2021;35:565–73.

13. Shah P, Thornton I, Turrin D, et al. Informed consent. Treasure Island (FL): StatPearls; 2023.

14. Takla A, Savulescu J, Wilkinson DJC, et al. General anaesthesia in end-of-life care: extending the indications for anaesthesia beyond surgery. Anaesthesia 2021;76:1308–15.

15. Truog RD, Waisel DB, Burns JP. DNR in the OR: a goal-directed approach. Anesthesiology 1999;90:289–95.

16. Truog RD, Waisel DB, Burns JP. Do-not-resuscitate orders in the surgical setting. Lancet 2005;365:733–5.

17. American College of S. Statement on advance directives by patients: "do not resuscitate" in the operating room. Bull Am Coll Surg 2014;99:42–3.

18. Schwarze ML, Bradley CT, Brasel KJ. Surgical "buy-in": the contractual relationship between surgeons and patients that influences decisions regarding life-supporting therapy. Crit Care Med 2010;38:843–8.

19. Schwarze ML, Redmann AJ, Alexander GC, et al. Surgeons expect patients to buy-in to postoperative life support preoperatively: results of a national survey. Crit Care Med 2013;41:1–8.

20. Goswami P. Advance Care Planning and End-Of-Life Communications: Practical Tips for Oncology Advanced Practitioners. J Adv Pract Oncol 2021;12:89–95.

21. Blackwood DH, Vindrola-Padros C, Mythen MG, et al. Advance-care-planning and end-of-life discussions in the perioperative period: a review of healthcare professionals' knowledge, attitudes, and training. Br J Anaesth 2018;121:1138–47.

22. Nurok M, Green DS, Chisholm MF, et al. Anesthesiologists' familiarity with the ASA and ACS guidelines on Advance Directives in the perioperative setting. J Clin Anesth 2014;26:174–6.

23. Services CfMaM. Subpart I - Advance Directives. 2023. Available at: https://www.ecfr.gov/current/title-42/chapter-IV/subchapter-G/part-489/subpart-I. [Accessed 26 September 2023].

24. Shapiro ME, Singer EA. Perioperative Advance Directives: Do Not Resuscitate in the Operating Room. Surg Clin North Am 2019;99:859–65.

25. Burkle CM, Swetz KM, Armstrong MH, et al. Patient and doctor attitudes and beliefs concerning perioperative do not resuscitate orders: anesthesiologists' growing compliance with patient autonomy and self determination guidelines. BMC Anesthesiol 2013;13:2.

26. Yamamoto K, Yonekura Y, Hayama J, et al. Advance Care Planning for Intensive Care Patients During the Perioperative Period: A Qualitative Study. SAGE Open Nurs 2021;7. 23779608211038845.

27. Blackwood DH, Walker D, Mythen MG, et al. Barriers to advance care planning with patients as perceived by nurses and other healthcare professionals: A systematic review. J Clin Nurs 2019;28:4276–97.

28. Fleuren N, Depla M, Janssen DJA, et al. Underlying goals of advance care planning (ACP): a qualitative analysis of the literature. BMC Palliat Care 2020;19:27.

29. Cooper Z, Corso K, Bernacki R, et al. Conversations about treatment preferences before high-risk surgery: a pilot study in the preoperative testing center. J Palliat Med 2014;17:701–7.

30. Brovman EY, Pisansky AJ, Beverly A, et al. Do-Not-Resuscitate status as an independent risk factor for patients undergoing surgery for hip fracture. World J Orthop 2017;8:902–12.

31. Brovman EY, Walsh EC, Burton BN, et al. Postoperative outcomes in patients with a do-not-resuscitate (DNR) order undergoing elective procedures. J Clin Anesth 2018;48:81–8.

32. Kazaure H, Roman S, Sosa JA. High mortality in surgical patients with do-not-resuscitate orders: analysis of 8256 patients. Arch Surg 2011;146:922–8.

33. Saager L, Kurz A, Deogaonkar A, et al. Pre-existing do-not-resuscitate orders are not associated with increased postoperative morbidity at 30 days in surgical patients. Crit Care Med 2011;39:1036–41.

34. Scarborough JE, Pappas TN, Bennett KM, et al. Failure-to-pursue rescue: explaining excess mortality in elderly emergency general surgical patients with pre-existing "do-not-resuscitate" orders. Ann Surg 2012;256:453–61.

35. Siracuse JJ, Jones DW, Meltzer EC, et al. Impact of "Do Not Resuscitate" Status on the Outcome of Major Vascular Surgical Procedures. Ann Vasc Surg 2015;29:1339–45.

36. Speicher PJ, Lagoo-Deenadayalan SA, Galanos AN, et al. Expectations and outcomes in geriatric patients with do-not-resuscitate orders undergoing emergency surgical management of bowel obstruction. JAMA Surg 2013;148:23–8.

37. Walsh EC, Brovman EY, Bader AM, et al. Do-Not-Resuscitate Status Is Associated With Increased Mortality But Not Morbidity. Anesth Analg 2017;125:1484–93.

38. Wenger NS, Greengold NL, Oye RK, et al. Patients with DNR orders in the operating room: surgery, resuscitation, and outcomes. SUPPORT Investigators. Study to Understand Prognoses and Preferences for Outcomes and Risks of Treatments. J Clin Ethics 1997;8:250–7.

39. Murphy P, Kreling B, Kathryn E, et al. Description of the SUPPORT intervention. Study to Understand Prognoses and Preferences for Outcomes and Risks of Treatments. J Am Geriatr Soc 2000;48:S154–61.

40. Cooper Z, Koritsanszky LA, Cauley CE, et al. Recommendations for Best Communication Practices to Facilitate Goal-concordant Care for Seriously Ill Older Patients With Emergency Surgical Conditions. Ann Surg 2016;263:1–6.

41. Clemency MV, Thompson NJ. "Do not resuscitate" (DNR) orders and the anesthesiologist: a survey. Anesth Analg 1993;76:394–401.

42. Clemency MV, Thompson NJ. "Do not resuscitate" (DNR) orders in the perioperative period–a comparison of the perspectives of anesthesiologists, internists, and surgeons. Anesth Analg 1994;78:651–8.

43. Clemency MV, Thompson NJ. Do not resuscitate orders in the perioperative period: patient perspectives. Anesth Analg 1997;84:859–64.

44. La Puma J, Silverstein MD, Stocking CB, et al. Life-sustaining treatment. A prospective study of patients with DNR orders in a teaching hospital. Arch Intern Med 1988;148:2193–8.

45. Engle RL, Mohr DC, Holmes SK, et al. Evidence-based practice and patient-centered care: Doing both well. Health Care Manage Rev 2021;46:174–84.

46. Hickey TR, Cooper Z, Urman RD, et al. An Agenda for Improving Perioperative Code Status Discussion. A A Case Rep 2016;6:411–5.

47. Lilley EJ, Cooper Z, Schwarze ML, et al. Palliative Care in Surgery: Defining the Research Priorities. Ann Surg 2018;267:66–72.

48. Lilley EJ, Khan KT, Johnston FM, et al. Palliative Care Interventions for Surgical Patients: A Systematic Review. JAMA Surg 2016;151:172–83.

49. Paul Olson TJ, Brasel KJ, Redmann AJ, et al. Surgeon-reported conflict with intensivists about postoperative goals of care. JAMA Surg 2013;148:29–35.

50. Schwarze ML, Brasel KJ, Mosenthal AC. Beyond 30-day mortality: aligning surgical quality with outcomes that patients value. JAMA Surg 2014;149:631–2.

51. Redmann AJ, Brasel KJ, Alexander CG, et al. Use of advance directives for high-risk operations: a national survey of surgeons. Ann Surg 2012;255:418–23.

52. Mendiratta P, Schoo C, Latif R. Clinical frailty Scale. Treasure Island (FL): StatPearls; 2023.

53. Slaets JP. Vulnerability in the elderly: frailty. Med Clin North Am 2006;90:593–601.

54. Lubben J, Blozik E, Gillmann G, et al. Performance of an abbreviated version of the Lubben Social Network Scale among three European community-dwelling older adult populations. Gerontol 2006;46:503–13.

55. Sherbourne CD, Stewart AL. The MOS social support survey. Soc Sci Med 1991; 32:705–14.

56. Cella D, Riley W, Stone A, et al. The Patient-Reported Outcomes Measurement Information System (PROMIS) developed and tested its first wave of adult self-reported health outcome item banks: 2005-2008. J Clin Epidemiol 2010;63: 1179–94.

57. Chapman R. Expected a posteriori scoring in PROMIS((R)). J Patient Rep Outcomes 2022;6:59.

58. Gerritsen RT, Jensen HI, Koopmans M, et al. Quality of dying and death in the ICU. The euroQ2 project. J Crit Care 2018;44:376–82.

59. Gerritsen RT, Koopmans M, Hofhuis JG, et al. Comparing Quality of Dying and Death Perceived by Family Members and Nurses for Patients Dying in US and Dutch ICUs. Chest 2017;151:298–307.

60. CAPC. CAPC Clinical. Training. Available at: https://www.capc.org/. [Accessed 26 September 2023].

61. VitalTalk. VitalTalk. Available at: https://www.vitaltalk.org/. [Accessed 26 September 2023].

62. Labs A. Serious Illness Care. Available at: https://www.ariadnelabs.org/serious-illness-care/. [Accessed 26 September 2023].

63. Respecting Choices. Available at: https://respectingchoices.org/types-of-curriculum-and-certification/. [Accessed 26 September 2023].

64. EPEC: Education in Palliative and End-of-Life Care. Available at: https://www.bioethics.northwestern.edu/programs/epec/about/index.html. [Accessed 26 September 2023].

65. Miller DC, McSparron JI, Clardy PF, et al. Improving Resident Communication in the Intensive Care Unit. The Proceduralization of Physician Communication with Patients and Their Surrogates. Ann Am Thorac Soc 2016;13:1624–8.

66. Szmuilowicz E, Neely KJ, Sharma RK, et al. Improving residents' code status discussion skills: a randomized trial. J Palliat Med 2012;15:768–74.

67. Waisel DB, Ruben MA, Blanch-Hartigan D, et al. Compassionate and Clinical Behavior of Residents in a Simulated Informed Consent Encounter. Anesthesiology 2020;132:159–69.

68. Back AL, Arnold RM, Baile WF, et al. Efficacy of communication skills training for giving bad news and discussing transitions to palliative care. Arch Intern Med 2007;167:453–60.

69. Back AL, Fromme EK, Meier DE. Training Clinicians with Communication Skills Needed to Match Medical Treatments to Patient Values. J Am Geriatr Soc 2019;67:S435–41.
70. Truog RD, Fried TR. Physician Orders for Life-Sustaining Treatment and Limiting Overtreatment at the End of Life. JAMA 2020;323:934–5.
71. Zambouri A. Preoperative evaluation and preparation for anesthesia and surgery. Hippokratia 2007;11:13–21.

Perioperative Care of the Patient with Directives Limiting Life-Sustaining Treatments

Tera Cushman, MD, MPH[a],*, Elizabeth Hays, MD[a],
Andrea K. Nagengast, MD[b]

KEYWORDS

- Advance directive • Resuscitation orders • Surgical procedures • Operative
- Anesthesiology • Personal autonomy

KEY POINTS

- For patients who have requested limitations to life-sustaining treatments, all providers caring for patients should understand goals of care and implications of the limitations on clinical options and decision making, particularly when surgery and anesthesia are being considered.
- The preoperative surgical clinic visit and preoperative medicine clinic visit represent the best initial opportunity to discuss life-sustaining medical therapy (LSMT) in the context of surgery, describe likely perioperative and postoperative LSMT, identify a surrogate decision maker, and elicit patient preferences.
- A central repository of advance care plan data in the electronic medical record may improve ease of access to and leverage of previous LSMT conversations.
- Failure to respect patient autonomy has significant medicolegal implications and has led to significant financial liability. Perioperative providers should consider the worst-case clinical scenario and its implications and plan care accordingly.
- It is important to acknowledge that these conversations and decisions are challenging and do not always have a satisfactory conclusion. The authors encourage open consultation with colleagues and the patient/surrogate to achieve the most medically reasonable path forward that respects patient self-determination.

[a] Department of Anesthesiology & Perioperative Medicine, Oregon Health & Science University, 3181 Southwest Sam Jackson Park Road, Portland, OR 97239, USA; [b] Portland VA Medical Center, 3710 Southwest US Veterans Hospital Road, Portland, OR 97239, USA
* Corresponding author. Department of Anesthesiology & Perioperative Medicine, Oregon Health & Science University, Kohler Pavilion 5006A, 3181 Sam Jackson Park Road, Portland, OR 97239.
E-mail address: cushmant@ohsu.edu
Twitter: @teracushman (T.C.)

Anesthesiology Clin 42 (2024) 393–406
https://doi.org/10.1016/j.anclin.2023.12.005
anesthesiology.theclinics.com
1932-2275/24/© 2023 Elsevier Inc. All rights reserved.

INTRODUCTION

Perioperative care requires multiple specialties collaborating to achieve high-quality care designed to fulfill each patient's goals. Because no one medical practitioner can do this alone, the responsibility is shared for the essential underpinnings of high-quality team-based care, including sound communication, patient-centeredness, and improving safety. This approach to care is particularly important when caring for a patient for whom there are limitations on implementation of life-sustaining therapies. As part of this process, it is critical for all providers to uphold central principles of biomedical ethics throughout the arc of perioperative care and decision making.[1]

Legislative bodies and landmark court cases have thoroughly established patients' rights to refuse life-sustaining medical therapy (LSMT). This right extends through the perioperative period. Professional society guidelines consistently and clearly recommend that limits to LSMT during the perioperative period be addressed and discussed in a patient-centered manner before surgery, and that patient wishes guide care both during and after surgery. However, perioperative providers may reasonably feel that they face a gauntlet of questions and potential contradictions in managing limits to LSMT perioperatively. Who should start the necessary conversations? What LSMT might be necessary to undergo a procedure safely? How should patients with limits to LSMT be counseled about perioperative risk and particularly the risk of morbidity and dependence after surgery? Do the values and goals that inform a patient's desire to limit LSMT outside the operating room (OR) apply when the patient is scheduled to undergo a surgical procedure under anesthesia? Whose responsibility is it to ensure that this shared decision-making process occurs, and that the patient's goals remain central to decisions during the course of care?

In this review, the authors discuss potential strategies, best practices, important points of collaboration, and potential pitfalls in perioperative management of directives limiting life-sustaining treatments at each stage in the perioperative course focusing particularly on the roles of surgeon, preoperative physician, and anesthesiologist in this management.

LONGITUDINAL CONSIDERATIONS

Decisions about acceptable care may be significantly influenced by the sociocultural and spiritual history of the groups to which an individual belongs. Provider awareness of cultural influences is important when engaging in LSMT discussions with patients and their families. Numerous studies have shown that Black and Hispanic patients nearing end of life are much less likely to use hospice care and much more likely to seek life-prolonging interventions versus palliative interventions.[2–4] Part of this pattern may be explained by profound and understandable mistrust of medical institutions among Black and other minoritized Americans resulting from a long history of horrific treatment and ongoing stark health outcome disparities. Indeed, Black patients nearing end of life are less likely than white patients to have their documented care preferences followed by their care providers.[5] There is likely also an intersectional component with spiritual traditions in Black and Hispanic/Latino communities that significantly influences approach to LSMT conversations and decisions.[6] Collective family decision making may be more common in families with Asian, Latino, and Indigenous backgrounds.[7] The authors strongly encourage adopting the practice of cultural humility and curiosity when approaching all patients, while also acknowledging that there is considerable variation within minoritized communities and that each patient should be approached as an individual in the present moment. These considerations are longitudinal, and providers all along the surgical care process should engage in LSMT preference conversations with a critical awareness of their own biases and acknowledgment of the need to address the patient's goals of care in a culturally sensitive and respectful manner.

PREOPERATIVE AND PLANNING PHASE
Surgery

Surgeons are the first and often the last point of patient contact in perioperative care pathways, with nearly all other perioperative practitioners providing episodic care (**Table 1**). The structure of the American College of Surgeons Geriatric Surgery Verification Program (ACS-GSV) standards reflects this longitudinal relationship by defining optimal resources for the care of surgical patients over age of 75 from the preoperative visit to the final discharge and postacute care follow-up.[8] Although not all patients with limits to LSMT are over age 75 and not all patients over the age of 75 wish to limit LSMT, there is substantial commonality in optimal approach to preoperative shared decision making for these patients. Section 5 of the ACS-GSV standards includes and emphasizes the importance of a preoperative discussion of overall health goals, treatment goals, and anticipated impact of surgical care on functional status, independence, and symptom burden. This section of the ACS-GSV specifically defines a standard for reviewing resuscitation status and any existing advance directive (AD) preoperatively. It also emphasizes the need to determine and to develop an advance care plan (ACP) in patients who do not have these already. This particular requirement addresses the notably low rate of documented ACP in older adults with multiple chronic conditions before high-risk surgery reported by Tang and colleagues.[9] ACS-GSV Section 5 also mandates identification and education/preparation of a health care representative or surrogate decision-maker (SDM) and requires an explicit discussion of the patient's desire for individual forms of LSMT if the surgery is to be followed by a planned intensive care unit (ICU) admission.

Cooper and colleagues[10] describe an excellent framework for preoperative patient-surgeon communication with seriously ill older patients, which in the authors' opinion is recognized as current best practice. Their recommendations include establishing a shared understanding of current medical condition and prognosis, describing the benefits and burdens of both surgical and nonsurgical options (including palliative treatments), eliciting and understanding patient goals and priorities, and finally, recommending a course of treatment most likely to achieve the patient's goals while aligning with their stated values.[10] Their recommendations include establishing a shared understanding of current medical condition and prognosis, describing the benefits and burdens of both surgical and nonsurgical options (including palliative treatments), eliciting and understanding patient goals and priorities, and finally, recommending a course of treatment most likely to achieve the patient's goals while aligning with their stated values.

Gaps in end-of-life communication training for physicians remain a major barrier to widespread adoption of these best practices. Procedural specialties, such as surgery and anesthesiology, appear to lag behind other specialties in serious illness communication training and comfort with end-of-life discussions. Studies suggest that medical house officers have significantly greater comfort and experience in conducting goals of care discussions than surgical house officers, and attending surgeons harbor conflicting feelings about ADs in high-risk surgical patients.[11,12] In a study of patients who died in a tertiary hospital, Morrell and colleagues[13] found

Table 1
Perioperative best practices for management of limits on life-sustaining medical therapies

Role	Preoperative Clinic Visits	Preoperative Holding Area	Operating Room	Postanesthesia Care Unit	Inpatient Ward/ICU	Postdischarge Care
			Phase of Perioperative Care			
Surgeon	• Identify patients with preferences for limited LSMT (ie, existing Portable Order for Life Sustaining Treatment [POLST] or previous DNR code status) • Address overall health goals, treatment goals, and anticipated impact of surgical & nonsurgical treatments • Review code status & advance care plan, discussing implications in the context of planned anesthesia and surgery • Specifically discuss LSMT indications & limitations as well as acceptability of LSMT with patients for whom an ICU admission is planned postoperatively • Identify and document surrogate	• If elective surgery, offer patient and/or SDM opportunity to reaffirm or change their original surgical decision making and make sure all questions/ uncertainties are addressed • If patient desires limitations to life-sustaining medical therapy (LSMT), ensure all member of OR team are aware of this limitation • If any OR team member is uncomfortable with desired care limitations, assist with reasonable effort to find replacement	• Include any limits to standard LSMT in preprocedure team pause • Collaboratively work to abide by patients' wishes regarding LSMT	• Ensure that postoperative management of any surgical complications is in accordance with current limits to LSMT • Involve patient and/or SDM (as applicable) in decisions on postoperative management particularly when clinical changes arise • Revisit limits to LSMT as postoperative care progresses, particularly after any major clinical status change		• Communicate anticipated postoperative management and discharge plan to primary care provider (PCP) • Assist patient or SDM in making any desired changes to advance directive, POLST, or other durable documentation of LSMT limits • Encourage early follow-up with PCP

decision maker (SDM). Provide education to patient and SDM to facilitate mutual understanding of patient's goals
• Document all above discussions and results of the shared decision-making process

Preoperative medicine clinic	• Identify and document SDM. Provide education to patient and SDM to facilitate mutual understanding of patient's goals • Review existing advance care plan and support upload to EMR. Offer education on advance care planning if none established and support completion of ACP • Review & document code status and any other desired limitations to LSMT. Educate patients on what LSMT may be indicated after surgery. Document all above discussions

(continued on next page)

Table 1
(continued)

	Phase of Perioperative Care				
Role	Preoperative Clinic Visits	Preoperative Holding Area	Operating Room	Postanesthesia Care Unit	Inpatient Ward/ICU Postdischarge Care
Anesthesiologist	• Work with preoperative medicine clinic to optimize process of obtaining existing advance care plans and including them in local medical record • Establish departmental policies & procedures that respect patient autonomy on limits to LSMT • Ensure anesthesia provider education on types of advance care planning and how these are documented in the medical record	• Review advance directive, preoperative code status, or presence of other documented care limitations. • In patients with limits to LSMT, collaboratively determine mutually agreeable anesthetic plan with patient using a goal-directed or procedure-directed approach • Document results of discussion, to include what changes (if any) are made to LSMT limits during perioperative period AND how long these changes will apply • If any OR team member is uncomfortable with desired care limitations, make reasonable effort to find replacement	• Include any limits to standard LSMT in preprocedure team pause • Collaboratively work to abide by patients' wishes regarding LSMT • Ensure that any break providers are aware of and comfortable with limits to LSMT	• Include limits to LSMT in sign-out to PACU nurse, taking special care to specify when and if limits to LSMT will revert to preoperative status • Ensure that medical management of any postanesthetic complications is in accordance with preagreed limits to LSMT • Involve patient and/or SDM (as applicable) in decisions on postanesthesia management particularly if clinical changes arise	

Preoperative/PACU nursing staff	• Review & document advance directive, preoperative code status, or presence of other documented care limitations • Confirm SDM and ensure that their contact information is available for OR staff • Include LSMT limits and SDM contact information in handoff to operating room nurse		• Ensure that nursing interventions and escalation of treatment are in accordance with preagreed limits to LSMT • Inform medical decision-makers (SDM, surgeon, and anesthesiologist as applicable) early of any clinical changes to allow collaborative decision making
Operating room nurses	• Confirm SDM and best method of reaching them intraoperatively • If any OR team member is uncomfortable with desired care limitations, make reasonable effort to find replacement	• Collaboratively work to abide by patients' wishes regarding LSMT • Ensure that any break providers are aware of and comfortable with limits to LSMT	• Include LSMT limits and SDM contact information in SBAR to PACU nurse
Postoperative consultant services			• Ensure that recommendations and medical management decisions made by consultant service are in accordance with current limits to LSMT • Involve patient and/or SDM (as applicable) in decisions on invasive treatments managed or recommended by consultant service

patients admitted to a surgical service had nearly twice the mean time from admission to Do-Not-Resuscitate (DNR) order as patients admitted to a medicine service.

Several tools and platforms have been developed to improve patient and provider engagement in and comfort with serious illness conversation and advance care planning. The PREPARE Web site—an interactive, patient-centered ACP Web site—shows promise in increasing ACP documentation compared with conventional ACP alone.[14] The US Department of Veterans Affairs National Center for Ethics in Health Care provides asynchronous, interactive, publicly available modules to health care practitioners seeking to gain greater skill and comfort with navigating these challenging topics.[15] Organizations such as ACP Decisions, VitalTalk, Center to Advance Palliative Care, Ariadne Labs, and Education on Palliative and End-of-Life Care at Feinberg School of Medicine all offer accredited CME modules and most also offer free online resources to support clinicians and patients in these conversations.

Preoperative Medicine Clinic

After a decision is made to proceed to surgery, most patients at the authors' institution are referred to the preoperative medicine clinic for risk stratification and medical optimization before surgery. The preoperative setting provides an additional valuable opportunity to review existing ACP documentation, to provide education that supports patients and surrogates in the care planning process, and to ground their decisions in the context of the planned surgery. This process is particularly salient for patients who have previously established preferences for limited LSMT. Even when surgery follows an expected course, patients undergoing most major surgery will require tracheal intubation and ventilator support while under general anesthesia, and, in some cases, postoperative care in the ICU. Some patients may require artificial nutrition, prolonged respiratory support, and hemodialysis as a result of a complex surgical procedure or unanticipated complication of care. Implementation of any of these life-sustaining therapies may conflict with a patient's prior stated preferences and should be addressed upstream. The Care Planning Umbrella framework developed by Hickman and colleagues[16] provides useful guidance for thinking about advance care planning as a process of preparing patients and their health care surrogates for medical decision making informed by personal values and understanding of the medical situation. They also emphasize that the care planning process is not static, but evolves over a lifetime, particularly when patients experience specific health events. Major surgery is a pivotal health event, and the preoperative setting is a valuable time to explore and contextualize health care values, particularly preferences for limited LSMT.

The first step of preoperative care planning is to review preexisting ACP documentation. This line of questioning is introduced as a standard part of the adult preoperative evaluation. Normalizing these questions from the beginning helps patients and families understand that the questions are important but routine and not reflective of a poor prognosis. The authors recommend beginning the discussion around preferred SDM. A modified Delphi panel of palliative care experts in 2017 highlighted the central value of identifying the SDM to successful advance care planning.[14] Having the SDM clearly and easily accessible in the chart supports the urgent decision making that occurs perioperatively, particularly in situations involving prolonged ventilator support or postoperative delirium when surrogate engagement is required. Also, the authors recommend reviewing existing ADs to clarify legal surrogates. This may also provide an opportunity to explore preferences around end-of-life care. With this background, it is important to educate patients and their surrogates about the limits of their ADs to guide complex decisions that may be required postoperatively. A qualitative analysis of physician attitudes regarding ADs for high-risk surgical patients published by Bradley and colleagues[12] described the ambivalence many perioperative clinicians feel about ADs. While they provide a useful framework to begin discussions about postoperative risks and care planning, they can be difficult to apply directly to the perioperative context. Finally, the authors recommend asking patients about preexisting preferences for selected, limited LSMT. These preferences may be documented in a Portable Order for Life Sustaining Treatment (POLST) or in DNR order from a previous hospitalization. To support this process, the electronic medical record (EMR) should ideally be configured to highlight existing ACP documents, such as the POLST and code status. Even when a previous DNR order exists, it must be reassessed with the patient before surgery, ideally by the surgeon and anesthesia teams. The preoperative clinician's role is to support this process by identifying existing preferences and preparing patients to make the decisions. In addition, involving SDM at this stage prepares them to step in later if needed. When patients choose to undergo major surgery, they are also choosing some amount of life-sustaining treatment in pursuit of a desired health goal. This trade-off should be made explicit. Educating patients and surrogates about the potential conflicts between their preferences for limited LSMT and necessary interventions supports goal-concordant care.

A comprehensive preoperative risk assessment may identify health conditions that pose significant risk for postoperative complications typically treated with LSMT. For example, patients with advanced chronic kidney disease may experience acute worsening owing to hypotension, sepsis, or obstruction and unexpectedly face the need for hemodialysis. Patients deserve the opportunity to prepare ahead for dialysis and to decide whether achieving the surgical goal warrants the risk of end-stage renal disease. Likewise, patients with chronic respiratory failure should understand the potential for prolonged and possibly indefinite postoperative ventilator support. Baseline heart and liver failure and even dementia increase the risk of postoperative complications requiring ICU level of care. During a comprehensive assessment, the preoperative clinician can quantify these risks and help patients and their surrogates understand how chronic health conditions may complicate their treatment course. Patient surrogates should be involved in these discussions so they can support decision making in the moment and be prepared to represent the patient's wishes if they are unable to speak for themselves in the future.

The final phase of preoperative care planning is documentation and communication to the larger care team. Ideally, a multidisciplinary team supports this valuable but labor-intensive process. At the authors' institution, they have had success with a quality improvement program focused on improving rates of SDM identification and documentation during the visit as well as improving rates of AD completion before surgery.[17] Based on the authors' quality improvement experience, they recommend the following to improve AD and SDM documentation:

- Prompt patients to bring or send in current ADs to add to the chart.
- Provide blank AD forms.
- Educate patients about ADs and encourage completion before surgery.
- Clearly document preferred SDM and where possible clarify whether preferred surrogate is also the legal designate according to state rules or existing power of attorney paperwork.

Preoperative providers should record complex care discussions regarding limited LSMT in a standard chart location so that the entire care team can easily review these previous discussions to inform future decision making. Direct patient quotes add nuance and demonstrate patient understanding and values. When a patient's preference for limitations to LSMT is discovered in the preoperative setting, the preoperative provider has a responsibility to alert the surgeon and anesthesiologist to allow for further discussion about the impact of this preference on their perioperative care.

PERIANESTHESIA PHASE

Anesthesiologists' work in the ORs requires both thorough planning and ample flexibility to meet the dynamic clinical challenges before them. In an ideal scenario, they meet patients desiring perioperative limits to LSMT in the pre-operative area after having reviewed documented LSMT conversations with primary care, preoperative medicine, and/or surgical providers, allowing them to conduct a targeted and informed discussion with the patient. At the authors' and many other institutions, all elective surgical patients who decline some or all blood products for religious or personal reasons have a dedicated preoperative clinic visit with the blood conservation team to review in detail what products they will and will not accept and sign corresponding consent forms. Refusal of other forms of LSMT is less well-protocolized at the authors' institution, but recent changes to the format of the preanesthesia workflow in the authors' EMR have significantly improved ease of access to documented ACP, ADs, SDM contact information, POLST form, and DNR order history. Development of a centralized repository of ACP information in the EMR is highly recommended and assists providers throughout the care continuum.

Conversations about the anesthetic plan in patients desiring limits to LSMT should ideally leverage previously documented conversations to discuss how these limits apply in the perioperative period. In the absence of this documentation, though, the American Society of Anesthesiologists (ASA) guidelines for care of patients who are DNR status still apply, and the acceptability of LSMT interventions must be revisited and discussed before each anesthetic.[18] Because many procedures routine to anesthetic practice represent resuscitative measures, it is important to devise a plan that both allows for the safe and ethical provision of anesthetic care and adequately respects the patient's right to self-determination. The following ASA guidelines provide a helpful framework on approaching these conversations: (1) Full attempt at resuscitation; (2) Limited attempt at resuscitation defined with regard to specific procedures; and (3) Limited attempt at resuscitation defined with regard to patient's goals and values.[18,19] Limited resuscitation that defines specific procedures provides greater clarity to the anesthesiologist but likely has less actual meaning to the patient. Conversely, limited resuscitation that hinges on patient goals and values is more likely to be patient-centered and goal-concordant but requires rapid application of medical decision making in a potentially dynamic and unpredictable clinical setting. At the authors' institution, the preanesthesia workflow provides each of these options in the anesthetic plan note along with a final option, which is full maintenance of the DNR order for the duration of the procedures. The authors recommend a standard method of documenting perioperative limits on LSMT in the EMR along with a corresponding free-text box to fully document the preanesthetic conversation and resulting plan.

Once a plan is determined by shared decision making, the patient-anesthesiologist dyad must then establish the planned duration of any changes to the patient's preoperative limits to LSMT in the perianesthesia period. Patients may not regain capacity until sometime after their general anesthesia, so plans developed between patient and anesthesiologist must extend at least until discharge from the Post-Anesthesia Care Unit (PACU). The anesthesiologist should then communicate the LSMT management plan to all OR team members (a responsibility they share with the surgeon, preanesthetic nurse, and circulating OR nurse, who also share responsibility for determining LSMT acceptability to the patient) and allow for transfer of care to another care provider should any team member have a personal moral objection to the planned perianesthesia limits to LSMT. Should the anesthesiologist likewise have a personal moral objection, they may also seek to transfer care in a nonjudgmental fashion to a colleague. However, as noted by the ASA guidelines, should alternate care providers be unavailable in a reasonable timeframe, the care should proceed with adherence to the patient's goals and wishes.[18]

Finally, the authors strongly recommend a priori mental planning on what actions will be taken should any feared complication occur. Confirmation of this plan should be communicated as part of the perioperative "time out." Before assuming care of a patient with maintained limits to LSMT, the anesthesiologist must clarify how to respond to unanticipated problems and potential "worst case" scenarios in a manner consistent with the patient's goals and requested limitations. Failure to appropriately respect patient autonomy has numerous consequences, including provider moral injury, patient and family grief, and significant medicolegal repercussions. In 2019, the first jury verdict for wrongful prolongation of life after ignoring a DNR order was awarded in Montana.[20] Many other similar suits for wrongful prolongation of life against wishes to limit LSMT have ended in large-dollar settlements before going to trial, and extensive case law exists supporting assault and battery charges when ADs and DNR orders are ignored.[21–23] The loss of community trust and impact of negative press should also not be underestimated.[24] Anesthesiologists are experts and leaders in resuscitation. Expertise inescapably carries responsibility, and assuming care of patients with limits to LSMT brings with it the responsibility to plan and envision when to stop rescue efforts if necessary to respect the patient's self-determination right.

POSTPROCEDURAL CARE

After the brief but significant physiologic changes that occur during and after surgery and anesthesia, clinical status and patient capacity should be reassessed to determine if any change in the LSMT limits is appropriate. LSMT interventions that a patient previously envisioned as acceptable may be unacceptable when they become a reality, and likewise, interventions that a patient initially declined may become acceptable and desired. Both decisions are valid, and postoperative management systems must be flexible enough to meet both scenarios. For any significant change in clinical status or initiation of postoperative LSMT in a patient with preoperative limits to LSMT, the authors strongly recommend checking in with the patient and/or SDM to establish the goals of the LSMT intervention, revisit their overall treatment goals, and discuss their current experience living with their condition.

For patients with defined limits to LSMT, any escalations in care represent an opportunity to reevaluate goals and future decision making. In these situations, additional consultant services involved in these decisions play pivotal roles in achieving goal-concordant care. The potential role of consultants can be illustrated by the increasing interest in palliative care education among nephrologists and development of serious illness communication tools tailored to nephrologists.[25–28] Early use of palliative care consultant services can be a valuable resource to help guide conversations around care goals and symptom management. Anesthesiologists can provide useful insight if they are consulted for participation for repeat procedures.[29] The authors encourage intensivists, surgeons, and other physicians with a longitudinal relationship be compassionate with themselves if they find it difficult to let go of LSMT options with a patient whom they have accompanied on an intense care journey. Consultant services and noninvolved colleagues can provide outside perspective and ease potential moral injury around decisions to forgo LSMT in these scenarios.[30,31]

SUMMARY

The patient arriving for surgery is most knowledgeable about their goals of care and what interventions are consistent with these goals, assuming there has been sufficient opportunity to engage in discussions with providers about plans of care, risks, benefits, and alternatives. Many, although not all, patients want to prioritize goals other than longevity. Providers must determine the optimal treatment recommendations for their patients to ensure that care is ethical, patient-centered, and evidence-based for those patients who request limitations to LSMT. Although conversations around perioperative LSMT management can be complex, challenging, and time-intensive, systems and practices to ensure patient-centeredness and mutual understanding improve both patient and provider experience of care.

CLINICS CARE POINTS

- Like most patient safety issues, perioperative management of limits to life-sustaining medical therapy requires a multidisciplinary approach in which all care providers share responsibility (please see **Table 1**).

- Sociocultural factors significantly influence patient preferences around life-sustaining medical therapy. Awareness of both historic and ongoing racial/ethnic and gender disparities in care is vital to approaching these life-sustaining medical therapy discussions empathetically with minoritized/marginalized groups. Early discussions of spiritual background may also significantly guide and inform discussions around life-sustaining medical therapy limits.

- The preoperative surgical clinic visit and preoperative medicine clinic visit represent the best initial opportunity to discuss life-sustaining medical therapy in the context of surgery, describe likely perioperative and postoperative life-sustaining medical therapy, and elicit patient preferences.

- The easiest and perhaps most vital component of preoperative preparation for patients with limits to life-sustaining medical therapy is identification and education of a surrogate decision maker.

- A central repository of advance care plan data in the electronic medical record may improve ease of access and leverage of previous life-sustaining medical therapy conversations.

- In determining which life-sustaining medical therapy limits will extend through the perianesthesia period, either a procedure-directed approach or a goal-directed approach is acceptable (although goal-directed may be more patient-centered). Full maintenance of Do-Not-Resuscitate or other limits to life-sustaining medical therapy should also be an option if medically reasonable.

- Failure to respect patient autonomy has significant medicolegal implications and has led to significant financial liability. The authors encourage perioperative providers to envision the worst-case scenario and plan accordingly.

- Postoperative clinical changes represent important moments to reconsider approach to life-sustaining medical therapy for patients with preoperative limits.

- Postoperative consultants may represent a useful outside perspective to help guide postoperative life-sustaining medical therapy decisions.

- It is important to acknowledge that these conversations and decisions are challenging and do not always have a satisfactory conclusion. The authors encourage open consultation with colleagues and the patient/surrogate decision-maker to achieve the most medically reasonable path forward that centers and respects patient self-determination.

DISCLOSURE

The authors have nothing to disclose.

REFERENCES

1. Beauchamp TL, Childress JF. Principles of biomedical ethics. 7th edition. New York: Oxford University Press; 2013.
2. Lin P-J, Zhu Y, Olchanski N, et al. Racial and ethnic differences in hospice use and hospitalizations at end-of-life among Medicare beneficiaries with dementia. JAMA Netw Open 2022;5:e2216260.
3. Ornstein KA, Roth DL, Huang J, et al. Evaluation of racial disparities in hospice use and end-of-life treatment intensity in the REGARDS cohort. JAMA Netw Open 2020;3:e2014639.
4. Samuel-Ryals CA, Mbah OM, Hinton SP, et al. Evaluating the contribution of patient-provider communication and cancer diagnosis to racial disparities in end-of-life care among Medicare beneficiaries. J Gen Intern Med 2021;36:3311–20.
5. Mack JW, Paulk ME, Viswanath K, et al. Racial disparities in the outcomes of communication on medical care received near death. Arch Intern Med 2010;170:1533–40.
6. Gazaway S, Chuang E, Thompson M, et al. Respecting faith, hope, and miracles in African American Christian patients at end-of-life: moving from labeling goals of care as "aggressive" to providing equitable goal-concordant care. J Racial Ethn Health Disparities 2023;10:2054–60.
7. Kwak J, Haley WE. Current research findings on end-of-life decision making among racially or ethnically diverse groups. Gerontol 2005;45:634–41.
8. American College of Surgeons. Optimal Resources for Geriatric Surgery: 2019 Standards. Available at: https://www.facs.org/-/media/files/quality-programs/geriatric/geriatricsv_standards.ashx. Accessed March 10, 2021.
9. Tang VL, Dillon EC, Yang Y, et al. Advance care planning in older adults with multiple chronic conditions undergoing high-risk surgery. JAMA Surg 2019;154:261–4.
10. Cooper Z, Koritsanszky LA, Cauley CE, et al. Recommendations for best communication practices to facilitate goal-concordant care for seriously ill older patients with emergency surgical conditions. Ann Surg 2016;263:1–6.
11. Kelley AS, Gold HT, Roach KW, et al. Differential medical and surgical house staff involvement in end-of-life decisions: a retrospective chart review. J Pain Symptom Manag 2006;32:110–7.
12. Bradley CT, Brasel KJ, Schwarze ML. Physician attitudes regarding advance directives for high-risk surgical patients: a qualitative analysis. Surgery 2010;148:209–16.
13. Morrell ED, Brown BP, Qi R, et al. The do-not-resuscitate order: associations with advance directives, physician specialty and documentation of discussion 15 years after the Patient Self-Determination Act. J Med Ethics 2008;34:642–7.

14. Sudore RL, Heyland DK, Lum HD, et al. Outcomes that define successful advance care planning: a Delphi panel consensus. J Pain Symptom Manag 2018;55:245–55.e8.

15. US Department of Veterans Affairs National Center for Ethics in Health Care. Goals of Care Conversations Skills Training for Clinicians. 2019. Available at: https://www.ethics.va.gov/GoCC.asp. Accessed September 22, 2023.

16. Hickman SE, Lum HD, Walling AM, et al. The care planning umbrella: the evolution of advance care planning. J Am Geriatr Soc 2023;71:2350–6.

17. Sweet AL, Brasel KJ, Hays ZE, et al. Advance care planning documentation in older adults undergoing evaluation at a preoperative medicine clinic: a single-center retrospective chart review. Perioperative Care and Operating Room Management 2022;26:100245.

18. Committee on Ethics and Professionalism. Ethical Guidelines for the Anesthesia Care of Patients with Do-Not-Resuscitate Orders or Other Directives That Limit Treatment. 2018. Available at: www.asahq.org/standards-and-guidelines/ethical-guidelines-for-the-anesthesia-care-of-patients-with-do-not-resuscitate-orders-or-other-directives-that-limit-treatment. Accessed February 6, 2019.

19. Truog RD, Waisel DB. Do-not-resuscitate orders: from the ward to the operating room; from procedures to goals. Int Anesthesiol Clin 2001;39:53–65.

20. O'Donnell vs. Harrison, No. CDV 2017-850. Montana, USA: Montana District Court, Lewis & Clark County; 2019.

21. Saitta NM, Hodge SD. What are the consequences of disregarding a "do not resuscitate directive" in the United States? Med Law 2013;32:441–58.

22. Pope TM. Legal briefing: new penalties for ignoring advance directives and do-not-resuscitate orders. J Clin Ethics 2017;28:74–81.

23. Pope TM. Clinicians may not administer life-sustaining treatment without consent: civil, criminal, and disciplinary sanctions. J Health Biomed Law 2013;9:213–96.

24. Span P. The patients were saved. That's why the families are suing. The New York Times; 2017. Available at: https://www.nytimes.com/2017/04/10/health/wrongful-life-lawsuit-dnr.html. Accessed January 8, 2020.

25. Combs SA, Culp S, Matlock DD, et al. Update on end-of-life care training during nephrology fellowship: a cross-sectional national survey of fellows. Am J Kidney Dis 2015;65:233–9.

26. Koncicki HM, Schell JO. Communication skills and decision making for elderly patients with advanced kidney disease: a guide for nephrologists. Am J Kidney Dis 2016;67:688–95.

27. Beben T, Rifkin DE. Recognizing our limits: deficiencies in end-of-life education for nephrology trainees. Am J Kidney Dis 2015;65:209–10.

28. Schell JO, Arnold RM. NephroTalk: communication tools to enhance patient-centered care. Semin Dial 2012;25:611–6.

29. DeVoe JE. Dad's last week. Ann Fam Med 2016;14:273–6.

30. Zib M, Saul P. A pilot audit of the process of end-of-life decision-making in the intensive care unit. Crit Care Resusc 2007;9:213–8.

31. Radcliffe C, Hewison A. Use of a supportive care pathway for end-of-life care in an intensive care unit: a qualitative study. Int J Palliat Nurs 2015;21:608–15.

End-of-life Care in the Intensive Care Unit and Ethics of Withholding/ Withdrawal of Life-sustaining Treatments

Andrea Cortegiani, MD[a,b],*, Mariachiara Ippolito, MD[a,b],
Sebastiano Mercadante, MD[c]

KEYWORDS

- End of life • Intensive care • Life-sustaining treatments • Palliative care

KEY POINTS

- End of life in the intensive care unit (ICU) can be stressful for patients, families, and clinicians.
- Most deaths in the intensive care unit follow a limitation of life-sustaining treatments mainly in the forms of withholding and withdrawal.
- Withholding and withdrawal of life-sustaining treatments must follow the evaluation of the appropriateness of support, shared goals of care with patients and families, and consensus among the ICU team.
- Their application is highly variable according to geographic location, and ethical, spiritual moral, and religious factors as long as provider experience.
- Palliative care aimed at optimizing patients' comfort, and communication with relatives and facilitating eventual bereavement must accompany the limitation of life-sustaining therapies.

INTRODUCTION

Critical care involves the most invasive environment in the hospital. Many activities in intensive care units (ICUs) can be traumatic, due to loss of autonomy, mind-altering

[a] Department of Precision Medicine in Medical, Surgical and Critical Care Area (Me.Pre.C.C.), University of Palermo, Palermo, Italy; [b] Department of Anesthesia Analgesia Intensive Care and Emergency, University Hospital Policlinico 'Paolo Giaccone', Via del vespro 129, Palermo 90127, Italy; [c] Main Regional Center of Pain Relief and Supportive/palliative Care, Nutrition (S.M.), La Maddalena Cancer Center, Via San Lorenzo, 312/D, Palermo 90146, Italy
* Corresponding author. Department of Surgical, Oncological and Oral Science, University of Palermo, Via del vespro 129, Palermo 90127, Italy.
E-mail address: andrea.cortegiani@unipa.it

Anesthesiology Clin 42 (2024) 407–419
https://doi.org/10.1016/j.anclin.2024.02.008
1932-2275/24/© 2024 Elsevier Inc. All rights reserved.

anesthesiology.theclinics.com

medication, noise pollution, disrupted sleep–wake cycles, venous and arterial line insertion, ventilation, vasopressors/inotropes, and hemofiltration.[1–3] A significant proportion of patients in ICU have a background of frailty, with poor bodily reserve to deal with persistent insults to organ function. ICU patients, including those with cancer, sepsis, or acute respiratory insufficiency, have particularly high rates of hospital death, and patients who need mechanical ventilation have mortality rates of more than 50%.[4] In a consensus on the basic definitions relating to end-of-life therapy in ICU patients, the list of comorbidities associated with medical futility included heart failure, advanced cancer, and failure of more organs. The greatest differences among the participants focused on identifying therapeutic procedures not recommended in end-of-life therapy.[5] In a retrospective analysis of administrative data, it was found that 20%, of patients in the United States died using ICU services. The doubling of persons over the age of 65 years by 2030 will require a system-wide expansion in ICU care for dying patients, unless the health care system pursues rationing, more effective advanced care planning, and increases capacity to care for dying patients in other settings. Of interest, ICU deaths account for a disproportionate percentage of spending, as about 60% of terminal admissions in ICU accounted for more than 80% of all terminal inpatient costs.[6] On the other hand, burnout and moral distress among ICU clinicians are commonly associated with end-of-life issues.[7] Moral distress causes clinicians to be dissatisfied with their work.[8] It has been estimated that 66% to 89% of intensive care nurses have provided futile treatment in their careers. Clinicians estimated that, on average, 20% of patients in ICUs units receive futile therapy.[9] Thus, end-of-life issues are an inherent component of ICU care. ICU competencies should include the provision of end-of-life care in addition to life-sustaining care and intensive treatment must be balanced with an understanding of its limitations, potential futility, and prolongation of distress.[1] Several studies exist in the literature related to how to approach the care of the dying patient clinically and ethically in the ICU, although there are no reliable estimates of the magnitude of this health issue. The aim of this article is to illustrate the major end-of-life issues in ICU and the general principles, practice, and ethics of limitation of life-sustaining treatments in the form of withholding and withdrawal.

DISCUSSION
End of Life Issues in Intensive Care Unit

Nature of the problem
In the last 30 years, palliative care has evolved as a specialty to address end-of-life issues and related concepts, including minimization of suffering, moral distress of health care professionals, and psychosocial support of patients, families, and caregivers, even in ICU patients. Palliative care is a holistic patient-centered care, focusing on symptom management, standardized assessment of care goals, and attention to the psychosocial needs of patients and families. Palliative care may overlap with the most aggressive of curative ICU care.[10] The intensity of curative and palliative care should be titrated to the goals and needs of every patient and patient family. The family may receive bereavement support even after the patient's death. Regretfully, dying patients often receive interventions they do not want, failing to improve outcomes.[11] Decisions to shift medical management to focus on end-of-life care can involve withholding or withdrawing life-sustaining treatments, either in ICU or on hospice transfer. A randomized cross-over study showed that early palliative care team involvement after ICU admission leads to a reduced incidence of intubation, tracheostomies, and readmissions.[12] Palliative care providers can clarify and reassess patient goals and wishes by advocating against unnecessary or unwanted procedures, thus preventing

overuse. In randomized controlled trials, consultation or involvement of an ethics team, that was able to identify the patient's values and preferences, decreased the number of days of mechanical ventilation, nutrition, and hydration as well as the overall hospital and ICU lengths of stay and quality of communication. Health care providers, patients, and patient family members were largely satisfied with the consult, would seek the consult again, recommending it to others.[13–17] Notably, such palliative care-related interventions resulted in fewer tests, procedures, interventions, less time in hospital, thus, decreasing overuse of resources and improving the health care quality.[18,19] Palliative care interventions have been reported to increase the percentage of ICU patients with do-not-resuscitate (DNR) status, as well as the number of patients in whom support has been withdrawn, and those whose end-of-life care wishes are known and documented at the time of patient death. Thus, palliative care does not advocate an alternative type of care. Rather, it ensures the care provided reflects the goals and wishes of the patient and decreases the misuse of health care resources. Moreover, palliative care teams may promote team collaboration, facilitating communication between health care providers, thus relieving the ICU team from some of that care burden, limiting moral distress and burnout.[18] However, it is important that the voice of the palliative care teams is in line with the one from the ICU caring team to avoid confusion and increased stress among family members. A multicenter randomized clinical trial demonstrated that family meetings led by palliative care specialists increased post-traumatic stress disorder symptoms in relatives of patients with chronic critical illness compared to routine family meetings led by the ICU teams. The application of palliative care in ICU has been adopted and tested in research as "consultative model," external palliative care teams that deal with palliative care needs in the ICU, or as "integrative model" where ICU teams address them directly. It has been advocated that a "mixed model", where the ICU (for all cases) and palliative care teams (especially for difficult cases) work together, may achieve the best results for patients and families.[20] Whatever the approach, it is pivotal that ICU teams improve their knowledge and skills regarding palliative care application in critically ill patients.[10,21]

End-of-life decisions depend on culture, religion, and geographic location. The differing legal and cultural frameworks prevent uniform recommendations.[22,23] The transition from active, invasive interventions to "no escalation" and comfort care is often fraught with conflict and moral distress, as well as misunderstandings and uncertaintis.[24–27] Compassionate end-of-life care is crucial in the ICU setting. In the last years it has been underlined the relevance of providing good quality end-of-life care in ICU. Patient- and family-centered care has emerged as a universal need for end-of-life care in ICU. The palliative care approach is aimed to improve the experience of patients and their families when active treatment has failed, other than providing symptom control.[19] Forward-thinking discussions among patients, next-of-kin, and staff are of paramount importance to ensure ongoing care prioritizes patients' best interests. An early involvement in these discussions is crucial.[1]

End-of-life issues still present several moral, legal, and practical challenges to ICU clinicians.[28] Several key ethical concepts have been introduced to clinical practice, including the moral equivalence of different types of limitations of life-sustaining treatments, as well as the difference between intended and foreseen circumstances. It is difficult to define what is the best interest of a patient, but above all it cannot be done in isolation. A shared decision-making process consists of two-way communication, with the aim of providing informed decision-making, and establish patient and next-of-kin values, gathering insight from caregivers who understand the patient's life, wishes, and medical condition. Communication is a difficult process, as it involves multiple conversations. Receiving information on poor prognosis or imminent death may be traumatic for next-of-kin to process. Next-of-kin commonly ask about the likelihood of recovery and the consequences of further procedures. Challenges arise when the relatives request invasive treatments that are not clinically indicated, or when discontinuing life support is in conflict with religious beliefs. A recent multicenter prospective observational study performed in the United States showed a high prevalence of discordance (1 of 3 cases) between patients/surrogates and staff about appropriateness of treatment. Indeed, disagreement was associated with prognostic discordance and lower patient/surrogate satisfaction and trust in ICU team.[29] Transitioning the model of care may be highly traumatic, requiring back-and-forth discussions. Having multiple discussions over a period of time may be helpful in explaining the clinical situation, reinforcing the goals and limitations of care and addressing questions or misunderstandings. Reapproaching discussions can give relatives time to reflect, after an initial psychological shock. Longer bedspace time may provide emotional space and improve recognition of a patient's condition. During these initial discussions, ICU physicians may specifically ask about plans for withholding or withdrawing life-sustaining treatments. This advance planning should be discussed at the time of admission to ICU to establish wishes on limits, or ceilings of care.[30] A multiple source multicenter study performed in 11 ICUs in France demonstrated the stringent need for goals of care discussion and the fear for their choices not be respected and are among the 15 most common preoccupations of ICU patients at high risk of dying.[31] The timing of these discussions is largely based on "prognostication" rather than patient-focused factors.[32,33] Timeliness of end-of-life care decisions is often clinician-dependent, and is affected by variable experience in communication training and in evaluating critical care prognosis.[34] Discussions should have a clear structure, establishing what is known, and laying out medical details that may be difficult to understand, requiring clarification and allowing time to address questions or clarify misunderstandings. The burden of these emotional conversations can take a toll, so that ICU teams should establish clear networks where staff can support each other or seek counseling to senior colleagues.[30] Research has shown satisfaction of caregivers with end-of-life care in the ICU setting is higher than on medical wards. This demonstrates that decisions regarding care provided in the intensive care setting are largely well considered in the context of patients' overall well-being.[35] Thus, compassionate care should be placed at the heart of any ICU management.

Ethics of Withdrawing/Withholding Support

Considerations

Limitation of life-sustaining treatments occurs in around 12% of ICU admissions worldwide[36] and in approximately 80% of cases of ICU deaths in Western countries.[2] Despite withdrawal and withholding of life-sustaining treatments in ICUs occurring more frequently over the years, a reduction in ICU mortality has progressively been registered.[2] Indeed, as technological and medical progress improves, long intensive care stay may be required, but often results in persistent disability, with uncertain efficacy related to long-term survival and quality of life. ICU physicians are usually skilled in identifying treatments that are not beneficial for long-term outcomes or not in line with patients and/or family wishes but only result in short-term prolongation of life. This trend in ethical practices seems to reflect the principle of allowing unavoidable deaths to occur, without prolonging agony or ICU stay. This trend has been proactively pursued by professional societies, that have issued recommendations and guidelines,[37,38] by institutions that have issued specific laws and regulations, and by the scientific community, that has produced updated data.[36] Steps toward reducing the use of potentially inappropriate treatments come not without efforts, both on the side of health care providers and institutions, but also for caregivers of dying people, who are more and more deeply involved in shared decision-making nowadays, as the principle of autonomy took over the old paternalistic medical approach in most countries. It is indeed challenging to distinguish treatments with at least some chances of beneficial effects but no effects on survival, from effective interventions and from completely futile interventions. The complexity of the issue is even greater if we take into account the number of health care providers, with different perspectives and roles, involved in the care of a critically ill patient, and the wide range of personal beliefs and backgrounds (eg, religious, emotional) that both patients and their caregivers may have.[39] The aim of this section of the review was to summarize the basic principles and data available regarding the ethics of withdrawing/withholding support.

Definitions

Definitions of withholding and withdrawal of life-sustaining treatments and of other key aspects of end-of-life have been recently produced by a world-wide consensus (the WELPICUS study) after a long period of terminology confusion.[5] Withdrawal of life-sustaining treatments refers to the decision to actively stop a life-sustaining intervention presently being given. Withdrawal of care may involve, for example, invasive mechanical ventilation, renal replacement therapy, and vasopressors. "Withholding life-sustaining treatments" regards a decision not to start or increase (eg, dose or level of intensity) a life-sustaining intervention, such as not performing cardiopulmonary resuscitation (CPR) after cardiac arrest. It includes both the decision not to initiate certain treatments (eg, intubation and invasive mechanical ventilation), even though available, or to avoid an escalation of treatment (eg, increase the dosage of vasopressors). Life-sustaining treatments include CPR, endotracheal intubation, and mechanical ventilation, vasopressor therapy, nutrition, dialysis, blood products, antibiotics, and intravenous fluids. Both withholding and withdrawal are performed for treatments that are considered prolonging patients' dying process without offering a benefit and/or not in line with the patient's wishes or goals. Despite being both legal in many parts of the world and considered ethically equivalent in Western countries, the prevalence of withdrawal and withholding practices differ and may have different implications for health care providers both in practical terms and in emotional burden.[40,41] Indeed, in some countries, withholding may be acceptable, while withdrawing is illegal or unethical regardless of the consent. The context may also be slightly different for the two procedures. Withdrawing occurs when the treatment is ongoing without clear signs of clinical response. This implies an *active* act of commission that makes patients, families, or even some health care workers feel uncomfortable in front of this decision. On the other hand, withholding requires the physician an a priori estimate of the effect and a decision not to start certain treatments from the beginning or not to increase the intensity of the treatments (a *passive* act of commission).[40] Both practices often occur after trials of full care, that is the decision to use a certain intensity of care for a brief time, in order to test its efficacy while further data are collected to consider the appropriateness of full-code. Withdrawal is often decided due to an ongoing worsening of the patient's condition over time, while withholding may occur at earlier stages, based on prognosis, except for cases regarding withholding of escalation of treatment. Notably, the real ethical or legal difference between the two practices can be questioned considering the whole clinical course of a critically ill patient, during which life-sustaining therapies may be not started, not escalated, or subsequently suspended at different times without meaningful difference on clinical ground.[42] Both forms of limitation took place after life supports start to be considered disproportioned to the prognosis *quoad vitam* and/or *valetudinem* considering shared goals of care between treating clinicians and the patient/family.

It is important that both withholding and withdrawing are well discussed within the team of care and to the caregivers as procedures aimed to relieve symptoms and remove burdens related to futile interventions. According to recommendations from the WELPICUS study, life-sustaining treatments should generally be withheld or withdrawn only after obtaining agreement from the patient and/or the surrogate decision maker or the family. However, the practices can be permitted even in cases when this agreement cannot be achieved.[5] Importantly, the decision should not be mistaken either for missed care, that is, patient care that is omitted or delayed or partially completed. Indeed, they should not be confused with active shortening of the dying process, defined as a circumstance in which an act with the specific intent of hastening death or shortening the dying process.[5]

Thus, decision-making in these challenging situations should be active and taken with professional responsibility, ensuring that all patients receive equitable care and, to the extent possible that minimize the risk of subjective biases, under the principle of autonomy, beneficence, nonmaleficence, and justice.[43]

Current evidence

Although interest in withdrawal and withholding has been well described in recent studies, it must be acknowledged that evidence on the topic has a long history. Indeed, a study published in 1997 had already shown a positive trend toward withdrawal and withholding procedures in ICU, describing an increase in such procedures from 1987–88 to 1992–93 in 2 study centers.[44] Decisions to forgo life-sustaining therapies were investigated in a secondary analysis of the SAPS3 database. It showed that 36.2% of ICU deaths occurred after limitations of treatment in the 282 study ICUs. The analysis also pointed out that organizational factors, such as the number of nurses, the availability of an ED, and the presence of full-time intensivists were independently associated with the incidence of decisions to withdraw or withhold therapies.[45] A study performed in 43 ICUs in France showed that the most common claimed rationales to justify withholding or withdrawing by clinicians were no additional information needed for decision making, limited subsequent functional autonomy, absence of curative strategy, presence of an advanced or terminal disease and no response to medical therapy.[46] The most recent and large evidence on withdrawal and withholding practices worldwide comes from the ETHICUS II study, a large multicenter prospective observational study performed in 199 ICUs in 36 countries, showing that limitation of life-sustaining treatment occurs nowadays in around 11.8% of ICU admissions. The most common form of limitation was withholding (44%) followed by withdrawal (36%) while shortening of the dying process was uncommon, with withholding life-sustaining procedures being the most common choice, followed by withdrawing life-sustaining treatment (0.5%). The study also identified factors associated with treatment limitations, such as age, diagnoses, and local end-of-life legislation.[36] Specifically, each 1 year increment was associated with a 1% odds increment for treatment limitations. Moreover, having a chronic condition (ie, cancer, respiratory, muscular, neurologic, cognitive) or an acute neurologic diagnosis were associated to higher chance of receiving treatment limitations. Treatment limitations were much more common in Northern Europe, Australia/New Zealand, and North America than in Africa, Latin America, and Southern Europe. Southern Europe and Latin America had the lowest rate of withdrawal and reluctance to apply limitations. The median time to the first limitation was 2 days. Surprisingly, 1 in 5 patients who received limitations survived at hospital discharge. Survival was lower after withdrawing (11.5%) than withholding (28%). The important geographic variability in the decision of withholding and withdrawing had been also demonstrated by a previous secondary analysis of an international study (ICON) conducted in 730 ICUs in 82 countries. The decision was significantly less common in low/middle compared to high gross national income countries (6% vs 12% of the 9524 included critically ill patients).[47] Notably, greater disease severity, presence of 2 or more organ failures, severe comorbidities, medical and trauma admissions, and admission from the emergency department (ED) or hospital floor were independently associated with the decision to apply withholding/withdrawal of life-sustaining therapies, after which almost 30% of patients were alive at hospital discharge.[47]

Evidence on which other variables impact decision-making related to withdrawal and withholding care is still being accumulated, though recent data suggest that socioeconomic and demographic factors may be associated with decisions to limit treatment.[48] Nevertheless, one of the analyses conducted in a study assessing 51 audiotaped physician–family conferences about major end-of-life treatment decisions at 4 hospitals has shown that lower family educational level seems to be associated with less-shared decision-making.[49] The study also showed that only 2% of decisions involved definitive shared decision-making, with the assessment of the family's understanding of the decision frequently missing (25%). Such data document a persistent barrier to communication and shared decision-making. The effects of implementing the contacts between the patient, family, and hospital staff were investigated by the landmark SUPPORT study in 1995,[11] whose phase II was a multicenter RCT. The study showed no improvement in patient–physician communication and other study outcomes, including physicians' knowledge of their patient's preferences not to be resuscitated (adjusted ratio, 1.22; 95% CI, 0.99–1.49).

In addition to what is described, guidelines and guidance documents also have been published in many countries, aiming at guiding local centers in implementing such practices on the basis of the growing evidence on the topic and to provide practical support to health care operators involved.[4,50] Notably, no international evidence-based guidelines have been published to date. It is reasonable to believe that national regulations and the highly variable local practices can be barriers to adoption of international guidelines.

Application

Withholding or withdrawing may relate to respiratory, cardiovascular, renal, or even nutritional support, use of antibiotics or blood products administration and often require technical competencies and experience, in addition to nontechnical skills (eg, communication). Doing so should also include palliative care support to ensure the comfort and dignity of the patient.

The team should continue to manage symptoms (eg, pain, dyspnea, anxiety, and discomforts), reach an effective communication with caregivers and provide support for coping with the procedure and the loss, maintaining the patient's dignity, ensure a safe professional environment for all the operators involved.

The practical implications of withdrawal and withholding practices are different. Indeed, to withhold invasive mechanical ventilation may include the choice not to intubate a patient with respiratory failure, or not to admit a patient to an intensive care unit, thus establishing that the appropriate maximum intensity of care has been reached. On the other hand, withdrawing an invasive mechanical ventilation assumes that the team will be ready (ie, technically and emotionally) to perform a terminal extubation as an active medical procedure.

For example, core competencies and technical skills for the procedures of withdrawal include[50]

- Assessment of pain during the procedure using standardized scoring systems;
- Assessment of agitation during the procedure using standardized scoring systems;
- Provision of medications in advance for the management of expected symptoms;
- Provision of additional pharmacologic support for uncontrolled symptoms (eg, increase dosage or administer bolus of benzodiazepine for breakthrough agitation; inhaled to treat postextubation stridor in conscious patients).

Each center may have peculiarities and the implementation of local formal protocols is suggested.[50] This is important also because evidence suggests an important variability in application of limitations between ICUs in the same country and even between physicians within the same ICU.[51] Protocols may guide the order of stepwise withdrawal (eg, vasopressors/inotropes first, then mechanical ventilation, and lastly airway), and help identifying the noncomfort interventions that should be interrupted, such as blood transfusions, nutrition, and antibiotics. A personalized approach should be always taken into account, aiming to ensure patient's comfort as the primary goal. Exceptions should be considered case by case (eg, extubation is preferable at the end of a wean, but avoidance is also acceptable). In addition, a supportive environment should be promoted toward health care operators involved in all the steps of such procedures, to ensure they are not deeply affected by these decisions and can safely improve their coping mechanisms.

Controversies

Despite progress in knowledge, competencies, laws, and data availability, withholding and withdrawal life-sustaining treatments remain ethically and logistically complex even in the most experienced centers and variability between providers remain high.[51] Problems and issues may arise in different moments of a patient's trajectory of care, for example, from intensivist consultations to assess ICU admission to patient's death. Pre-ICU admission issues can regard disagreements with non-ICU physicians on withholding decisions (eg, to do not intubate a patient, to do not admit a patient to ICU, to candidate a patient for palliative care).

The use of a "surprise question" may help interprofessional communication and limit the overestimation of the outcomes. Non-ICU physicians, who are usually less trained in end-of-life care, can be posed the question if they would be surprised in case of patient's death in the subsequent 12 months. A positive answer may help open honest discussions with colleagues and caregivers on reasonable outcomes. Indeed, many families have unrealistic expectations regarding ICU admission and ICU stay, which should be specifically addressed with constructive communication. A recent cluster randomized trial demonstrated that early palliative care consultation within 48 hours from ICU admission may increase DNR/DNI orders and transfers to hospice care while reducing overall ventilator-days, tracheostomies, and ICU readmission compared to standard care. These data suggest that early multidisciplinary discussion with physicians with expertise in palliative care may help defining more appropriate trajectories of care after ICU admission.[12]

Similar difficulties may take place inside the ICU, especially along death trajectories that have been described as "prolonged dwindling" or in the case of patients with previous ICU admissions and successful discharges. In such cases, the high risk of treatment failure is difficult to be understood by families and caregivers and disagreements may occur.[29] Moreover, different professional age and working experience may hamper comprehension of such trajectories, and lead to disagreements within the team of care. Despite complexity, consensus among the ICU team about the options and the recommended plan should be achieved before anyone approaches the patient or family to apply/discuss limitations of life-sustaining treatments.[40] Attitudes toward withholding and withdrawal can be different between providers inside each ICU, and this can be emotionally stressful for providers at bedside who are in charge of applying limitations, especially if they feel themselves *alone* in that task. It is important to consider, discuss, and apply limitations of life-sustaining therapies as a shared *team decision*. It has been recommended to document the decision to withhold or withdraw life-sustaining treatments in the medical records, as long as its rationales and the persons involved in such decision.[5] Efforts should be made to share clear information among the whole ICU team on which limitations of treatments have been applied in that particular case, avoiding generic "no escalation" orders.[26] Disagreements can also derive from differences in nursing and medical approaches toward the patient.[21] Indeed, nurses may have a more holistic background, while physicians have only recently started to be trained on the uncertainty of death and on end-of-life ethics and may be more focused on acting against the disease. In line of these difficulties and potential issues, guidelines recommend the availability of an experienced physician, nurse, and respiratory therapist for all the cases of limitations of life-sustaining therapies and their presence at bedside in cases anticipated to be difficult to manage.[50]

Lack of structured training contributes to slow improvement in the field of medical ethics and palliative care and to suboptimal application in clinics.[43,52] Concerning this aspect, a recommendation with high grade of consensus of the WELPICUS study stated that health care professionals should receive training in the core end-of-life skills so they can become experts in decision-making at the end of life in accordance with local cultural and legal norms.[5] Legal aspects also often are listed as obstacles in performing withdrawal and withholding, despite many countries having specific legal provisions that outline the circumstances under which withdrawal and withholding of life-sustaining treatments are permissible, and this also confirms the need for specific training to be provided to health care operators.

SUMMARY

End-of-life decisions depend on culture, religion, and geographic location. Compassionate end-of-life care is crucial in the ICU setting and patient- and family-centered care has emerged as a universal need for end-of-life care in ICU. The transition from full-code treatments to "no escalation" and comfort care, together with withdrawing and withholding life-sustaining treatments are essential phases to provide compassionate and patient-centered care in the ICU. Specific competencies, training, and experience are needed to implement such procedures, offering physicians an opportunity to go beyond the impotence generated by unavoidable death and to focus on patients' dignity and wishes. They should be seen as a "limitation" of not proportioned support. Incorporating palliative care into the process may support patients and their families.

CRITICS CARE POINTS

Key practical steps before applying limitations of life-sustaining therapies in the ICU
1. Comprehensive clinical judgment about the appropriateness of life support in light of clinical course, response to therapies, and most probable prognosis;

2. (Re)discussion of goals of care considering patient's wishes, eventual medical advance directives, family opinions, after readily and clearly understood explanations of clinical conditions.
3. Discussion of the case among the ICU team, involving both physicians and nurses as long as other key health care professionals involved in patient care (eg, phycologists, respiratory therapists).
4. Plan actions with the head of the team and share them with the whole multidisciplinary team. Any *stress trigger*, uncertainty, or doubt of any type (ethical, moral, religious, or legal) by any member of the team and by patient and family should be promptly discussed and solved before taking any step ahead; Experienced personnel should lead the plan.
5. Document the decision to withhold or withdraw life-sustaining therapies in the medical records as long as the rationales and the persons involved in this decision.

DISCLOSURE

All authors have nothing to disclose.

REFERENCES

1. Abeywickrema M, Turfrey D. Compassionate end-of-life care in the intensive care unit involves early establishment of treatment goals. J Patient Exp 2022;9. 23743735221089452.
2. Sprung CL, Ricou B, Hartog CS, et al. Changes in end-of-life practices in european intensive care units from 1999 to 2016. JAMA, J Am Med Assoc 2019; 322(17):1692–704.
3. Vincent J-L, Marshall JC, Namendys-Silva SA, et al. Assessment of the worldwide burden of critical illness: the intensive care over nations (ICON) audit. Lancet Respir Med 2014;2(5):380–6.
4. Truog RD, Campbell ML, Curtis JR, et al. Recommendations for end-of-life care in the intensive care unit: A consensus statement by the American College of Critical Care Medicine. Crit Care Med 2008;36(3):953–63.
5. Sprung CL, Truog RD, Curtis JR, et al. Seeking worldwide professional consensus on the principles of end-of-life care for the critically ill. The Consensus for Worldwide End-of-Life Practice for Patients in Intensive Care Units (WELPICUS) study. Am J Respir Crit Care Med 2014;190(8):855–66.
6. Angus DC, Barnato AE, Linde-Zwirble WT, et al. Use of intensive care at the end of life in the United States: an epidemiologic study. Crit Care Med 2004;32(3):638–43.
7. Papazian L, Hraiech S, Loundou A, et al. High-level burnout in physicians and nurses working in adult ICUs: a systematic review and meta-analysis. Intensive Care Med 2023;49(4):387–400.
8. Hamric AB, Blackhall LJ. Nurse-physician perspectives on the care of dying patients in intensive care units: collaboration, moral distress, and ethical climate. Crit Care Med 2007;35(2):422–9.
9. Damps M, Gajda M, Słotny L, et al. Limiting futile therapy as part of end-of-life care in intensive care units. Anaesthesiol Intensive Ther 2022;54(3):279–84.
10. Mercadante S, Gregoretti C, Cortegiani A. Palliative care in intensive care units : why , where , what , who , when. How 2018;1–6.
11. Connors AF. A Controlled Trial to Improve Care for Seriously Ill Hospitalized Patients. JAMA 1995;274(20):1591.
12. Ma J, Chi S, Buettner B, et al. Early Palliative Care Consultation in the Medical ICU: A Cluster Randomized Crossover Trial. Crit Care Med 2019;47(12):1707–15.

13. Schneiderman LJ, Gilmer T, Teetzel HD, et al. Effect of ethics consultations on nonbeneficial life-sustaining treatments in the intensive care setting: a randomized controlled trial. JAMA 2003;290(9):1166–72.
14. Lautrette A, Darmon M, Megarbane B, et al. A communication strategy and brochure for relatives of patients dying in the ICU. N Engl J Med 2007;356(5):469–78.
15. Kentish-Barnes N, Chevret S, Valade S, et al. A three-step support strategy for relatives of patients dying in the intensive care unit: a cluster randomised trial. Lancet (London, England) 2022;399(10325):656–64.
16. Campbell ML, Guzman JA. Impact of a proactive approach to improve end-of-life care in a medical ICU. Chest 2003;123(1):266–71.
17. Curtis JR. Treece PD., Nielsen EL., et al. Randomized Trial of Communication Facilitators to Reduce Family Distress and Intensity of End-of-Life Care. Am J Respir Crit Care Med 2016;193(2):154–62.
18. Aslakson R, Pronovost PJ. Health care quality in end-of-life care: promoting palliative care in the intensive care unit. Anesthesiol Clin 2011;29(1):111–22.
19. Aslakson R, Cheng J, Vollenweider D, et al. Evidence-based palliative care in the intensive care unit: a systematic review of interventions. J Palliat Med 2014;17(2):219–35.
20. Curtis JR, Higginson IJ, White DB. Integrating palliative care into the ICU: a lasting and developing legacy. Intensive Care Med 2022;939–42. https://doi.org/10.1007/s00134-022-06729-7.
21. Effendy C, Yodang Y, Amalia S, et al. Barriers and facilitators in the provision of palliative care in adult intensive care units: a scoping review. Acute Crit Care 2022;37(4):516–26.
22. Chakraborty R, El-Jawahri AR, Litzow MR, et al. A systematic review of religious beliefs about major end-of-life issues in the five major world religions. Palliat Support Care 2017;15(5):609–22.
23. Hartog CS, Maia PA, Ricou B, et al. Changes in communication of end-of-life decisions in European ICUs from 1999 to 2016 (Ethicus-2) - a prospective observational study. J Crit Care 2022;68:83–8.
24. St Ledger U, Reid J, Begley A, et al. Moral distress in end-of-life decisions: A qualitative study of intensive care physicians. J Crit Care 2021;62:185–9.
25. Frisella S, Bonosi L, Ippolito M, et al. Palliative Care and End-of-Life Issues in Patients with Brain Cancer Admitted to ICU. Med 2023;59(2). https://doi.org/10.3390/medicina59020288.
26. Batten JN, Blythe JA, Wieten SE, et al. "No Escalation of Treatment" Designations: A Multi-institutional Exploratory Qualitative Study. Chest 2023;163(1):192–201.
27. Dahill M, Powter L, Garland L, et al. Improving documentation of treatment escalation decisions in acute care. BMJ Qual Improv Reports 2013;2(1). https://doi.org/10.1136/bmjquality.u200617.w1077. u200617.w1077.
28. Azoulay E, Timsit J-F, Sprung CL, et al. Prevalence and factors of intensive care unit conflicts: the conflicus study. Am J Respir Crit Care Med 2009;180(9):853–60.
29. Wilson ME, Dobler CC, Zubek L, et al. Prevalence of Disagreement About Appropriateness of Treatment Between ICU Patients/Surrogates and Clinicians. Chest 2019;155(6):1140–7.
30. Kentish-Barnes N, Meddick-Dyson S. A continuum of communication: family centred care at the end of life in the intensive care unit. Intensive Care Med 2023. https://doi.org/10.1007/s00134-023-07005-y.

31. Kentish-Barnes N, Poujol A-L, Banse E, et al. Giving a voice to patients at high risk of dying in the intensive care unit: a multiple source approach. Intensive Care Med 2023;49(7):808–19.

32. Gutierrez KM. Prognostic categories and timing of negative prognostic communication from critical care physicians to family members at end-of-life in an intensive care unit. Nurs Inq 2013;20(3):232–44.

33. You JJ, Dodek P, Lamontagne F, et al. What really matters in end-of-life discussions? Perspectives of patients in hospital with serious illness and their families. C Can Med Assoc J 2014;186(18):E679–87.

34. Visser M, Deliens L, Houttekier D. Physician-related barriers to communication and patient- and family-centred decision-making towards the end of life in intensive care: a systematic review. Crit Care 2014;18(6):604.

35. Rolnick JA, Ersek M, Wachterman MW, et al. The Quality of End-of-Life Care among ICU versus Ward Decedents. Am J Respir Crit Care Med 2020;201(7): 832–9.

36. Avidan A, Sprung CL, Schefold JC, et al. Variations in end-of-life practices in intensive care units worldwide (Ethicus-2): a prospective observational study. Lancet Respir Med 2021;9(10):1101–10.

37. Bosslet GT, Pope TM, Rubenfeld GD, et al. An official ATS/AACN/ACCP/ESICM/SCCM policy statement: Responding to requests for potentially inappropriate treatments in intensive care units. Am J Respir Crit Care Med 2015;191(11): 1318–30.

38. Vergano M, Bertolini G, Giannini A, et al. Siaarti recommendations for the allocation of intensive care treatments in exceptional, resource-limited circumstances. Minerva Anestesiol 2020;86(5):469–72.

39. Catalisano G, Ippolito M, Marino C, et al. Palliative care principles and anesthesiology clinical practice: current perspectives. J Multidiscip Healthc 2021;14: 2719–30.

40. Bandrauk N, Downar J, Paunovic B. Withholding and withdrawing life-sustaining treatment: The Canadian Critical Care Society position paper. Can J Anaesth 2018;65(1):105–22.

41. Levin PD, Sprung CL. Withdrawing and withholding life-sustaining therapies are not the same. Crit Care 2005;9(3):230–2.

42. Vincent J-L. Withdrawing may be preferable to withholding. Crit Care 2005;9(3): 226–9.

43. Porta L, Mauri E. A narrative review on palliative care in the emergency department: dealing with the uncertainty of death. Emerg Care J 2023;19(1):31–6.

44. Prendergast TJ, Luce JM. Increasing incidence of withholding and withdrawal of life support from the critically ill. Am J Respir Crit Care Med 1997;155(1):15–20.

45. Azoulay É, Metnitz B, Sprung CL, et al. End-of-life practices in 282 intensive care units: Data from the SAPS 3 database. Intensive Care Med 2009;35(4):623–30.

46. Lesieur O, Leloup M, Gonzalez F, et al. Withholding or withdrawal of treatment under French rules: a study performed in 43 intensive care units. Ann Intensive Care 2015;5(1):56.

47. Lobo SM, De Simoni FHB, Jakob SM, et al. Decision-Making on Withholding or Withdrawing Life Support in the ICU: A Worldwide Perspective. Chest 2017; 152(2):321–9.

48. Strandberg G, Lipcsey M. Association of socioeconomic and demographic factors with limitations of life sustaining treatment in the intensive care unit. Intensive Care Med 2023. https://doi.org/10.1007/s00134-023-07177-7.

49. White DB, Braddock CH, Bereknyei S, et al. Toward shared decision making at the end of life in intensive care units: Opportunities for improvement. Arch Intern Med 2007;167(5):461–7.
50. Downar J, Delaney JW, Hawryluck L, et al. Guidelines for the withdrawal of life-sustaining measures. Intensive Care Med 2016;42(6):1003–17.
51. Mark NM, Rayner SG, Lee NJ, et al. Global variability in withholding and withdrawal of life-sustaining treatment in the intensive care unit: a systematic review. Intensive Care Med 2015;41(9):1572–85.
52. Cortegiani A, Russotto V, Raineri SM, et al. Attitudes towards end-of-life issues in intensive care unit among Italian anesthesiologists: a nation-wide survey. Support Care Cancer 2018;26(6):1773–80.

Brain Death
Medical, Ethical, Cultural, and Legal Aspects

Matthew W. Pennington, MD, PhD[a],
Michael J. Souter, MB, ChB, FRCA, FNCS[b,c],*

KEYWORDS

• Brain death • Medical ethics • Irreversibility • Transplantation

KEY POINTS

- Brain death resulted from technological innovations in critical care, driven by resource implications and regulation of organ procurement.
- Although brain death is frequently associated with physiologic collapse and endocrine failure, this has not always occurred, especially in children. There have been no credible instances of recovery.
- There is a significant confusion of terminology and usage in both the lay public and health care professions, which have contributed to family disbelief and rejection of the diagnosis.
- The diagnosis has ethical implications, which include elements of beneficence, non-maleficence, and social justice, but there are may also be cultural barriers complicating communication, understanding, and agreement.
- Criticisms of biological and medicolegal inconsistency have arisen; however, no valid alternatives have achieved any degree of acceptance.

BACKGROUND

The premise for neurologic criteria that define death arose consequent to innovation in critical care in the 1950s—specifically with the development of cardiovascular and respiratory support of the neurologically devastated patient who would previously have died of their disease process and where such patients neither displayed or recovered any function of the central nervous system (excluding the spinal cord).[1]

This created a twofold dilemma: (1) the continued delivery of care to those who did not demonstrate any recovery and (2) the consumption of resources that could

[a] Department of Anesthesiology & Pain Medicine, University of Washington, University of Washington Medical Center (Montlake), Box 356540, 1959 NE Pacific Street, Seattle, WA 98195, USA; [b] Department of Anesthesiology & Pain Medicine, University of Washington, Box 359724, Harborview Medical Center, 325 Ninth Avenue, Seattle, WA, USA; [c] Department of Neurological Surgery, University of Washington, Box 359724, Harborview Medical Center, 325 Ninth Avenue, Seattle, WA, USA
* Corresponding author. Department of Anesthesiology & Pain Medicine, University of Washington, Box 359724, Harborview Medical Center, 325 Ninth Avenue, Seattle, WA.
E-mail address: msouter@uw.edu

Anesthesiology Clin 42 (2024) 421–432
https://doi.org/10.1016/j.anclin.2023.11.003
1932-2275/24/© 2023 Elsevier Inc. All rights reserved.

anesthesiology.theclinics.com

(especially in the early days of critical care) frustrate access to care for those patients who may have had potential for recovery.

An added layer of stressful complexity was the absence of legal and ethical structures to guide responses in these situations. Physicians expressed concerns of their vulnerability to charges of murder.

The continued challenges to the fundamental cardiorespiratory mechanisms of mortality had at the same time provoked discussions on life and existence and concern about the appropriateness of continued technological support in the absence of recovery. Pope Pius XII addressed this in part with a 1957 decree that physicians were not obliged to deliver extraordinary care[2]—defined subsequently as associated with "excessive expense, pain, or other inconvenience"… without "reasonable hope of benefit."[3] This was followed by the conceptualization of "hopeless care" by Ayd in 1962, with advocation for withdrawal of support where death appeared inevitable.[4] In 1968, the 22nd World Medical Assembly met in Sydney released a declaration on human death which included the statement that death "lies not in the preservation of isolated cells but in the fate of a person."[5] This declaration included an important bio-philosophical concept—that of death presenting as a continuum of cellular loss, organ dysfunction, and eventual mortality of the organism. Progression along that continuum will inevitably pass a tipping point of irreversibility, with brain death considered as such.

Concurrently, advances in immunologic treatment rendered organ transplant a feasible therapeutic practice. Its previously limited scale had been constrained in scope and access by only being feasible in those patients succumbing to cardiorespiratory arrest in circumstances where procurement could swiftly be mobilized. The developing awareness of "brain death" as a putative entity created some challenges in ethically regulating who made the diagnosis and when the approach for procurement was made, with a transplant surgeon at a conference in 1966 describing the criteria he used in diagnosis of brain death and the subsequent retrieval of organs from beating heart patients.[6]

The Harvard Criteria were devised to provide some structural basis to that diagnostic process, as well as offering justification for the termination of care—and importantly providing one of the first articulations of what became known as the dead donor rule—where vital organs should not be removed from living patients, but may permissibly be removed from the dead.[7]

As such, the Harvard criteria were conceptually supportive of the ethical principles of utilitarianism and social justice, coupled with a deontological and beneficent effect by both reducing distress to health care staff and the aggregate level of suffering and financial burden experienced by families.

In the United States, the Presidents Commission reviewed criteria to afford a standard definition of death.[8] This was subsequently encoded that the same year into the Uniform Determination of Death Act (UDDA, 1981), adopted in concept by all 50 states of the United States. Death was defined as the *irreversible* loss of function of the cardiorespiratory function or the *irreversible* loss of function of the entire brain, including the brain stem. The United Kingdom and some other countries chose more circumspect criteria—based on the permanent loss of function of the brain stem. Diagnostically, the criteria for each are essentially identical.

DISCUSSION
Biological Argument for Brain Death

Neuronal tissue has no intracellular energy stores; with the consequence, the cessation of function follows cessation of blood flow carrying oxygen and nutrients. This cessation of function includes the generation of electrical activity but also the basic metabolic maintenance of the cell. The empirical support for this concept is provided by the evidence of brain necrosis in states such as ischemic stroke, profoundly severe and prolonged hypoxia, and extreme intracranial hypotension. Neurons can also be killed by mechanical factors (eg, the shearing of acceleration/deceleration injuries) as well as hypoxia and hypotension altering the threshold of viability—all of which render neurons more susceptible to death and/or apoptosis.

Understanding death of the brain is predicated on understanding its essential functionality. At the most basic level, it constitutes a predominantly integrative processing of sensory and environmental stimuli to in turn effect reactions, which themselves confer a survival advantage for the organism. Higher orders of function allow endocrinological and homeostatic regulation, whereas increasing complexity of neuronal communication is associated with sapience. Conversely, damage to the brain will initially impinge on higher level functions and with increasing severity be associated with degradation of homeostasis and ultimately a loss of receptivity and response to stimuli.

In the early clinical observations of injury guiding the formulation of brain death criteria, there was also empirical evidence that widespread systemic collapse followed on the heels of the diagnosis of brain death. This was thought originally to be an inevitability but is now understood as constituting a combination of the physiologic derangements directly consequent to the *cause* of injury (hypotension, hemorrhage, hypoxia, hypercarbia), endocrinological dysfunction (loss of much of the hypophyseal-pituitary adrenal axis), and the inflammatory activation initiated by the original disease process, but subsequently amplified by the release of chemical mediators from dead and dying brain tissue.[9]

As such, with improved therapies in endocrinology, fluid and electrolyte therapy, and treatment of inflammation, the "inevitability" of physiologic collapse of the whole organism became less evident, and in some cases (especially in pediatric cases), it failed to manifest entirely. This has been taken by some to impute that brain death is not equivalent to systemic death in that it does not inevitably precede the other. Alternatively, one might argue that the "distance" along the continuum of mortality, from "tipping point" to the endpoint of systemic death, has merely been extended.

The "entire brain" definition

Nevertheless, the emphasis on the loss of function of the entire brain remained in force, with implications that persisting pituitary function would contradict a diagnosis of brain death. However, pituitary perfusion derives from both extracranial and intracranial supplies, consequent to the embryologic development and migration of the pituitary from pouch of Rathke in the roof of the pharynx. This, in part, explains the variability in the expression of diabetes insipidus after brain death.

Even with complete interruption of blood supply to the brain, at some stage (measured in days), the consequent inflammation and edema will subside, and cerebral perfusion may again ensue—but by this stage the metabolic insult is so pronounced that neurons are either dead or dying—to be eventually replaced by calcification or fibrosis. The deficit of neurologic function is persistent, however.

In circumstances of partial perfusion (eg, to pituitary), some endocrine function may persist, with evidence of sexual maturation in children pronounced brain dead, but who are subsequently ventilated over the longer term. The reaction to and integrative processing of stimuli to evoke a response remains absent. Despite this, the definition of brain death in applying to the "whole brain" has generated criticism that in such cases, death has not in fact occurred.[10] Some newer guidelines have specifically stated that persisting pituitary function does not exclude a diagnosis of brain death.[11]

The higher brain definition

Some have proposed that persistent "loss of the person" is in itself sufficient to declare brain death. Veatch has passionately argued that the required qualifications and nuances in navigating the entire brain diagnosis have rendered it implausible and suggests an alternative based on the permanent loss of the integrative function of mind and body.[12] Critics of this "higher function" approach make the case that either the persistently vegetative state or minimally conscious states may be conflated into this diagnosis.[13] Anencephaly also presents a further alternative challenge in defining the difference between life and death in circumstances where technological supplementation of function can perpetuate physiology.

The "integrative whole brain" definition

Bernat takes a more nuanced view where he distinguishes the higher brain definition from that of "whole brain function," but with the caveat that within the whole brain there is a *critical* threshold of neurons which must cease functioning in order to induce the permanent cessation of *critical* functions of the organism as a whole.[13] Essentially, not every neuron needs die for there to be an "irreversible loss of function of the entire brain." While conceptually attractive, it has not really answered the concerns surrounding the whole brain definition in that the definition of *criticality* requires some qualification of time scale and perspective.

The brain stem definition

The brain stem criteria arose from the descriptive case series by Mohandas and Chou, detailing their use of clinical criteria of brain stem examination to declare brain death.[14] While very similar to the Harvard criteria, they identified the need for etiologic preconditions, a basic apnea test, and the irrelevance of spinal reflexes, together with concerns on the utility of EEG. The principle of the brain stem as a key mediator of whole brain function was further refined by Pallis, based on the role of the brain stem in the transfer of essential information into and out of the cerebral hemispheres, along with hosting the reticular activating system as a crucial component of consciousness. He further developed the principle outlined in the Declaration of Sydney, saying:

> The irreversible cessation of heartbeat and respiration imply the death of the patient as a whole. They do not necessarily imply the immediate death of every cell in the body. The irreversible cessation of brain stem function implies the death of the brain as a whole. It does not necessarily imply the immediate death of every cell in the brain.[15]

While initially dissimilar, the clinical approach to the diagnosis of brain death in the United Kingdom and United States has largely converged to the UK practice, whereas the differences remaining are predominantly philosophic and semiotic, as detailed by Wijdicks.[16] Nevertheless, few countries outside the United Kingdom have adopted a brain-stem death standard.

Psychosocial Argument for Brain Death

Entwined within these biologic definitions is the concept of loss of self or personhood via the loss of brain function. The most extreme instance of loss of brain function is decapitation, and even though, it is technically possible to maintain physiologic function in the bodies of decapitated animals; few would describe these physiologic preparations as still being alive, although mechanistically there is no difference between this state and that of brain dead animals. In a noted thought experiment, Shewmon in fact proposed that if body and head were divided and function maintained in each, the identity of the person would be with the head.[17]

From a decidedly more humanistic perspective, since Quinlan,[18] there has been recognition of the concept of permanent unresponsiveness as an undesirable mode of existence for many—evidenced by significant growth in the frequency of withdrawal of therapy as the mode of death within intensive care units. Although this is often based on principles of autonomy of choice—especially in relation to advance directives—these attitudes and practices are in themselves Western (and predominantly North American) in many respects, and as such may have their own ethnocentric bias that precludes translation to other countries and cultures.

Despite that caveat, the persistent loss of higher functions and the facility to communicate is often seen as an "existence without meaning," which begs the question as to whether the persistence equates to permanence. The irreversibility inherent within a diagnosis of brain death would offer some support of the concept, irrespective of concerns surrounding residual pituitary function. There are no credibly reported instances of recovery of correctly diagnosed brain death.[19]

Veatch has termed brain death in such circumstances as "the irreversible loss of that which is essentially significant to the nature of man,"[20] which in its simple brevity summates the concept, but frustrates on the details of what is truly significant in living, which may have answers that differ across different cultures.

In consequence, Truog and others have made the case that consequently death is now a social construct, with sufficient confusion about thresholds of irreversibility in either cardiocirculatory or neurologic death to frustrate exact biological definitions before decomposition.[21] He argues that society, rather than the medical profession, should determine what it means (and requires) to be considered alive and its converse.

However, varying statements have been made about the lay public's comprehension of what brain death truly means. There is increasing evidence that considerable confusion persists on the understanding of both the biology and legal status of brain death.[22]

Brain death is almost always an acute diagnosis; consequently, there is often some element of rejection of the diagnosis, as part of a denial mechanism inherent within grieving.[23]

Coupled with increasing use of the flawed medium of the Internet as an information source, the current skepticism of science and "known fact" serves to increase the burden of families in untangling misinformation from what is established and remains validated as physiologic fact. The earlier overstatement of the inevitability of physiologic collapse after brain death has not helped any premise of scientific authoritativeness, especially as families are often eager to seize on any uncertainty or discordant element to deny the consequences of devastating brain injury.

These individual family experiences may present as part of the public dialogue, but the fact remains any societal decision would be taken in abstract, which offers a considerable challenge in improving the contemporary publics education and understanding.

Legal Rationales Around Death

Most countries in the world have adopted neurologic criteria of death that allow removal of therapeutic care.[24] There is, however, some variation in the accommodations to be made for religious grounds—most notably in the United States where the state of New Jersey allows for the rejection of the diagnosis on religious grounds, whereas California and Illinois say that religious objections should be taken into account. Other states, such as Nevada, have reacted differently to challenges by strengthening use of neurologic criteria by explicit referral to the American Academy of Neurology guidelines as the standard by which brain death is diagnosed.[25]

Some commentators have noted that enduring concerns around the diagnosis of brain death are largely a North American problem, deriving from a more fundamental culturally based mistrust of the biological sciences among sections of the general public and their legislative representatives.[26]

Nevertheless, the persisting criticism within the United States has been sufficient to provoke consideration of revision of the UDDA—a process which is currently ongoing.[27] Although this may offer some more concrete legal support to the satisfaction of definitive criteria equating to death (as in Nevada), it also carries the risk of paradoxically increasing variability, if, for example, religious exceptions are introduced. This could lead to the same person being dead in one state and alive in another (as in the case of Jahi McMath who was declared dead in California, but considered alive within the state of New Jersey, when subsequently transferred there).

Truog has suggested that the apparent inconsistencies between biologic diagnoses and the UDDA be resolved with the adoption of brain death as a "legal fiction"—in other words an operative concept in law that need not directly relate to the biological facts.[28] While interesting, this suggestion has not gained much traction.

Ethical Reasoning Around Brain Death

One of the roles of Bioethics is to address conflict in a way that settles questions by what is right, moral, and agreed on. A moral space is a domain in which some number of people are addressing ethical questions and pursuing answers to immediate considerations. The clinical space around a neurologically deceased patient is almost always a moral space, as patients (through directives or remembered wishes), next of kin or legal representatives, and clinicians are dealing with a rare circumstance that is likely to be novel to many of the parties involved. This circumstance occupies a cognitive region that is at once highly technical and informed by moral considerations that may derive from an enormous spectrum of belief, education, and tradition.

In the absence of moral clarity or consensus, it is tempting and yet sometimes counterproductive to fall back solely on the application of protocols and policies, without consideration of the human being at the heart of the situation. It may be better to treat these processes as cognitive aides that allow one to develop a sufficient moral consensus with the other parties involved. A review of ethical principles can help develop the clinician's ability to understand the dimensions of the situation and navigate toward that consensus with those other parties.

Deontological analysis is complicated by varying perceptions of what is right, and to whom, as well as what is likely an evolving understanding of the physical reality of a clinical situation. For ease of argument at this point, we will suppose that the diagnosis of brain death has been made in a technically correct fashion. The perpetuation of care in such circumstances may be the impulse of the patient's family, in line with many belief structures that justify this from some irreducible right and wrong. The justification for continuing care, here, would be in the broad category of beneficence. Hope and belief does not restore the neurologic function of a loved one, though, and the result of this approach may be criticized in perpetuating false hope and failing non-maleficence. This hard bedside reality is likely to present a challenge to any untested belief structure, and the experience is undeniably intense for patient families who may experience the moral burden of their evolving understanding in complex ways. Little has been done to quantify or understand the *total summative* burden of grief and emotional consequences of such. Therefore from the family side, non-maleficence and beneficence are difficult to establish and may in fact vary over time.

The cultural considerations may be more evident in the pluralistic society of the United States but also serve to emphasize that although death is an ancient and familiar concept, brain death is relatively recent in historic terms and is very much a product of Western enlightenment thought as it developed through the prior two centuries. This cultural force can be considered a natural product of its place and time, but it has had cascading effects on how Western societies subsequently regard the existential question of being human and alive.

The dominant culture has many reasons to be invested in the concept of brain death as universal: a legally definable fact of nature and an objective point in an individual's life at which their rights and the rights of their representatives change with respect to the prerogatives of society at large. The confluence of this broad interest in the concept's existence and force, its deterministic origins in a narrow scientific discipline, the demonstrable fact of the misassumptions about its nature consequences, and its origin as a solution of necessity to the problem of resource limitation should give one pause in too rapidly navigating its specifics at the bedside—especially within a multicultural society, where deontological clarity may be less evident, and good faith not universally assumed.

At the same time, there are more moral agents in the room than just patient families. Physicians and nurses report moral distress as a consequence of continuing to deliver care to someone they understand to be dead. This has both direct and indirect consequences, the former to the individuals of the health care team, and the latter to the health care system in that moral distress is associated with burnout in both physicians and nurses,[29,30] which may impact the provision of care for others.

This aspect of social or distributive justice is the more utilitarian application of biomedical ethics and would certainly also be conflicted by the continued consumption of resources in perpetuating care indefinitely, as well as the frustration of access in areas where critical care is in high demand. It is important to point out that this was one of the initiating considerations of the Harvard Committee[7] and subsequently of the President's Commission.[8]

How should the medical practitioner proceed in such circumstances, when the underlying legitimacy of a brain death as a concept is in question by a patient's representatives? First, it is critically important to acquaint oneself with and understand legal statute in one's immediate vicinity in its effect on practice. Many consider that much of the initial rejection of brain death as a diagnosis is the rejection of the non-recovery of the patient. There are few instances where objections arise due to the goal of simple existence (with the previously noted caveats of culture and religion—especially non-western—offering some limitations to the breadth of that observation). In many ways, the problem is a consequence of a sophistication of technology that challenged the traditional perspectives on what death is and means.

At the same time, that rejection of irreversibility is interesting when innovations in cardiovascular technology have progressed to the point that as Racine says "...the irreversibility of the cessation of cardiocirculatory function is likely even more questionable than that of the brain."[26] An increasingly voiced concept informing such considerations is that of "all human death ultimately being brain death"—whether it is anoxic damage sustained from intracranial hypertension or the cessation of perfusion after cardiopulmonary arrest.[31]

Returning to the central issue of the patient, the narrative ethics approach offers some benefits in addressing the questions and conflicts arising from the diagnosis of brain death. Using techniques that have been identified as beneficial in palliative care, the family and possibly the carers are encouraged to tell their stories of the patient and in that way develop shared understanding of the patient's ideas and responses to life, its challenges, and its joys.[32] A critical component of this approach is that it does not attempt a reduction to values or virtues immediately, but it gives room to explore the lived experience of the moral agents involved. The narrative approach operates from the primacy of longitudinal experience, perspective, and developed understanding of the world as the basis by which diverse people approach decisions, action, and conflict resolution in the present, with a strong emphasis on the empathy required of the listeners. It is an ethics practice of mutual education and collaboration more than an ethics of deduction or elaboration of rules and tie-breakers. It asks the question "how did we get here?" as the prerequisite to answering and not simply begging the question "what do we do now?"[33]

A critical tool within the narrative ethical approach is the acknowledgment and critical analysis of master narratives. A master narrative is the name for a story or set of stories that reflect the underlying predominant belief structure as it pertains to a moral question—providing a thought template to approaching questions of morality that may be considered an archetype of a culture. They are a shared idea that provides an interpretive framework as well as instruction on one's interaction with the world at large, as experienced by one's fellows. People apply these master narratives frequently with varying levels of introspection and critical evaluation. This is appealing on face value, but master narratives are, by their nature, majoritarian, and in-group defining, and may consequently be difficult to challenge. Importantly, they may not represent the experience of racial or cultural minorities, and a technique to avoid majoritarian excess becomes mandatory. This tool in narrative ethics is the counternarrative or stories and story fragments that represent the experience of marginalized people subject to dominance or underrepresentation. We have found it productive to use the moral space around brain death as an opportunity to develop counternarratives in a place and time dedicated to that purpose. This has the potential to give some measure of justice to the people involved and can additionally be morally enriching for the clinician. This is additionally a way for patient families to expand their own thought structures in a way to accommodate the declaration of brain death in a way organic to their experience. An understanding of the master narrative is vital for both creating the protected space and time for developing and hearing out relevant counternarratives, as well as understanding the challenges in avoidance of manipulation while maintaining empathetic authenticity.[34]

The master narrative of brain death has penetrated the popular consciousness to such a degree that most families will arrive with some notion of what brain death is. Most will associate it with terminality and irreversibility. Many will associate it with a state of distaste or revulsion, or consider it a state against nature, to be hastened through en route to a state more consistent with visible deterioration of the body. Many will use the words "brain dead" to describe any state to which they ascribe these properties, though these might be states of severe or even modest disability, temporarily reduced consciousness, dementia, aphasia, developmental delay, or other neurologic impairment. It is not unheard of for clinicians to express themselves similarly. The master narrative has overwhelmingly set the scene around brain death as being one of negative experience, moral hazard, and nonspirituality. This is only partly mitigated by a master narrative on the value of organ donation.

A key challenge in these circumstances is that of not using the counternarrative to deny the reality of brain death and its irreversibility, but rather to listen to the story of this individual patient and understand the impact of this diagnosis on their family. This may aid in staging the progression of informing the family, with options to involve them in key clinical examination[35] or the inclusion of cultural mediators.[36] Ideally, the process is collaborative.

From any ethical perspective, the goal in such circumstances is to minimize unnecessary grief and suffering of families while remaining within the more broadly defined dictates of statute and societal necessity.

The Future and Implications

Capron described the determination of death as being "at once well settled and persistently unresolved."[37] As has been noted previously, there is ongoing discussion surrounding the legal definition of death amid possible changes to individual state legislation, as well as a revision of the UDDA. The religious and cultural questions surrounding the diagnosis of brain death are very much a product of their respective communities, and although global harmonization is a valid aspiration, the reality may be something else.

The impact on organ donation cannot be ignored in this analysis but should be considered in a secondary fashion to satisfy the ethical imperative of the dead donor rule. In other words, the question of death must be answered first and separately.

Some have advocated the abandonment of the diagnosis of brain death given the failure of exact agreement between biological and medicolegal criteria.[38] The consequences of rejecting the basis of brain death are not trivial, however, in considering the immediate harm to life and health in reducing an already limited pool of donated organs, with an anticipated increase in the number of patients dying while awaiting transplantation. The rejection of brain death would also seem to prohibit the ongoing adoption of the practice of normothermic regional perfusion, where after circulatory arrest has occurred and death is declared, circulatory perfusion is restored with extracorporeal support, with the active exception of the cerebral circulation which is clamped and divided before reperfusion. This essentially transforms the donor after circulatory death into the donor after brain death. An alternative proposal is the abandonment of the dead donor rule.[39] It seems unlikely that society is ready or willing to take that step, but that assumption remains unproven either way, at this point.

The abandonment of the diagnosis altogether seems unlikely, and perhaps, as Truog and others have suggested, the probable course may simply be that we continue with the status quo, using the current diagnosis and law, and dealing with the (relatively) infrequent problems on an individual basis.[40]

SUMMARY

We have discussed the biological premise for brain death with its psychosocial aspects and the critiques arising from apparent medicolegal inconsistencies. Much of the intolerance of the current state could conceivably be classed as arising more from academic circles, based on their rejection of "flawed thinking," rather than any apparently widespread rejection by the public overall—supporting what may be considered as the current social construct of "accidental pragmatism."[26]

As previously stated, a significant proportion of the immediate reaction to the diagnosis is a rejection of the removal of hope and as such, may be mitigated by thoughtful and compassionate communication over time, building trust in the intention and integrity of the team in their attention to appropriate detail and the validity of their conclusions.

What is certain amid the current uncertainty is that the discussion will continue to evolve, necessitating continued attention to that most basic of existential puzzles— "what makes me alive?"

CLINICS CARE POINTS

- The diagnosis of brain death originated conceptually in response to technological innovations within critical care, with concern for regulation of that resource as well as the developing field of organ transplantation.

- Definitions have centered on the loss of functions of the brain, with the majority of the world looking to the whole brain standard, although some focus on function of the brain stem. The former has complicated cases where residual pituitary function has persisted.

- Although diagnostic authority originally centered on the inevitability of systemic physiologic collapse, evolving experience has demonstrated does not always occur, particularly with pediatric patients.

- There are, however, no credibly reported instances of recovery of correctly diagnosed brain death.

- The ethical environment is complex, requiring careful consideration of beneficence and non-maleficence—especially with regard to the family left grieving—as well as social justice in the implications for health care resources (including organ transplantation).

- Those considerations should include appropriate recognition of cultural barriers and the necessity for extended communication strategies to maintain family inclusion amid diversity.

- Although relying on legal statute may satisfy the minimums, our duty of care to patients would argue for extending that care to their families, in compassionately communicating and collaborating in their education and acceptance of the finality of the diagnosis.

DISCLOSURE

Dr MJ Souter is Medical Director for LifeCenter Northwest, which provides salary support to the University of Washington. Dr Souter is a consultant for Teleflex Medical Inc.

REFERENCES

1. Wertheimer P, Jouvet M, Descotes J. [Diagnosis of death of the nervous system in comas with respiratory arrest treated by artificial respiration]. Presse Med 1959; 67(3):87–8. A propos du diagnostic de la mort du systeme nerveux dans les comas avec arret respiratoire traites par respiration artificielle.
2. Pius Xii Pope. The Prolongation of Life. The National Catholic Bioethics Quarterly 2009;9(2):327–32.
3. Kelly G. Preserving life. Linacre Q 1957;24(1):1.
4. Ayd FJ Jr. The hopeless case: medical and moral considerations. JAMA 1962; 181(13):1099–102.
5. Gilder SS. Twenty-second world medical assembly. Br Med J 1968;3(5616):493–4.
6. Machado C. The first organ transplant from a brain-dead donor. Neurology 2005; 64(11):1938–42.
7. A definition of irreversible coma. Report of the ad hoc committee of the harvard medical school to examine the definition of brain death. JAMA 1968;205(6): 337–40.
8. Defining Death: A Report on the Medical, Legal and Ethical Issues in the Determination of Death, 1981. United States: President's Commission for the Study of Ethical Problems in Medicine and Biomedical and Behavioral Research, 1981.
9. Barklin A. Systemic inflammation in the brain-dead organ donor. Acta Anaesthesiol Scand 2009;53(4):425–35.
10. Nair-Collins M, Miller FG. Current practice diagnosing brain death is not consistent with legal statutes requiring the absence of all brain function. J Intensive Care Med 2022;37(2):153–6.
11. Shemie SD, Wilson LC, Hornby L, et al. A brain-based definition of death and criteria for its determination after arrest of circulation or neurologic function in Canada: a 2023 clinical practice guideline. Can J Anaesth 2023;70(4):483–557.

Une définition cérébrale du décès et des critères pour sa détermination après l'arrêt de la circulation ou de la fonction neurologique au Canada : des lignes directrices de pratique clinique 2023.

12. Veatch RM. The impending collapse of the whole-brain definition of death. Hastings Cent Rep 1993;23(4):18–24.

13. Bernat JL. A defense of the whole-brain concept of death. Hastings Cent Rep 1998;28(2):14–23.

14. Mohandas A, Chou SN. Brain death. a clinical and pathological study. J Neurosurg 1971;35(2):211–8.

15. Pallis C. ABC of brain stem death. from brain death to brain stem death. Br Med J 1982;285(6353):1487–90.

16. Wijdicks EFM. The transatlantic divide over brain death determination and the debate. Brain 2011;135(4):1321–31.

17. Shewmon DA. Caution in the definition and diagnosis of infant brain death. In: Monagle JF, Thomasma DC, editors. Medical ethics: a guide for health professionals. Rockville, MD: Aspen Publishers; 1988. p. 38–57.

18. Falck DP. In re Quinlan: one court's answer to the problem of death with dignity. Wash Lee Law Rev. Winter 1977;34(1):285–308.

19. Wijdicks EF, Varelas PN, Gronseth GS, et al, American Academy of Neurology. Evidence-based guideline update: determining brain death in adults: report of the Quality Standards Subcommittee of the American Academy of Neurology. Neurology 2010;74(23):1911–8.

20. Veatch RM. The whole-brain-oriented concept of death: an outmoded philosophical formulation. J Thanatol 1975;3(1):13–30.

21. Truog RD. Commentary: defining death: definitions, criteria, and tests. Camb Q Healthc Ethics 2019;28(4):642–7.

22. Jones AH, Dizon ZB, October TW. Investigation of public perception of brain death using the internet. Chest 2018;154(2):286–92.

23. Truog RD, Morrison W, Kirschen M. What should we do when families refuse testing for brain death? AMA J Ethics 2020;22(12):E986–94.

24. Wahlster S, Wijdicks EF, Patel PV, et al. Brain death declaration: PRACTICES and perceptions worldwide. Neurology 2015;84(18):1870–9.

25. Biel S, Durrant J. Controversies in brain death declaration: legal and ethical implications in the ICU. Curr Treat Options Neurol 2020/03/18 2020;22(4):12.

26. Racine E. Revisiting the persisting tension between expert and lay views about brain death and death determination: a proposal inspired by pragmatism. J bioeth Inq 2015;12(4):623–31.

27. Lewis A, Bonnie RJ, Pope T, et al. Determination of death by neurologic criteria in the united states: the case for revising the uniform determination of death act. J Law Med Ethics 2019;47(4_suppl):9–24.

28. Truog RD, Miller FG. Changing the conversation about brain death. Am J Bioeth 2014;14(8):9–14.

29. Xue B, Wang S, Chen D, et al. Moral distress, psychological capital, and burnout in registered nurses. Nurs Ethics 2023;0(0). https://doi.org/10.1177/0969733023 1202233. 09697330231202233.

30. Dzeng E, Curtis JR. Understanding ethical climate, moral distress, and burnout: a novel tool and a conceptual framework. BMJ Qual Saf 2018;27(10):766–70.

31. Manara AR. All human death is brain death: the legacy of the Harvard criteria. Resuscitation 2019;138:210–2.

32. Brody H, Clark M. Narrative ethics: a narrative. Hastings Cent Rep 2014;44(s1):S7–11.

33. Lindemann H. Damaged identities, narrative repair. Ithaca: Cornell University Press; 2001.

34. Mitchell C. Qualms of a Believer in Narrative Ethics. Hastings Cent Rep 2014; 44(s1):S12–5.

35. Tawil I, Brown LH, Comfort D, et al. Family presence during brain death evaluation: a randomized controlled trial. Crit Care Med 2014;42(4):934–42.

36. Lele AV, Brooks A, Miyagawa LA, et al. Caseworker cultural mediator involvement in neurocritical care for patients and families with non-english language preference: a quality improvement project. Cureus 2023;15(4):e37687.

37. Capron AM. Brain death — well settled yet still unresolved. N Engl J Med 2001; 344(16):1244–6.

38. Truog RD. Is it time to abandon brain death? Hastings Cent Rep 1997;27(1):29–37.

39. Miller FG, Truog RD, Brock DW. The dead donor rule: can it withstand critical scrutiny? J Med Philos 2010;35(3):299–312.

40. Truog RD. The uncertain future of the determination of brain death. JAMA 2023; 329(12):971–2.

Ethics Consultation in Anesthesia Practice

Andrew P. Notarianni, MD

KEYWORDS

- Ethics in anesthesiology • Ethics in critical care • Ethics consultation
- Surgical ethics • Perioperative goals of care • Surgery at the end of life

KEY POINTS

- The anesthesiologist confronts several ethical challenging during the course of perioperative care, often having to address conflicts between ethical principles to determine the best clinical management.
- The ethics consultation can serve as a valuable supportive team in the perioperative setting when conflict arises.
- Modern anesthesia care has expanded greatly into the intensive care unit and into mechanical circulatory support, encountering special ethical challenges.
- Surgical care at the end of life may raise important ethical concerns regarding patient autonomy, capacity, and ongoing care in the face of medical futility.
- The anesthesiologist occupies a special space in patient allyship, providing a unique and valuable perspective into health and surgical disease in the perioperative setting.

INTRODUCTION

As the global population ages, patients present to the operating room and surgical intensive care unit (ICU) with more advanced medical and surgical disease.[1] Progress in surgical technique and medical therapy have lessened the physiologic burden of many surgeries and minimally invasive options, such as transcatheter valve replacement, and have substantially altered the risk calculus for procedural decision-making.[2] As clinical care has advanced, however, chronic medical illness remains prevalent and patients increasingly present for procedural and surgical intervention with life-limiting diagnoses and/or advanced care goals such as "do not resuscitate."[3–5] Anesthesiologists frequently find themselves at the crossroads of these mounting pressures, often without the benefit of establishing care with the patient until immediately preprocedure. As the boundaries and capabilities of anesthetic care and critical care anesthesiology expand so too do the specialty's needs for support in ethical decision-making.[3,6,7]

Department of Anesthesiology, Yale University School of Medicine, 333 Cedar Street, TMP 3, PO Box 208051, New Haven, CT 06520-8051, USA
E-mail address: Andrew.Notarianni@yale.edu

Anesthesiology Clin 42 (2024) 433–443
https://doi.org/10.1016/j.anclin.2024.01.001
1932-2275/24/© 2024 Elsevier Inc. All rights reserved.
anesthesiology.theclinics.com

Anesthesiologists play a vital role in protecting the patient's interests during the periprocedural period, especially during urgent or emergent situations. As Lewis and Yeldo point out, there are many pressures confronting the perioperative physician to "get the case done" and, in some cases, potentially compromise the best interests of the patient in doing so. These pressures may be a result of secondary gain in the form of case productivity on the part of the institution or surgical team or due to the lack of understanding on the part of other providers of the implications of comorbid medical disease on anesthetic management.[7]

To address some of these challenges, ethics consultation can be a valuable tool in decision-making in the perioperative setting. Unfortunately, given the time-sensitive nature of many of the most challenging ethical situations in the anesthesiology, it is critical that the anesthesiologist be familiar with the logistics of this process and be able to navigate the principles of medical ethics in the perioperative setting independently when needed. The anesthesiologist is able to provide a unique and valuable vantage to the patient in the surgical setting as an expert consultant, making critical recommendations in the evaluation of both the comorbid medical disease and anticipated perioperative management strategies. This counsel may greatly inform the independent patient's decision-making about their own care. The specialty's medical skill and expertise can thus help patients make better decisions for themselves by offering a fuller appreciation of the implications of pursuing (or foregoing) anesthesia and surgery and provide a deeper appreciation for procedural expectations than can either the surgical or medical teams alone.

Many situations encountered by the contemporary anesthesiologist, such as surgery at the end of life, advanced care wishes for limited intervention, and extracorporeal support modalities, highlight these concepts.[1] An understanding of the nature of the ethical consultation is helpful to the practicing anesthesiologist and some familiarity with the ethical underpinnings should be considered essential for the responsible care of these difficult cases.[8]

THE PERIOPERATIVE ETHICS CONSULTATION

The health-care ethics team exists to assist patients and their surrogates, and the health-care team, by serving as an authority on ethics to clarify morally ambiguous situations in health-care decision-making, provides an unbiased approach to ethical medical decision-making and resolves professional and patient conflict without resorting to the courts.[9–12] This service is an adjunct to the everyday ethical decision-making performed by health-care providers during the delivery of routine care.[12] The team is appointed by the health-care institution to address specific, nonroutine ethical concerns raised during the delivery of care.[11] The ethics consultation service consists of professionals with training and competencies in ethics that enable the team serve as an institutional authority in this domain.[12] Medical specialists frequently participate in these teams; however, the health-care ethics team will be expected to consult on clinical situations across many subspecialties and care areas. Therefore, specialized clinical training in the medical specialty requesting consultation cannot be considered an expectation. Much has been written regarding the models, structure, composition, and competencies necessary for a functional ethics consultation service.[9–12] A full review of these attributes is beyond the scope of this article. However, several key characteristics of these teams may have a major impact on anesthesiologists encountering ethical challenges in the perioperative setting.

When considering an institutional ethics consultation service from the vantage of anesthesiology, individual anesthesiologists and departments should ask themselves how well the institutional ethics team is aware of and can accommodate the unique demands of the perioperative setting. Three special areas of concern immediately arise: the need for advanced knowledge in a specialized care environment, accessibility, and time-sensitivity. The accessibility of the ethics team and how quickly it can assess a new concern will determine how well the team can evaluate and offer guidance on urgent or emergent cases. As perioperative ethical issues may present suddenly and with limited context, each department of anesthesiology is vulnerable to being underserved by the ethics team. This is recognized as a particular challenge and threat in rural and smaller sized institutions in which there are limited resources available to address complex ethical situations.[13] Smaller ethics teams or even individuals serving as the ethics consultation for select circumstances may be advantageous in this regard because they may be able to evaluate and "weigh in" more rapidly, even in urgent circumstances. Given the unique and specialized care delivered in anesthesiology, the time that a nonanesthesiologist provider will require to understand and process the immediate care needs or clinical questions unique to the perioperative setting further compounds the urgency around time sensitivity. Furthermore, the health-care ethics team may be limited in the information they receive before the patient arrives in the care of the anesthesiologist. For example, the surgical team may have limited insight into the ways in which a patient's medical disease will influence surgical course, and similarly, the medical team may not fully appreciate the full implications of surgical intervention. It has been noted that not all members of the ethics team need to be experts in the care area requesting the consultation[10] but they must have competency in the basic medical framework of the illness. Special experts in advanced knowledge domains, such as intraoperative care, surgical critical care, and extracorporeal mechanical support need not be standing members of the ethics team but should be available to the team to help process complex or subspecialty specific disease topics.[9,10]

Anesthesiology by its very nature is a multidisciplinary endeavor, interfacing with nearly the full breadth of clinical medicine and surgery. Given the knowledge gaps of medical and surgical team members in the perioperative arena and the growing role of the specialty in the management of critically ill patients and those requiring mechanical support, anesthesiology clearly has the potential to contribute much to the ethics consultation in the perioperative setting. It is clear that a clinical ethics team requires significant ongoing time and personnel investment. Staff members participating in ethics consultation must also take care to distinguish these efforts and separate them from any clinical role in the care of the patient, thus further straining the clinical care team in resource-limited settings.[11]

Despite these challenges in addressing the need for practitioners' knowledgeable about ethical issues, particularly in the perioperative and critical care settings, participation of anesthesiologists in the health-care ethics teams has the potential to address many of the most pressing ethical issues developing in the perioperative period. Because the anesthesiologist will be participating in the care of the patient, no additional time is required to understand the clinical circumstances and implications of anesthetic and surgical care. Accessibility is improved because there are existing relationships between members of the surgical and anesthesiology teams that facilitate communication and shared decision-making. Finally, anesthesiologists are trained in emergency care requiring rapid decision-making. Urgent clinical scenarios are frequently encountered and the need to reach a decision under time pressure is understood, helping the ethics team work on the timeline demanded by the clinical scenario. Given these advantages, each department of anesthesiology should carefully consider the benefits offered by departmental participation in the health-care ethics team with the associated costs of dedicating their own staff time to the requisite training and ongoing participation.

Ethics teams have been demonstrated to aid in resolving patient–provider conflict, interprofessional conflict, and in reducing nonbeneficial care, all of which would be of direct benefit to individual anesthesiologists, anesthesiology departments, and health-care institutions.[3,14] The discussion in later section will highlight special situations and circumstances in anesthesiology care that warrant special ethical consideration. The reader should rightly question how the ethical challenges in these areas could be better served with the active participation of anesthesiologists on the institutional ethics team and if the benefits of this participation are greater than the costs of participation. Anesthesiology departments should also consider how these potential benefits of minimizing unhelpful care, prolonged ICU stays, improved throughput, and improved conflict resolution grow the department's presences as a positive force within the larger institution.

THE CONTEXT OF ETHICS CONSULTATION IN ANESTHESIA PRACTICE

Many questions remain ill-defined in the role of the ethics consultation in anesthesiology and surgical practice. Few studies and explorations exist to detail the formal ethical consult in acute care anesthesiology. Further, there exists a general lack of insight into the understanding of what prompts ethics consultations in surgical populations and how they differ from medical populations.[14] To better define the context of the ethics consultation in surgery, Meredyth and colleagues examined a series of 548 consecutive ethics consultations at their own institution. Surgical patients were found to account for approximately 25% of the overall volume of ethics consultations. They found no statistically significant differences in demographic data across medical and surgical patients receiving a consultation. Surgical patients did have significantly longer lengths of stay, a slightly longer length of stay before consultation, a greater proportion of consultation requests from the ICU, and a significantly lower incidence of do not resuscitate (DNR) or do not intubate (DNI) code status.[14] Of interest, although not reaching statistical significance, there were trends regarding the indication for ethic consultation suggesting a greater frequency of consultation from surgical teams pertaining to concepts of futility and informed consent. Review of the surgical consultations suggested a recurrent theme of family requests for the termination of ongoing care that the surgical or intensive care team considered premature or ill-advised. The perceived, although not explicit, necessity of "buy-in" from the perspective of the surgeon or care team, regarding "routine" and "nonroutine" postoperative care for major procedural intervention in the medically vulnerable, was cited as significant and potentially informing factor. Moreover, worthy of note, "communication" was implicated in up to 40% of ethics consultations in perioperative setting, far greater than observed in the medical cohort.[14] This finding underscores the study's other findings and suggests that communication deficiencies drive provider–family discord disproportionately in the surgical setting. Resolving conflict through clear communication, a major strength of the ethics consultation, may therefore be a particularly helpful in this setting.

Perioperative Do Not Resuscitate Wishes

Another unique consideration in the perioperative setting concerns the implications of "do-not-resuscitate" and other advanced expressed desires that limit the provision of anesthetic care. Many elements of the periprocedural period set the anesthetic and surgical arenas apart from other care areas. The inherit potential of even the most "routine" anesthetic to lead to an acutely unstable clinical situation stands in contradistinction to the medical specialties, where most medical emergencies are precipitated by the underlying medical condition and not the active role of the practitioner. Not surprisingly then, caring for a patient with "do-not-resuscitate" orders can be quite uncomfortable for the responsible anesthesiologist and surgeon because a terminal event may be directly related to the active anesthetic care delivered, or the surgical procedure, rather than the underlying medical illness. In this situation, the options for the anesthesiologist's corrective action are limited.[15] At the same time, because anesthesia-related emergencies occur in a highly resourced and monitored setting, they are more often rapidly and fully reversible with standard anesthetic care—creating an ethical challenge when caring for a patient with a preexisting do not resuscitate order.[4,7,15]

The patient's surgical disease and anticipated perioperative course may greatly influence the procedural risk calculus, medical-surgical recommendations, and inform the perioperative code status discussions. For example, the presenting surgical illness may enjoy a favorable outlook with a relatively minor intervention. In this case, it may be appropriate for the anesthesiologist to council the patient to consider rescinding care directives such as "do-not-resuscitate" or "do-not-intubate" to allow for the necessary anesthetic care (such as intubation for general anesthesia) for a lesser magnitude, curative surgical procedure. Conversely, there may be situations in which the magnitude of surgical illness makes survival with an acceptable quality of life very unlikely even with timely surgical intervention. How then, do the anesthesiologist and the surgeon council the patient (or medical decision-maker) in the setting of uncertain outcome and even uncertain diagnosis, leading to the surgery? In these situations, can informed consent be a reasonable expectation and obtained at all if concrete expectations for perioperative course remain uncertain?[4,16]

It is widely agreed that shared decision-making should guide these clinical conversations[1,8,17] but as Schuijt details, shared decision-making exists on a spectrum between fully patient-driven decision-making and physician-driven decision-making.[17] Although decisions are infrequently made at either extreme of the spectrum, the balance of responsibility for individual medical decisions may skew significantly toward the patient or toward the physician in clinical cases. Similarly, in medically frail and older patients, understanding and insight into the nature of the injury may be impaired due to underlying cognitive decline or medical illness.[1] Focusing on goals of care and establishing them early on may be one of the most helpful tactics in these conversations and can inform both elective and urgent procedural decision-making.[17] This may also be helpful should an ethics consultation be sought later in the hospital course.[17] By establishing goals of care early in the encounter, the anesthesia and surgery teams can more effectively advocate for the best individual treatment plan and also develop preliminary contingency planning such as for the potential loss of capacity. Scenario planning may be very helpful in this setting, providing a "best-case, worse case" framework to guide these conversations, facilitating the further illumination of goals of care and informing planning for the end of life.[1,2,17]

At all times, the anesthesiologist should focus on improving the quality of care delivered in such circumstances of great vulnerability. It is critical that the anesthesiologist remain an active and out-spoken member of the perioperative care team to ensure the periprocedural care is delivered in accordance with the patient's own wishes and with respect their person.[7,18]

Ethics Consultation in Intensive Care in Practice

An increasing number of anesthesiologists now serve at least a part of their clinical time in the ICU. Given the nature of the conflicts at the end of life and the high-acuity of acute care surgery, it may not be surprising that three-quarters of all ethics consults for surgical patients may originate in the ICU.[14] Unfortunately, despite this disproportionate need, work remains to be done in determining the best use of the ethics consultation in the ICU.

New insights into strategies to facilitate and extend the role of the ethics consultation in intensive care are likely to be helpful. A better understanding of the optimal timing of consultation may also provide benefit with some small studies suggesting a benefit for early engagement.[19,20] Many approaches have been proposed and used such as the institutional prereview and examination of common perioperative ethical challenges.[21] Commonly cited challenges include limited capacity for decision-making, consent under duress or pain, surgical futility, and the lack of assent of a patient with limited formal decision-making capacity to an appointed decision-maker's procedural choices.[5,22,23] In addition, participation of family members and others in these difficult discussions can have an impact on patient and/or surrogate decision-making. Proposed strategies recommended for ethics experts to address these issues away from the bedside may include educational sessions or discussions with staff, clarification regarding specific topics relevant to the institution and clinical unit through the preemptive distribution of information and literature, and the development of institutional policy.[21] When posed with a clinical case presenting ethical concerns, the ethics team is well equipped to assist the ICU team in many ways including analysis of the problem, mediation of conflict, and facilitation of understanding. Not infrequently, the clinical and ethical needs of the patient, family, and medical team my shift over the course of the consultation as the medical or surgical course evolves.[21] The ethics team can also provide significant benefit to the care team by leading or facilitating retrospective case reviews to aid in guiding future care when encountering a new clinical challenge institutionally, as was demonstrated dramatically during the recent coronavirus pandemic.[21] Finally, a major recurring theme in the literature is the value of the ethics team in helping to push shared decision-making to the forefront of the care team's mind and strengthen the alignment of the medical or surgical therapy with the patient's own goals of care. This has been demonstrated consistently in those studies reviewing interviews of the care team and patient families.[1,5,20]

One very important area of active study is whether the ethics consultation can actually affect the care itself delivered in the ICU, rather than just mediate in times of conflict. In a small, randomized trial Schneiderman and colleagues sought to investigate whether ethics consultations in the ICU could reduce nonbeneficial treatments received by patients. They defined nonbeneficial treatment as treatment or time in the ICU delivered to patients that do not survive to hospital discharge. They also asked, "do patients, families, and health-care workers feel that the ethics consultation was helpful?" Although only 70 patients were enrolled there were statistically significant differences observed in ICU days, artificial nutrition, and days on the ventilator. Analysis of family members' responses to the ethics consult revealed favorable attitudes toward the consultation with greater than 70% positive responses in all domains with family members describing the consult as "helpful," "educational," "fair," and "supportive." Interestingly, but perhaps not surprisingly, 40% of respondents reported "strongly agree" when asked if the process was stressful, although 75% reported they would seek an ethics consultation again if in similar circumstances in the future. Health-care workers also reported favorable responses toward the consultation with 87% reporting they would seek an ethics consultation again in similar circumstances and 98% reporting that they would recommend the consultation to others.[24]

Lessons learned during the coronavirus pandemic regarding uncertainty of care and futility brought the ethics consultation into new light for many ICUs.[25] As more institutions realize the inherit value of and gain experience with the ethics consultation in intensive care, interest in greater and earlier participation in this care area is likely to increase.[26]

Special Topic: Mechanical Circulatory Support

Because anesthesiology expands past the traditional bounds of the operating room into new high-acuity settings such as critical care, serious new ethical challenges are frequently encountered. Anesthesiology participation in those units extending mechanical circulatory support (MCS) deserves special mention. Perhaps, no unit more frequently encounters the need for ethics consultation on a case-per-case basis than these cardiothoracic and medical ICUs where anesthesiologist intensivists have become integral members of the MCS team determining candidacy, participating in cannulation, and supporting day-to-day management. Extracorporeal support (extracorporeal membrane oxygenation [ECMO]) represents an extraordinary and often underappreciated broad spectrum of situations where bodily survival is most often wholly dependent on the extracorporeal device. Although the ECMO circuit is supportive, it is not curative. Physiologic recovery or bridge to durable therapy (such as transplantation or permanent ventricular assist device) is requisite for survival. Because of the constant, extreme threat to life and uncertainty of both the outcome and the timeline until the outcome becomes clear, these increasingly used modalities are worthy of special support and consideration from the healthcare ethics team.

When the option for ECMO is presented, the patient, or more often the surrogate decision-maker, is often faced with a choice to pursue highly intensive life-sustaining ECMO support, continue maximal medical therapy, or transition goals of care to comfort. This decision-making can also be very complex for the medical care team because the optimal implementation for ECMO and the specific patient populations that stand to benefit from it are still being elucidated.[27] Age, medical comorbidity, and, perhaps most importantly, an identified and reversible insult play major roles in anticipated outcome in ECMO.[28] Unfortunately, even with the aid of risk calculators, predicting survival is difficult and outcomes data remain extremely dynamic in contemporary practice. Rapid advancement in techniques and expansion of ECMO-capable centers will continue to make it difficult to set expectations for outcomes.[20] Additionally, patients and/or decision-makers are often presented with ECMO as an option only when survival with maximal medical therapy alone seems extremely unlikely and ECMO is "the only chance" for hope of recovery. Presented with such a "choice," it is fair to question whether true and uncoerced decision-making can occur in this situation.[29]

Peetz and colleagues have recently reviewed the challenges of informed consent in the setting of extracorporeal support, illuminating several critical issues. These include the entrustment of care to the "judgment" of "expert" care team members, time pressure due to the nature of the emergency where delay may rightly be expected to eliminate hope for survival, therapeutic misconception regarding the goals or capabilities of ECMO (life-sustaining vs curative), complexity of decision-making, and lack of information to guide decision-making given the current uncertainty of outcomes in extracorporeal support.[16] A final but no less-consequential consideration is that most patients requiring ECMO are too sick to provide consent to therapy directly; surrogate decision-makers are frequently called on to help guide medical decision-making, often under extreme duress.[27] In light of the complexity of this highly intensive care, it can be nearly impossible for even the closest surrogate decision-maker to anticipate any individual patient's wishes or, in many cases, represent the patient's perspective rather than their own when confronted with life-death decisions. It is likely that even patients with capacity cannot be expected to fully grasp the consequence of decision-making under these conditions as has been demonstrated in other vulnerable groups.[30]

Many strategies have been proposed and implemented to aid families and care teams in medical decision-making for ECMO patients. One such effort used by centers extending extracorporeal support has been the automatic consultation of the palliative care team and/or an automatic ethics consultation on cannulation. Wirpsa studied just such a protocol in their institution and thoroughly investigated the impact of the ethics consultation in a series of 68 patients.[20] In addition to investigating patient outcomes, they subdivided the ethical concerns across extracorporeal support runs and closely analyzed interviews the medical staff caring for these patients. A standard consultation template was devised with close records kept of the reason for consult, clinical narrative, ethical analysis, and recommendations in each case. Interviews were conducted with members of the care team including physicians, fellows, advanced practice providers, and nurses at the conclusion of the study period. Interview topics included the nature of the conflicts leading to consultation, usefulness, and impact of the ethics consultation.

In this study, all 20 members of the care team considered the protocol a positive intervention. Two significant benefits noted by these team members were the involvement of the ethics team before it became clear that hope of recovery had been lost and that the involvement of the ethics team was "no longer seen as a failure."[20] One other interesting strategy used in this study was to rate the patient's decision-maker at the beginning of the consultation on a 5-point scale regarding their understanding of and insight into their own ethical role, their partnership role in shared decision-making with the health-care team, and ECMO as a time-limited trial. Patient decision-makers scoring 4 to 5 on this scale were deemed to have a high level of insight and understanding into the clinical situation. They represented more than half of the cases of consultation. Although this study was limited in scope, it adds to a body of literature supporting a greater, integrated role of ethics specialists in these complex patients.[19,27]

The coronavirus proved a major accelerant to the wider adoption of ECMO. No longer limited to major referral centers, previously concentrating experience and resource, the major ethical challenges posed by ECMO can now be expected in smaller, less-experienced centers.[31] Given the large investment in launching these programs, it is unlikely that institutions new to ECMO support will discontinue their programs, and the roles of the ethics team will likely see continued expansion in ECMO programs large and small due to these inherit challenges with the modality.

SUMMARY

The health-care ethics team can play a vital role in mediating conflict in the periprocedural period. As anesthesiology expands beyond the classic bounds of the operating room, new ethical challenges are encountered. The unique role, insight, and training of the anesthesiologist allows for a holistic evaluation of and special allyship with the surgical patient that can greatly inform shared decision-making. An understanding of the role and utility of the ethics consult in anesthesia care during times of moral or ethical conflict can be of great help mediating conflict in this inherently interdisciplinary space. Future expansion of anesthesiology presence on institutional health-care ethics teams has the potential to improve these critical efforts by providing expert insight into these highly complex clinical areas.

CLINICS CARE POINTS

- The health-care ethics team exists to assist patients and their surrogates, and the health-care team, by serving as an authority on ethics to clarify morally ambiguous situations in health care decision-making, provides an unbiased approach to ethical medical decision-making and resolves professional and patient conflict.

- Ethics consultations for surgical patients are more likely to be requested in the intensive care setting. Length of stay seems longer and the incidence of DNR or DNI status seems lower than medical patients receiving ethics consultation. Demographics do not seem to differ from medical patients.

- The surgical intensive care setting has a relatively high utilization of ethics consultation. There is evidence to suggest the engagement of the ethics team can significantly alter nonbeneficial care in this setting, decreasing the length of stay and days on the ventilator in this setting.

- Extracorporeal mechanical support utilization is rapidly expanding but presents many challenges to traditional concepts of informed consent, resource utilization, and futility. Early or automatic involvement of the ethics team has been helpful in small studies and may have the potential to mitigate these ethical concerns.

DISCLOSURE

Dr A.P. Notarianni reports no relevant commercial or financial disclosures relevant to the topic.

REFERENCES

1. Jablonski SG, Urman RD. The Growing Challenge of the Older Surgical Population. Anesthesiol Clin 2019;37(3):401–9.
2. Saeed S, Skaar E, Romarheim A, et al. Shared Decision-Making and Patient-Reported Outcome Measures in Valvular Heart Disease. Front Cardiovasc Med 2022;9:863040.
3. Aulisio MP, Chaitin E, Arnold RM. Ethics and palliative care consultation in the intensive care unit. Crit Care Clin 2004;20(3):505–23, x-xi.
4. Sumrall WD, Mahanna E, Sabharwal V, et al. Do Not Resuscitate, Anesthesia, and Perioperative Care: A Not So Clear Order. Ochsner J. Summer 2016;16(2):176–9.
5. Kalra A, Forman DE, Goodlin SJ. Medical decision making for older adults: an international perspective comparing the United States and India. J Geriatr Cardiol 2015;12(4):329–34.
6. Schmitz D, Duewell M. Ethics Consultation-A Blind Spot of Philosophy in Bioethics? Am J Bioeth 2022;22(12):47–8.
7. Lewis MC, Yeldo NS. The Ethics of Surgery at End of Life. Anesthesiol Clin 2019;37(3):561–71.
8. Williams SP, Howe CL. Advance directives in the perioperative setting: Managing ethical and legal issues when patient rights and perceived obligations of the healthcare provider conflict. J Healthc Risk Manag 2013;32(4):35–42.
9. Tarzian AJ, Asbh Core Competencies Update Task F. Health care ethics consultation: an update on core competencies and emerging standards from the

American Society For Bioethics and Humanities' core competencies update task force. Am J Bioeth 2013;13(2):3–13.

10. Aulisio MP, Arnold RM, Youngner SJ. Health care ethics consultation: nature, goals, and competencies. A position paper from the Society for Health and Human Values-Society for Bioethics Consultation Task Force on Standards for Bioethics Consultation. Ann Intern Med 2000;133(1):59–69.

11. ASf Bioethics, Humanities. Improving competencies in clinical ethics consultation: an education guide. Chicago, IL: American Society for Bioethics & Humanities; 2012.

12. American Society for B, Humanities, Arnold RM, et al. Core competencies for healthcare ethics consultation. 2nd edition. Chicago, IL: American Society for Bioethics and Humanities; 2011. p. 60, iii.

13. Nelson WA, Rosenberg MC, Mackenzie T, et al. The presence of ethics programs in critical access hospitals. HEC Forum 2010;22(4):267–74.

14. Meredyth NA, Fins JJ, de Melo-Martin I. Ethics Consultation in Surgical Specialties. HEC Forum 2022;34(1):89–102.

15. Truog RD. "Do-not-resuscitate" orders during anesthesia and surgery. Anesthesiology 1991;74(3):606–8.

16. Peetz AB, Sadovnikoff N, O'Connor MF. Is informed consent for extracorporeal life support even possible? AMA J Ethics 2015;17(3):236–42.

17. Schuijt HJ, DPJ Smeeing, Verberne WR, et al. Perspective; recommendations for improved patient participation in decision-making for geriatric patients in acute surgical settings. Injury 2023;54(10):110823.

18. Mohr M. [Ethical conflicts during anesthesia. "Do not resuscitate" orders in the operating room]. Anaesthesist 1997;46(4):267–74. Ethische Konflikte wahrend der Anasthesie. "Do not resuscitate"–Verfugungen im Operationssaal.

19. Massutta D. Moral Distress, Ethical Environment, and the Embedded Ethicist. J Clin Ethics. Winter 2017;28(4):318–24.

20. Wirpsa MJ, Carabini LM, Neely KJ, et al. Mitigating ethical conflict and moral distress in the care of patients on ECMO: impact of an automatic ethics consultation protocol. J Med Ethics 2021. https://doi.org/10.1136/medethics-2020-106881.

21. Picozzi M, Gasparetto A. Clinical ethics consultation in the intensive care unit. Minerva Anestesiol 2020;86(6):670–7.

22. Wada K, Charland LC, Bellingham G. Can women in labor give informed consent to epidural analgesia? Bioethics 2019;33(4):475–86.

23. Ryan GL, Brandi K, Ethics C. Informed Consent and Shared Decision Making in Obstetrics and Gynecology. Obstet Gynecol 2021;137(2):E34–41.

24. Schneiderman LJ, Gilmer T, Teetzel HD. Impact of ethics consultations in the intensive care setting: a randomized, controlled trial. Crit Care Med 2000;28(12):3920–4.

25. Writing Committee for the R-CAPI, Higgins AM, Berry LR, et al. Long-term (180-Day) Outcomes in Critically Ill Patients With COVID-19 in the REMAP-CAP Randomized Clinical Trial. JAMA 2023;329(1):39–51.

26. Guidry-Grimes L, Warren M, Lipman HI, et al. Clarifying a Clinical Ethics Service's Value, the Visible and the Hidden. J Clin Ethics. Fall 2019;30(3):251–61.

27. Abrams D, Curtis JR, Prager KM, et al. Ethical Considerations for Mechanical Support. Anesthesiol Clin 2019;37(4):661–73.

28. Patel B, Davis RP, Saatee S. Mechanical Circulatory Support Devices in the Elderly. Anesthesiol Clin 2023;41(3):583–94.

29. Henry B, Verbeek PR, Cheskes S. Extracorporeal cardiopulmonary resuscitation in out-of-hospital cardiac arrest: Ethical considerations. Resuscitation 2019; 137:1–6.
30. Sudore RL, Landefeld CS, Williams BA, et al. Use of a modified informed consent process among vulnerable patients: a descriptive study. J Gen Intern Med 2006; 21(8):867–73.
31. Supady A, Combes A, Barbaro RP, et al. Respiratory indications for ECMO: focus on COVID-19. Intensive Care Med 2022;48(10):1326–37.

Public Good versus Private "Goods"

Ethical Implications of Drug Shortages on Anesthesiology Practice

Joel B. Zivot, MD, FRCP(C), MA, JM*

KEYWORDS

- Anesthesiology • Drug shortages • Bioethics • Rationing • Market failure
- Monopsony

KEY POINTS

- Drug shortages are common and impact anesthesiology.
- Attempts at ethical rationing represent a short-term fix but fail to address the underlying problems.
- Market failures in drug manufacturing are largely the root cause of drug shortages.

INTRODUCTION

The practice of medicine is a complex and ethical endeavor. Medical providers are committed to important and enduring values shared by our culture. Safe and reliable medical practice depends on reliable medical technology and the unfettered supply of needed supplies, equipment, and pharmaceuticals. Over the past few years, the availability of drugs critical to clinical practice has become an increasing challenge that impacts all aspects of the health care system with significant implications specific to the safe practice of anesthesia. Despite the general consensus that drug access is critical to the practice of anesthesia, it has been claimed that the problem of drug shortages is just too complex and multifactorial to understand or manage; in addition, and somewhat surprisingly disagreements about the definition of drug shortages continue and undermine attempts to address them.[1] While drug shortages have become the "new normal" it is better acknowledged as the normalization of deviance. Drug shortages are, in fact, solvable and are the direct result of a market failure[2] that resulted from many factors, including production problems, lack of production of low-cost drugs

Emory University School of Medicine, Emory Center for Ethics, Emory University, 200 Dowman Drive, Atlanta, GA 30322, USA
* Emory University Hospital, Department of Anesthesiology, 1364 Clifton Road, Atlanta, GA 30322.
E-mail address: jzivot@emory.edu

Anesthesiology Clin 42 (2024) 445–455
https://doi.org/10.1016/j.anclin.2023.12.001
1932-2275/24/© 2023 Elsevier Inc. All rights reserved.
anesthesiology.theclinics.com

in favor of high-priced proprietary drugs as well as industry changes including a contraction in the number of brand-named drug manufacturers and expansion of generic manufacturers of variable quality products. Contraction of the drug vendor supply has resulted in a corresponding shrinking of the manufacturing supply chain. When shortages occur because of production challenges, other manufacturers are unable to rapidly enter the market. The complexity and needed regulation of drug manufacturing blocks upward supply flexibility and in the worst-case scenario, the drug is simply not available at any price. A traditional bioethical approach to this problem has stemmed from an acceptance of drug shortages as the new reality. In some cases, less effective alternative drugs are used and, more importantly, implementation of rationing strategies.[3] Such a strategy is harmful to the common good and grants a needless pass to the underlying problem. Anesthesiology practice relies heavily on sterile injectable drugs, a critical component of the drug supply. An absence of these medications results in direct harm to both individual patients and the population and as such, constitutes a major medical ethical transgression, possible legal liability, and a public health emergency. The reality of drug shortages requires action. Ethical imperatives guide our actions toward understanding and rectifying the underlying cause.

THE NATURE OF ETHICS AND THE STRUCTURE OF ETHICAL ADJUDICATION

To understand how bioethics can help address how we effectively approach drug shortages and their impact on clinical practice, it is first necessary to understand the nature of ethical reasoning and the background and structure of ethical adjudication. Ethics is a philosophic study of morality[4] and can be described broadly as serving 2 purposes. First, its purpose is to justify and define moral obligations—what is morally wrong and what is morally right. Second, its purpose is to resolve particular moral problems, for example, under what circumstance is abortion morally justified? It must be stated that ethics is not a set of puritanical prohibitions preventing medical progress. Additionally, ethics and bioethics are not something intelligible only in the context of religion. The intersection of religion and medical practice is a subject all of its own. Ethics can work independently of religious belief. Bioethics is the branch of ethics that pertains to biomedical practice.

As we consider both the implications of drug shortages and how to address their impact in the clinical setting, it is helpful to review what role and value bioethics has on decision-making. Bioethics is a set of principles, both durable and modifiable. Some details of conduct will change, but the broad moral principles of medical practice endure. Public opinion will naturally evolve commensurate with the evolution and maturation of civil society. Bioethics tracks this to an extent, but some popular public ideas may still lie outside of bioethical medical practice. While bioethics is a practice concerned with ethical dilemmas around medical care, bioethics itself is not a profession, but provides important underlying principles upon which providers can effectively address challenging issues and situations arising in clinical practice. The Joint Commission on Accreditation of Health care Organizations requires hospitals to have a mechanism for adjudicating ethical issues involving patient care. It recommends creating a multidisciplinary ethics committee.[5] One does not need a license to practice bioethics or participate in determining how to address ethical challenges. Hospital ethics committees are generally populated by individuals of various backgrounds and various skills, including, but not limited to those with formal ethics training, but also relevant clinicians with broad experiences forming the foundation to address difficuilt issues. While these discussions by a hospital ethics committee can be very helpful in clarifying the ethical dilemmsa and providing advice and support, the ethics committee does not offer binding arbitration which represents an alternative method dispute resolution.[6] Conflicts at the bedside are not uncommon, but, in many situations, participation by a skilled adjudicator is more appropriate and effective than requesting an ethics committee reconcile differences of opinion. This is not to dismiss the value of bioethics and ethics committees, but unreasonable expectations on the authority and purpose of an ethics committee diminish the true benefit of bioethical thought. Bioethical reasoning is meant to be carried inside the practitioner and serve as a constant filter through which all medical acts must pass. The bioethical physician has an imperative to turn knowledge into individual action and, when necessary, broad policy.

DEONTOLOGY AND UTILITARIANISM

One way of dividing bioethical reasoning is to consider 2 schools of thought. On one hand, bioethics is considered under a system of rules. In this model, if a rule is broken, a bioethical violation has occurred. This idea is referred to as deontology and was first proposed by Immanuel Kant.[7] Every medical student learns the 4 rules promulgated by Beecham and Childress.[8] They are as follows

1. Do no harm (non-maleficence)
2. Do good (beneficence)
3. Autonomy
4. Social justice, distributive justice, (rationing)

It is noteworthy that rule #1 cautions against harm. The job of medicine is undoubtedly dangerous and dangerous practice is not only the result of technical shortcomings but also can occur from bioethical transgression. The problem of any rule-based system is the discovery of exceptions to rules, generally solved by writing more and more specific rules, or by ranking rules by some hierarchy. Detractors would say life and death decision making is too complex to be governed simply by written rules. Detractors will further argue that rule-based advocates are not realists and deontology is best left to the classroom and not the bedside.[9]

The other broad approach to ethics and the answer to the complexities of practice that make rules hard to apply is the concept known as "consequentialism." The best-known example of this is utilitarianism, proposed by JSMill and Jeremy Bentham. The classic utilitarian regards an action as right if it produces an increase in the average overall happiness of everyone affected and any alternative action is wrong if it does not. Utilitarianism has many advantages to medical decision-making. Utilitarianism has some serious shortcomings, however. Utilitarianism places no limits on the extent to which society may legitimately interfere with a person's liberties, provided overall average happiness is achieved. It is important to also recognize that a utilitarian approach to the idea of settling on the lesser of 2 evils still produces an evil result.[10]

As a practical approach, the combination of these 2 broad ideas might serve as the most effective way to navigate the daily work. It is also fair to acknowledge that what also concerns clinicians is what sort of decision-making will mitigate most strongly against legal risk. An understanding of criminal and civil wrongs is also worth a separate examination but beyond the scope of this article. Bioethical medical practice, born out of this discussion, will greatly reduce one's legal risk against negligence.[11]

ETHICAL RATIONING

Now that a background in bioethical discourse is established, it is possible to address more specifically the intersectional conflict between drug shortages and bioethics.

Rationing in a well-resourced western medical system is almost always the result of poor management decisions, or as an alternative, the result of priority setting strategies that focus on potentially arbitrary ranking of health care choices.[12] It is not the consequence of a truly depleted resource despite careful advanced planning and responsible resource stewardship. In the recent coronavirus disease (COVID) epidemic, rationing of mechanical ventilators became a widely considered policy.[13] Deeper analysis found that resource shortages could have been anticipated at early epidemic stages[14] and a rationing model that sought to remove mechanical ventilators from patients based on age or other factors, despite patient protestation, was ultimately unethical and legally unsupportable and very likely, unnecessary.[15] Designing an ethical rationing system when the underlying cause for drug shortages is known and fixable risks providing ethical cover for a broken and corrupted drug supply system. Though anesthesiologists widely acknowledge the presence of drug shortages, very few are willing to state that a patient under their care was directly harmed because of shortages. Any ethical rationing system must also inform patients in advance of procedures that some substitutions might occur because of shortages. For any patient to consent to treatment decisions, they must have all the needed facts. Practically, drug substitution at the bedside because of shortages proceeds on a more *ad hoc* basis. The ethical anesthesiologist would not knowingly put a patient at risk, even when shortages exist. Hospitals will scramble to search for other drug sources and OR pharmacy and bedside compounding may be implemented to stretch exisiting supply. Neither hospitals nor clinicians will consider withholding clinical services in spite of the drug limitations. They will and do identify alternatives, some of which impact management, but in most cases will do whatever is necessary to continue to provide safe care despite the shortages. From a utilitarian perspective, the greatest good favors making the best out of a difficult situation and continuing to provide care, but other mitigation strategies may also be considered.[16]

HOW DO DRUG SHORTAGES IMPACT HEALTH CARE AS A RIGHT RATHER THAN A PRIVILEGE?

Access to pharmaceuticals remains at the core of health care delivery. Drug shortages might violate a duty to deliver health care if we consider health care a right. The proper bioethical response to drug shortages requires an understanding of the structure of health care delivery to engage the rights/privilege question. The United States continues to struggle with the implementation of universal government run health care for all citizens. If health care is a right, then a corollary duty must exist to deliver that right. A 2022 Gallup Poll[17] found that 57% of Americans support universal government run health care but Americans continue to be divided sharply along party lines. Poling results found that 88% of Democrats, 59% of independents, and just 28% of Republicans think the government is responsible for health care delivery. This partisan view has been relatively stable for the last 2 decades. The US Supreme Court upheld the constitutionality of the Affordable Care Act (ACA)[18] reflecting the majority view on government health care coverage. The ACA contained provisions to make health care insurance coverage more affordable through subsidies and cost-sharing reductions based on income. The ACA also contains an individual mandate on the part of the citizen to purchase health insurance. Non-compliance was to be punishable by an internal revenue service (IRS) tax. The constitutionality of the individual mandate tax punishment was challenged, and the issue was ultimately resolved by leaving the individual mandate in place but imposing no IRS fine for non-compliance.[19] To a degree, this may be seen as a step forward in that health insurance was not available to many individuals prior to this act and the overall percentage of Americans with health insurance did rise slightly. From a cost perspective, the theory behind the individual mandate was to compel healthy people to buy insurance thereby capitalizing the market to cover the costs of caring for the sick. Requiring the purchase of health insurance is not the same as receiving health care and 7% of Americans remain uninsured.[20] This corresponds to 25 million citizens without health insurance.

DRUG SHORTAGES—PUBLIC GOODS AND PRIVATE GOODS

Reliable health care requires a reliable pharmaceutical supply. In economics, a pharmaceutical is a good. Goods are items that satisfy human wants, provide utility or usefulness, and in certain categories have limited availability. An economic good must also be capable of being transferred from one person to another or produced and consumed. Economic theory divides goods into 4 types based on excludability and rivalrousness. The 4 categories of goods are public, private, common resources, and club goods. For the purposes of discussion, we can focus on the difference between a public and a private good. A private good belongs to someone and the use of that good makes it unavailable to others. As an example, consider something desirable but in limited supply, like a car. A public good on the other hand is something that everyone can access. No one's individual use interferes with anyone else's capacity for use. Consider as an example, the air or a lighthouse or national defense. Public goods can become rivalrous and excludable when the demand because extremely high but under normal usage, public goods are accessible and useable by anyone.

If health care is a right, we aspire to provide it as a public good. If health care is a public good, pharmaceuticals are also public goods. With respect to a duty to deliver health care, federal law has existed since 1986 with the passage of the unfunded mandate of The Federal Emergency Medical Treatment and Labor Act (EMTALA).[21] This act requires any hospital that participates in Medicare to evaluate and stabilize any emergency medical condition of any individual that presents to the emergency room of that hospital, irrespective of their capacity to pay. In effect, EMTALA establishes a standard of care and the medical practice at the bedside must comport with this standard. In the setting of drug shortages, it may not be possible to deliver the proper standard of treatment making it impossible to follow federal law. A physician on duty in a hospital emergency room must deliver health care in the prevailing standard. Drug companies, purchasing groups, and wholesalers enter the drug production and delivery market voluntarily. Entry into the market does not carry a fiduciary obligation to supply all necessary medication without disruption apart from what might be in place in a contract between supplier and customer. Nevertheless, it may be stated that a stable and reliable drug supply is a public good.[22] In this regard, drugs should be manufactured even in the circumstance that a manufacturer leaves the market for reasons of a negative return on investment. If drugs are a public good, no reasonable barrier should exist on the part of any manufacturer wishing to enter the market to maintain drug supply.

MARKET INCENTIVES SHOULD DRIVE IN THE DIRECTION OF ROBUST SUPPLY (IMPACT OF ANTI-KICKBACK LEGISLATION)

In 1972, the US congress passed the first anti-kickback provision, 42 U.S.C. §1320a-7b, in the Social Securities Act of 1935. The purpose of this provision was to ban certain activities in the practice of medicine that would drive up the costs of federal payments through Medicare reimbursement. Prior to this provision, physicians were financially incentivized toward activities that were not necessarily in the interest of patients. The language of the provision specifically forbids kickbacks, bribes, or rebates, in the form of remuneration, in cash or in kind, in exchange for patient, product, or service referrals. From the perspective of the Federal Government, the likely intent was to control cost that appeared to have no natural control. From the perspective of duty-based ethics of Immanuel Kant,[23] in the absence of the anti-kickback rule, physicians might otherwise treat patients as a means to a financial end.

It is from a consequentialist or utilitarian perspective that concern was raised over the federal anti-kickback provision. In 1987, The Medicare and Medicaid Patient and Program Protection Act[24] was passed in response to industry confusion and uncertainty regarding the application of the statute. This act united the separate Medicare and Medicaid Anti-Kickback statutes into a single statute, created an intermediate sanction-program exclusion, and directed the United States Department of Health and Human Services to develop "safe harbors" (42 CFR § 1001.952) for certain payments and business practices that might otherwise violate the statute but should be permitted for the greater good with respect to health care. Within the list of safe harbors, Group Purchasing Organizations (GPOs) warrant special consideration.

GPOs are the purchasing arms of a group of businesses, in this case hospitals, that have joined together to create leverage in buying because of representing a portion of the market sufficient to warrant such leverage. Initially, GPOs served a valuable purpose by creating advantageous price contracting that might be otherwise not obtainable by individual hospitals. These purchasing entities were initially funded by hospitals and therefore were not in conflict with the anti-kickback statute. Through congressional lobbying, GPOs made the case that their fee should be collected directly from the vendor. The argument was made that this would allow smaller hospitals without the capital on hand to pay the GPO fee and presumably expand to provide service for the benefit of patients. Further, if GPOs collect fees directly from vendors, hospitals will have less incentive to join forces and form large anti-competitive organizations. It is unclear how much competition improves health care delivery from the patient's point of view. Nevertheless, GPO fee collection directly from the vendor would conflict with the anti-kickback statute in the absence of the safe harbor exemption. From a consequentialist view, the greater good argument[25] advanced in defense of the anti-kickback rule might be seen as reasonable from the perspective of cost. What is lost in this argument is that fundamentally, hospitals and drug manufacturers must maintain an uninterrupted supply of medication for health care delivery. The inexorable downward pressure on price, as set by the purchaser, has created a monopsony,[26] or a buyer's monopoly, and this has driven out redundancy in drug manufacturing. As price falls, manufacturers compensate by adopting a just in time production model which has the effect of improving a return on investment (ROI) by reducing the cost associated with carrying extra inventory on the shelf. Manufacturing a drug is a complex activity and requires a robust supply chain, as was, for example, acutely demonstrated in the recent COVID epidemic.[27] When manufacturers leave the market, the remaining production supply chain is also affected as each supply chain component runs in its leanest fashion to maximize its own ROI. The supply chain can also be disrupted by natural disasters, labor disputes, regulation, and licensing issues, to name a few. In solving drug shortages, any activity along the supply chain that can be shown to be a proximate cause of drug shortages should be removed. Consequentialism stipulates that all people should be considered in pursuit of the greatest good. In that regard, the present market has not shown itself to properly consider all individuals, most notably, the patient.

ADDRESSING THE DRUG SHORTAGE THROUGH THE GRAY MARKET

The term "black market" refers to methods of commerce that violate the law with respect to any component of that commerce. To further use this color analogy, the normal and lawful market might be referred to as white. The term "gray market"[28] describes commerce that though not illegal, does not follow the intended supply chain of that market. This term was originally coined by Premier Healthcare Alliance, which was a large group purchasing organization in the United States. Concern has been raised that secondary pharmaceutical distributors sell to hospitals at prices beyond what would be expected to cover costs plus "normal" profit, that is, the minimum level of profit needed for a company to remain competitive in the market. Further, concern also exists that pharmaceuticals will pass through different sellers, each taking some profit, and therefore elevating the final price paid by the end buyer. Secondary distributors play a small but important role in pharmaceutical distribution. Distributors, regardless of size, are regulated entities. Certain business practices, like price discrimination, are illegal. Price discrimination occurs when sales of identical goods and services are sold at different prices. The Robinson–Patman Act of 1936, 15 U.S.C. § 1, is federal law that prohibits anti-competitive practices, specifically, price discrimination. Price discrimination also occurs when the same price is charged to customers that have different supply costs. Ethical pricing is considered part of good markets. The basis of ethical pricing reflects a greater good standard. Secondary distributors, to a small degree, might adopt price-gouging tactics but no evidence exists that this is widespread. Further, it is unclear how a very small part of the market would influence manufacturers to leave the market or discourage sellers to such a degree that drugs are not available. Price discrimination may in fact be present in the manufacturing-distribution contract of the larger primary distributors. Manufacturers must sell to the large primary and smaller secondary drug distributors at the same price as they are in the same class of trade. Price contracting allows the primary distributor a chargeback to the manufacturer, effectively lowering the price differentially among manufacturers. The secondary distributor does not have the chargeback contract and has therefore paid a higher price for the same product. This higher price is now passed on, plus normal profit, to the final buyer. This creates an illusion of a price gouge but is the direct result of a form of price discrimination that creates a contract price available to the large distributor at or below cost. Manufacturers and the contracted distributor now must control a very large portion of the market to be profitable.

FAIR DISTRIBUTION POLICIES ARE INSUFFICIENT TO EESOLVE THE FUNDAMENTAL PROBLEM OF A LACK OF SUPPLY

In a normal market, manufacturing would logically increase to meet demand. Generic drug manufacturing contains several elements that prevent market responsiveness. In our present society, drug supply disruption is meant to be a "never" event. In that regard, manufacturers can't leave the market easily if normal profit is not achievable. The Food and Drug Safety and Innovation Act, S.3187, passed both the house and senate and was signed into law July 9th, 2012. This act requires manufacturers to provide earlier warning to the Food and Drug Administration (FDA) if shortages are anticipated. With this knowledge, the FDA can seek alternative supply. The FDA lacks federal authority to compel manufacturers to stay in the market. The FDA has authority to regulate manufacturers and inspect facilities in the public interest through the Current Good Manufacturing Practice [29] regulations for human pharmaceuticals. Manufacturing generic pharmaceuticals has become a costly and complex enterprise with exceedingly narrow margins, unlike manufacture of branded (ie, not generic) drugs which are protected by patent. In the circumstance of decreased supply, new manufactures of branded drugs are unable or unwilling to enter the market. The concept of distributive justice[30] supports the development of rationing and distribution policies within health care delivery entities, but rationing is only a temporary solution and fails to address the root cause. Hospitals have developed methods to obtain supply from many sources to meet demand. However, in the circumstance where supply is fixed, drug acquisition by one hospital will lead to a lack of that drug in another hospital. In health care, the question of a hospital catchment area must be addressed. In the mobile health care society, geography is no longer a barrier to access. Hospitals need to collaborate to create distributive justice solutions that reflect this reality.

A ROBUST AND FAIR COMPENSATED GENERIC DRUG MARKET IS AS IMPORTANT AS THE DRIVE TOWARD INNOVATION IN THE BRANDED DRUG MARKET

Pharmaceutical manufacturing is grounded on a financial model of drug innovation supported by the constitutionality of patent protection and exclusivity.[31] Patents allow a prolonged period of profit taking. Supporters of this system argue that the development of a new drug is extremely[32] costly and only through patent protection can a profitable business model be developed. The drive to innovation has created extremely powerful and valuable compounds that have use within health care delivery long after the patent has expired. Market forces have had a profound effect on driving prices down after the patent expires. The result has been that extremely useful compounds are manufactured at a lower and lower cost because of a Walmart effect[33] on pricing. Less money is available to manufacturers to maintain infrastructure and production is increasingly disrupted. In our present model of health care delivery, tension and conflict exist over which parts of health care should be subject to a bottom-line model and which parts are not. If pharmaceutical development and manufacturing are to be governed fundamentally by market forces, a business model must be put in place that will maintain the manufacturing of excellent quality generics. The business of medicine is caring for patients. To a major degree, health care practitioners depend on the pharmaceutical industry to provide the necessary drugs to meet the ethical obligation of health care delivery. From the perspective of the patient, timely access to that care can be a matter of life and death. Have patients benefitted by innovation in the drug development market? Undoubtedly, the answer is yes in the aggregate. However, the more pressing question might be in measuring the rate of innovation as measured, for example, by numbers of patents issued, patent citations, field trials, clinical trials, etc. and its relationship to the benefits of innovation.

Concern has been raised that the US Patent and Trademark Office grants patents that are only minor variants of previously patented drugs, so called "evergreening."[34] This raises the more general question of whether innovation is supply-driven, for example, by innovators pushing through new drugs to reap the potentially enormous benefits of a successful one, or demand-driven, for example, by the need to treat disease more effectively. The Drug Price Competition and Patent Term Restoration Act, informally known as the "Hatch-Waxman Act" [Public Law 98–417], is a 1984 United States federal law establishing an incentive for generic drug entry when branded drugs come off patent. Section 505(j) (2) (A) (vii) (IV), Paragraph IV, created the Abbreviated New Drug Application (ANDA) that allows 180-day exclusivity to companies that are the "first-to-file" an ANDA against holders of patents for branded counterparts. The ANDA only requires that the new drug be bio-equivalent to the branded alternative. Whether Hatch-Waxman encourages production entry is unclear since the landscape has been complicated by the practice of "reverse payments" and "pay for delay" paid by large branded pharmaceutical companies to other manufacturers wishing to enter the generic market.[35]

THE BIOETHICAL IMPERATIVE TO ACT

When a needed good, in this case a pharmaceutical, is in short supply, the simple and superficial approach is to create a rationing system that strives to provide a fair distribution to help the most people. Such a system draws from a utilitarian model of a greatest good but the risks and dangers of such a principle turned into policy raises a myriad of risks. From a deontological perspective, drug shortages should be a never event and the only pathway forward is to fix it, not make the best of it. Drug shortages are the result of a production market failure produced by purchasing contracts to get the best price for a buyer, even if it means the product becomes unavailable. Such a policy is short-sighted and likely harms patients. This market failure can be set on a remediation pathway by eliminating the safe harbor granted to purchasing groups. The result might be a rise in the drug sale price but a much more robust drug supply. Incentives and regulations to encourage manufacturing improvements as well as more manufacturers in the market will also produce downward price pressure. These solutions are the demand imperative of the ethical anesthesiologist. When it comes to drug manufacturing, it is necessary to strike the balance between innovation, good health, and human flourishing. Our ethical duty is to continuously remind ourselves that medical practice is an ethical endeavor, and we should seek to share a common value that puts the patient first. We are all the beneficiaries of good health and good health is priceless.

CLINICS CARE POINTS

- Developing a rationing plan during shortages is reasonable and possibly necessary but must comport with bioethical principles and the law.

- Hospital administration in collaboration with pharmacy services should keep the clinician informed about current and future shortages.

- Searching for additional drug supply, while reasonable, may help one hospital at the expense of another.

- Anesthesiologists should seek to understand legislative barriers and help identify ways to overcome them; they are also very effective advocates for addressing challenges in the pharmaceutical manufacturing marketplace.

DISCLOSURE

The author declares that he has no relevant or material financial interests that relate to the information described in this paper.

REFERENCES

1. Aronson JK, Heneghan C, Ferner RE. Drug shortages. Part 1. Definitions and harms. Br J Clin Pharmacol 2023;89:2950–6.
2. Khan R. "Unsustainable low prices causing generic drug market failure leading to supply chain distributions and shortages". Forbes; 2020.

3. Hantel A, Siegler M, Hlubocky F, et al. "Prevelance and severity of rationing during drug shortages" JAMA. Intern Med 2019;179(5):710–1.

4. Singer P. Practical ethics. Cambridge University Press; 2011.

5. Joint Commission on Accreditation of Healthcare Organizations. Accreditation manual for hospitals. Oakbrook Terrace, IL: Joint Commission on Accreditation of Healthcare Organizations; 1992.

6. Templin B. Contracts: a modern coursebook. Wolters Kluwer; 2019.

7. Barrow JM, Khandhar PB. StatPearls. StatPearls Publishing; 2023.

8. Page K. The four principles: can they be measured, and do they predict decision making? BMC Med Ethics 2012;13:10.

9. Alexander L. and Moore M., Deontological Ethics, The Stanford Encyclopedia of Philosophy (Winter 2021 Edition), Zalta E.N., editor. Available at: https;//plato.stanford.edu.archives/win2021/entries.ethics-deontological.

10. Sinnott-Armstrong W., "Consequentialism", The Stanford Encyclopedia of Philosophy (Winter 2023 Edition), Zalta E.N., Nodelman U., editor. Available at: https://plato.stanford.edu/archives/win2023/entries/consequentialism.

11. Card AJ. What Is Ethically Informed Risk Management? AMA J Ethics 2020; 22(11):E965–75.

12. Berezowski J, Czapla M, Manulik S, et al. "Rationing in healthcare – scoping review" Front. Public Health, Sec. Health Economics 2023;11.

13. Anderson DR, Aydinliyim T, Bjarnadóttir MV, et al. Rationing scarce healthcare capacity: "A study of the ventilator allocation guidelines during the COVID-19 pandemic". Prod Oper Manag 2023. https://doi.org/10.1111/poms.13934. Epub ahead of print. PMID: 36718234; PMCID: PMC9877846.

14. Turse, N. (2020). Donald Trump Says America's Ventilator Shortage Was "Unforeseen." Nothing Could Be Further From the Truth. The Intercept. https://theintercept.com/2020/03/24/donald-trump-says-americas-ventilator-shortage-was-unforeseen-nothing-could-be-further-from-the-truth/.

15. Zivot J. Coronavirus Disease 2019 Triage Teams: Death by Numbers. Crit Care Med 2020;48(8):1241–2.

16. Shukar S, Zahoor F, Hayat K, et al. Drug Shortage: Causes, Impact, and Mitigation Strategies. Front Pharmacol 2021;12:693426.

17. Brenan, M. (2023). Majority in U.S. still say Gov'T should ensure healthcare. Gallup.com. https://news.gallup.com/poll/468401/majority-say-gov-ensure-healthcare.aspx#:~:text=The%20latest%20findings%2C%20from%20Gallup's,40%25%20say%20it%20should%20not.

18. Blake V. The constitutionality of the Affordable Care Act: an update. Virtual Mentor 2012;14(11):873–6.

19. Justice Department reverses position on ACA's individual mandate | AHA News. (2021, February 10). American Hospital Association | AHA News. https://www.aha.org/news/headline/2021-02-10-justice-department-reverses-position-acas-individual-mandate#:~:text=The%20U.S.%20Court%20of%20Appeals,could%20survive%20without%20the%20mandate.

20. U.S. uninsured rate hits record low in first quarter of 2023 | Blogs | CDC. (2023). https://blogs.cdc.gov/nchs/2023/08/03/7434/#:~:text=7%25%20or%2025.3%20million%20Americans,the%20same%20period%20in%202022.

21. 42 U.S. Code § 1395dd - Examination and treatment for emergency medical conditions and women in labor United States Code, 2018 Edition, Supplement 3, Title 42-THE PUBLIC HEALTH AND WELFARE

22. Jamison DT, Breman JG, Measham AR, et al, editors. The International bank for reconstruction and development/the World bank. New York: Oxford University Press; 2006. Washington (DC).
23. Misselbrook D. Duty, "Kant, and deontology". Br J Gen Pract 2013;63(609):211.
24. 101 Stat. 680 - Medicare and Medicaid Patient and Program Protection Act of 1987. PUBLIC LAW 100-93-AUG.18, 1987, 100th Congress
25. Sinnott-Armstrong, Walter, "Consequentialism", The Stanford Encyclopedia of Philosophy (Winter 2023 Edition), Edward N. Zalta & Uri Nodelman (eds), forthcoming URL = <https://plato.stanford.edu/archives/win2023/entries/consequentialism/>.
26. Moliterno TP. Monopsony. In: Augier M, Teece DJ, editors. The palgrave encyclopedia of strategic management. London: Palgrave Macmillan; 2018. https://doi.org/10.1057/978-1-137-00772-8_586.
27. Socal MP, Sharfstein JM, Greene JA. The Pandemic and the Supply Chain: Gaps in Pharmaceutical Production and Distribution. Am J Publ Health 2021;111(4): 635–9.
28. Woodward C. Prices gone wild: grey market 'scalpers' scoring windfall in American drug market. CMAJ (Can Med Assoc J) 2012 Feb 7;184(2):E119–20.
29. 61 FR 52602 - Medical Devices; Current Good Manufacturing Practice (CGMP) Final Rule; Quality System Regulation
30. Lamont, Julian and Christi Favor, "Distributive Justice", The Stanford Encyclopedia of Philosophy (Winter 2017 Edition), Edward N. Zalta (ed.), https://plato.stanford.edu/archives/win2017/entries/justice-distributive/.
31. U.S. Const., art I, Sec. 8, Cla 8.
32. Wouters OJ, McKee M, Luyten J. Estimated Research and Development Investment Needed to Bring a New Medicine to Market, 2009-2018. JAMA 2020;323(9): 844–53. Erratum in: JAMA. 2022 Sep 20;328(11):1110. Erratum in: JAMA. 2022 Sep 20;328(11):1111. PMID: 32125404; PMCID: PMC7054832.
33. Fishman C. The Wal-Mart Effect and a Decent Society: Who Knew Shopping Was so Important? Acad Manag Perspect 2006;20(3):6–25. http://www.jstor.org/stable/4166248.
34. Collier R. Drug patents: the evergreening problem. CMAJ (Can Med Assoc J) 2013;185(9):E385–6.
35. School CL. FTC: 'Pay for delay' hinders competition in the pharmaceuticals market. Concord Law School; 2022. https://www.concordlawschool.edu/blog/news/ftc-pay-for-delay-pharmaceuticals-market/.

Medical Triage
Ethical Implications and Management Strategies

Gentle S. Shrestha, MD, FACC, EDIC, FCPS, FRCP (Edin), FSNCC (Hon), FNCS[a],*,
Denise Battaglini, MD, PhD[b],
Kanwalpreet Sodhi, DA, DNB, IDCCM, EDIC, FICCM[c],
Marcus J. Schultz, MD, PhD[d,e,f,g]

KEYWORDS

- Disaster • Catastrophe • Pandemic • Resource limitations • Scarcities
- Resource allocation • Medical triage • Triage

KEY POINTS

- Medical triage protocols are valuable tools to aid allocation of scarce resources during the time of disasters and pandemics.
- Existing triage protocols have several limitations.
- Incorporating the principles of ethics, learning from the pandemics and disasters in the past and multidisciplinary involvement of stakeholders can help to refine the existing triage protocols.

INTRODUCTION

In the twenty-first century, mass casualty incidents have become a global phenomenon due to an increasing vulnerability to disasters both natural and man-made. Mass casualty incidents can be either medical or public health emergencies, including natural events such as pandemics, earthquakes, and tsunamis, or man–made disasters such as wars, acts of terrorism, and air crash accidents. Climate change may exacerbate this in various ways. The American College of Emergency Physicians defines a medical disaster as a situation in which the "destructive effects of natural or

[a] Department of Critical Care Medicine, Tribhuvan University Teaching Hospital, Maharajgunj, Kathmandu, Nepal; [b] Department of Anesthesia and Intensive Care, IRCCS Ospedale Policlinico San Martino, Genoa, Italy; [c] Department of Critical Care, Deep Hospital, Ludhiana, India; [d] Department of Intensive Care, Amsterdam University Medical Centers, Location 'AMC', Amsterdam, the Netherlands; [e] Mahidol Oxford Tropical Medicine Research Unit (MORU), Mahidol University, Bangkok, Thailand; [f] Nuffield Department of Medicine, University of Oxford, Oxford, UK; [g] Division of Cardiothoracic and Vascular Anesthesia & Critical Care Medicine, Department of Anesthesia, General Intensive Care and Pain Management, Medical University of Vienna, Vienna, Austria
* Corresponding author.
E-mail address: gentlesunder@hotmail.com

Anesthesiology Clin 42 (2024) 457–472
https://doi.org/10.1016/j.anclin.2024.01.006

man–made forces overwhelm the ability of a given area or community to meet the demand for health care."[1]

Global experiences highlight the inadequacy of routine community capabilities and medical services in disaster settings, underscoring the need for systematic planning. Consequently, triage, particularly when facing limited resources is pivotal in averting mass casualties, usually demanding swift, objective, accurate, efficient, and, above all, ethical implementation. The word "triage" comes from the French word "trier," meaning "to sort," which originated as a method to evaluate and categorize the wounded in battle.[2] Triage prioritizes the likelihood of survival. However, when planning for triage in disasters, health care providers encounter unique challenges in clinical decision-making. These challenges include rationing—deciding who receives care and what type of care—imposing restrictions such as quarantine, and grappling with ethical dilemmas inherent in the practice of triage.[3]

From an ethical standpoint, triage serves as a classic example of distributive justice, exploring how benefits and burdens should be distributed within a population.[4] In emergency situations, a conflict arises between public health and clinical bioethics values. Physicians are faced with the dilemma of choosing between the utilitarian principle, that is, aiding those for whom they can do the most good and the egalitarian principle of justice, that is, assisting those with the greatest need, all while navigating the complexities of setting aside traditional Hippocratic ethics.[5–8]

As the world faces increasing numbers of challenges of responding to and rebuilding from unforeseen impacts of extreme natural disasters, which include recurrent infectious pandemics and catastrophes induced by the climate change, we bring attention to ethical considerations in triaging. This discussion holds relevance for both developed nations and resource-limited regions or countries aiming to enhance their preparedness for disaster events. In this review, our focus is on ethically evaluating triage systems to develop optimal management strategies in a just and ethical manner.

DEFINITIONS, OBJECTIVES, ETHICS, AND CHALLENGES

The primary purpose of medical triage is to determine priorities for access to care and treatment, particularly when using advanced and expensive diagnostic–therapeutic methods becomes necessary. Prioritization typically relies on specific triage protocols, crucial documents directing health care workers in making decisions on treatment distributions during shortages or critical emergencies.[9] The critical elements of a triage protocol and the ethical components that need to be incorporated in a triage protocol are discussed in the following section.

Ethical constraints are pivotal in medical triage. The decision-making process in medical triage should be dynamic, incorporating feedback, adapting to changing circumstances, and learning continuously from experiences, with a focus on ethical concerns and decision-making. Emergency medical services bear the responsibility of triaging, stabilizing, and transporting victims, playing a crucial role in planning a successful strategy to minimize the burden of mass casualty incidents. In addition, when faced with major disasters, all health care providers and systems must participate in the triage, management and care of victims, often in unfamiliar environments with limited resources. In addition, these services face challenging decisions, determining who receives immediate care and who may experience delays.[9–12]

The ethical principles guiding medical triage center on justice, nonmaleficence, and autonomy. Justice, essential for fair arbitration in the face of disputed claims, becomes especially important in mass casualty incidents, where the inability to treat everyone is a looming threat. The triage procedure should be fair and equitable, ensuring equal treatment for all patients based on their medical requirements rather than personal characteristics such as age, gender, race, or socioeconomic status. Preexisting disabilities present a significant challenge to prioritization in the context of mass casualty incidents, contributing to inequities based on social models that highlight discrimination. Therefore, medical triage should incorporate the principle of egalitarian justice. To achieve this, triage protocols can apply capability theory, acknowledging that disability may be perceived differently based on one's ability to adapt to a critical context. The ethical aspects of triage in patients with disabilities are discussed in the section on perspectives of different groups. The principle of non-maleficence underscores the obligation to prioritize individuals with a higher chance of survival in medical triage, acting to achieve overall well-being.[9]

The preservation of patients' autonomy is a crucial ethical imperative to pursue during mass casualty incidents. Inclusive decision-making, encompassing patients' preferences, values, and objectives, is essential.[9–12] Therefore, effective communication assumes a paramount role in medical triage. Clear and honest communication is vital in mass casualty incidents as a way to build trust and involve victims in decision-making whenever possible. Patients need to be informed about the triage process, decision-making criteria, and the rationale for resource distribution.[9] Importantly, individuals not prioritized during medical triage should receive ongoing follow-up to ensure appropriate care and support.[9–12]

Challenges in medical triage encompass various factors, including but not limited to scarcities in resources, time constraints, subjective decision-making criteria, ethical considerations, and emotional burden. Shortage in life-saving medical resources, such as personal protective equipment, ventilators, and supplies, became particularly evident during the recent coronavirus disease 2019 (COVID-19) pandemic. In response, numerous triage protocols were developed to minimize wasting and ensure effective resource allocation. Time constraints are a critical factor in medical triage, necessitating the swift evaluation of numerous patients to promptly identify potential life-threatening conditions to provide timely attention and treatment.[12]

Adequate preparedness of health care workers and the health care system by means of training, education, and simulation is pivotal for effective and ethical handling of the disaster. It is elaborated in the subsequent section on human factors, trainings, and simulations. Based on the increasing number of disasters, the health care system needs to implement better approaches to triage, including identifying existing resources, alternative sights of care, and other criteria to be better prepared to handle the future disasters and pandemics. The lessons learned from the recent pandemics and disasters are discussed in the Lessons learned from recent catastrophes section. Meanings and explanations of terms and principles related to ethics are summarized in **Box 1**.

CRITICAL ELEMENTS OF TRIAGE PROTOCOLS

Triage protocols play a pivotal role in efficiently allocating limited health care resources during mass casualty incidents. In health care, an array of triage protocols and systems are used, each customized to suit various care settings and scenarios (**Table 1**). All these protocols and systems share several common objectives: (1) they are designed to help health care providers and emergency responders prioritize patients based on the severity of their condition; (2) they involve the assessment of patients' vital signs, symptoms, and clinical criteria to assign a level of urgency or acuity to their condition; (3) they are typically designed to be scalable, allowing health care

Box 1
Glossary of terms and principles

Justice: fair solution of a disputed topic

Egalitarian justice: justice based on the principle that all individuals, with or without preexisting disability, are equal and deserve allocation of resources without discrimination

Nonmaleficence: preventing harm or minimizing harm in ethical decision-making

Autonomy: individual freedom and self-determination in personal choices and actions

Capability theory: fostering individuals' ability to lead a fulfilling and meaningful life—in the current context this applies to the individuals with a disability, whose perception and ability to adapt may vary from those without a disability

Patient-centered approach: approach that considers the unique preferences and values of an individual

Values: cultural criteria to differentiate between good or bad, moral or immoral, and desirable or undesirable; these criteria guide attitude and behavior

Societal values: collectively shared ideas by the members of a given society or culture

Dynamic adaptation: ability to change in response to evolving circumstances and evidences

providers to use them in various settings, from large-scale disasters to routine patient care in emergency departments or pre-hospital care by emergency medical services; and (4) they provide a standardized approach to patient assessment and triage, helping ensure consistency and uniformity in the decision-making process.

Table 1
Examples of triage protocols, for use in mass casualty incidents, in emergency departments, out-of-hospital crisis, and military[a]

START	Designed for use during mass casualty incidents and quickly categorizes patients into color-coded groups based on their treatment needs: immediate, delayed, minimal, and expectant
Triage Sieve	Modification of the START system, designed to further refine the initial assessment of patients during a mass casualty event; it uses specific criteria to categorize patients and allocate resources accordingly
MTS	Widely used in emergency departments in many countries, MTS categorizes patients into different priority levels based on the urgency of their condition, with a focus on ensuring that the most critical patients receive care first
ESI	ESI is an emergency department triage algorithm that assigns patients into five levels of acuity, with Level 1 representing the most critical cases and Level 5 being the least urgent
CTAS	Similar to the ESI, CTAS is a widely used system in Canada for prioritizing patients in emergency departments based on their acuity and needs
EMS	EMS personnel often use protocols to determine whether a patient should be transported to the hospital and, if so, to which facility; these protocols vary by region and are adapted to local needs
TCCC	Triage system usually employed by the military to prioritize wounded soldiers in combat situations

Abbreviations: CTAS, Canadian Triage and Acuity Scale; EMS, emergency medical services triage and transport decisions; ESI, Emergency Severity Index; MTS, Manchester Triage System; START, simple triage and rapid treatment; TCCC, tactical combat casualty care.
[a] This list of examples is not exhaustive; additional triage protocols for various scenarios can be found in the literature.

Table 2
Key ethical elements in the development of triage protocols, with examples from triage protocols for in the COVID-19 pandemic

Elements	Meaning	Aim	Examples From the COVID19 Pandemic
Utility	Maximizing the *overall* benefit for the *greatest* number of people	To make the most efficient and effective use of limited resources to achieve the best possible results in terms of saving lives and improving the outcome of individuals	In cases of oxygen scarcity during a pandemic and near-capacity health care facilities, health care providers may prioritize invasive ventilation over HFNO to optimize limited oxygen resources and maximize overall benefits
Maximization of benefits	Using resources to benefit patients with the *greatest need* and efficiently using resources to benefit patients with *the best prospects* of a good outcome	To ensure that resources are used efficiently and effectively to save lives and improve the outcome of patients	With the surge in critically ill patients requiring ventilators, but limited numbers of ventilators, health care providers may make decisions to prioritize to use them for patients who have the highest likelihood of recovery and the best prospects for long-term quality of life
Prioritization of clinical criteria	Use of clinical criteria to assess *the severity and outcome*	To ensure that medical resources are allocated in a way that maximizes the potential for positive outcomes	Patients who require ICU could be prioritized, or patients with no significant underlying health issues or comorbidities that could complicate their response to treatment may be given preference

Abbreviations: COVID–19, coronavirus disease 2019; HFNO, high-flow nasal oxygen; ICU, intensive care unit.
It is important to note that the choice of a triage protocol may vary based on the specific context and the level of care (eg, pre-hospital, emergency department and even within hospital wards like an intensive care unit).

In the development of triage protocols, key ethical elements include the principles of "utility," "maximization of benefits," and "prioritization of clinical criteria" (**Table 2**). "Utility" underscores the need to allocate limited resources in a way that maximizes overall benefits, aiming to save the most lives or achieve optimal health outcomes. "Maximization of benefits" focuses on efficiently using resources to benefit patients with the greatest need, ensuring that resources are allocated effectively. "Prioritization of clinical criteria" involves evaluating patients based on their condition severity, likelihood of survival, and expected response to treatment (**Table 3**).

These ethical elements can sometimes be in conflict with each other, particularly in situations of resource scarcity, such as during a pandemic. Balancing utility, maximization of benefits, and prioritization of clinical criteria can present ethical dilemmas. For example, a scenario may arise where allocating resources to a patient with a lower

Table 3
Frequently used scoring systems and criteria used in the "Prioritization of Clinical Criteria," with examples of challenges with these systems when using them in the COVID–19 pandemic[a]

System	Description	Purpose	Challenges in the COVID–19 Pandemic[b]
SOFA	Assigns scores based on physiologic parameters	Helping prioritize treatment in intensive care settings	COVID-19 patients can experience rapid clinical deterioration; SOFA is typically calculated over a 24-hour period and may not capture these sudden changes
APACHE	Assigns scores based on physiologic parameters and the medical history	Used to evaluate the severity of illness in critically ill patients, helping to assess prognosis and guide treatment decisions	Relying solely on APACHE may raise concerns of fairness and equity; in some cases, patients with higher APACHE, which could be related to comorbidities or chronic health conditions, may be at a disadvantage in resource allocation
CSF	Assesses the degree of frailty in patients based on criteria like mobility, independence, and cognitive function	Helps guide decisions about appropriate treatment and interventions	May raise ethical and value-based questions about prioritizing patients based on their age, frailty status, and potential for recovery; it can be perceived as discriminatory against older adults or individuals with preexisting health conditions

Abbreviations: APACHE, acute physiology and chronic health evaluation; CSF, Clinical Frailty Scale; COVID–19, coronavirus disease 2019; ICU, intensive care unit; SOFA, Sequential Organ Failure Assessment.
[a] The choice of scoring system and the specific criteria used may vary from one medical scenario to another, this table focuses on the COVID-19 pandemic.
[b] This list is not complete, there are certainly more challenges that can be managed.

likelihood of survival but a potentially higher quality of life could conflict with the goal of maximizing overall benefits by saving more lives. In addition, prioritizing clinical criteria may result in resource allocation decisions that seem unfair or even discriminatory, especially if certain individuals are disproportionately disadvantaged by the criteria used (**Box 2**).[9] Many factors can hinder effective implementation of ethical principles during medical triage (**Fig. 1**).

Managing these conflicts requires careful consideration, transparency, and the involvement of ethicists, health care professionals, and policymakers to develop and implement triage protocols that aim to strike a balance between these principles while addressing specific ethical concerns. It is essential to have clear and flexible guidelines in place to navigate these challenges and make informed decisions during times of resource scarcities.

There are several other challenges. One area of concern centers on the patient-centered approach. Many existing triage protocols may not adequately account for individual patient preferences, values, and unique circumstances. A shift toward a more patient-centered approach, which considers factors such as age, comorbidities, and patient input, could substantially augment both the ethical and practical aspects of triage decision-making. By factoring in these individual nuances, triage protocols can strive to provide more personalized and equitable care.

A second concern underscores the significance of understanding and incorporating community and societal values into triage protocols. These values, deeply ingrained in the fabric of our societies, can play a pivotal role in determining who should receive priority when critical resources, such as intensive care unit beds and ventilators, are in short supply. Integrating these values into the decision-making process ensures that resource allocation aligns with the collective moral compass, fostering a sense of equity and fairness.

Finally, a third area of focus emphasizes the need for dynamic adaptation. Triage protocols must be agile, capable of accommodating changing circumstances and

---

Box 2
Examining the ethics of clinical triage protocols and decision-making frameworks, with a focus on individuals with increased medical needs

During COVID-19 pandemic, authorities created and revised frameworks for guiding clinical decision-making and patient prioritization. Most if not all protocols emphasized a utilitarian approach.

This utilitarian perspective can inadvertently disadvantage certain groups. For instance, using the likelihood of survival as a criterion to exclude care for individuals with severe baseline cognitive impairment, inability to perform activities of daily living, advanced irreversible neurodegenerative disease, and decreased functional capacity raise concerns about the de-prioritization of individuals with increased medical needs.

The criteria like CFS and SOFA score are inaccurate in predicting COVID-19 mortality, as for predicting outcome in individuals with disabilities. The use of these scoring systems may result in higher scores for individuals with stable underlying disabilities that do not predict short-term mortality, potentially leading to the de-prioritization of individuals with increased medical needs.

Abbreviations: COVID–19, coronavirus disease 2019; CSF, Clinical Frailty Score; SOFA, Sequential Organ Failure Assessment

Adapted from Zhu J, Brenna CT, McCoy LG, Atkins CGK, Das S. An ethical analysis of clinical triage protocols and decision making frameworks: what do the principles of justice, freedom, and disability rights approach demand of us? BMC Medical Ethics. 2022 Feb;23:11.

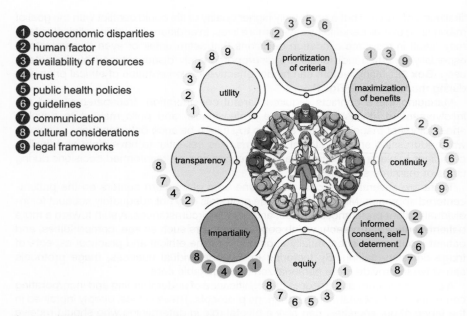

1 socioeconomic disparities
2 human factor
3 availability of resources
4 trust
5 public health policies
6 guidelines
7 communication
8 cultural considerations
9 legal frameworks

Fig. 1. Ethical principles to be considered during medical triage and management of patients (mentioned inside the colored circles) and the factors that can affect/hinder effective implementation of the principles (enumerated as one to nine and matched with the corresponding ethical principles).

emerging evidence. The pace of change during a pandemic or catastrophe can be staggering, demanding rapid adjustments to protocols in response to new information and evolving best practices. The ability to pivot and recalibrate is the key to maintaining the relevancy and effectiveness of triage protocols in the face of uncertainty.

PERSPECTIVES OF DIFFERENT GROUPS

Triage protocols and management must take into account the needs of diverse patient populations. One area of concern is how existing triage protocols take into account the needs of people living with disabilities. The management of this diverse population raises several concerns. They are at higher likelihood of being excluded from the care based on factors such as cognitive impairment, neurodegenerative disorders, and functional limitations that might suggest likelihood of higher mortality. Moreover, the people with disabilities often live in settings that might render them to be at higher risk of being affected during pandemics and disasters.

The World Health Organization considers disability to be a part of being a human. Several studies have demonstrated that the people with disability have very high level of capacity to adapt. Those people who have acquired disability can experience similar level of happiness and satisfaction as in the state prior to be disabled. Such experience of the disabled may differ vastly from those who are not disabled. Also, it is possible that those who are disabled since birth may have even stronger sense of satisfaction and bodily integrity. They could experience the surroundings, emotions, attachments, and so forth in their own way which can be of equal importance to those being experienced by other people without disability. Perhaps most important, the presence of disability may not necessarily translate into long-term poorer outcome and the scoring systems such as the Sequential Organ Failure Assessment (SOFA) score, which is used by existing triage protocols may be imprecise for evaluating people with disability. In order to address these valid concerns, the guiding principle of justice, which emphasizes on ethical obligation of fair settlement of controversial claims, need to be embraced. Involvement of disability right proponents, representatives from the disabled groups, and personalizing allocation of resources while dealing with the marginalized and disabled group of people can be a way forward (**Table 4**).

Pandemics and disasters create a situation when the conventional individual patient-based approach to care transitions (often very acutely) to the population-based approach for management of the patients. Depending on the magnitude of the surge, response strategy may shift from conventional approach maintaining the usual level of care to contingency approach and then to crisis response, often requiring deviation from standards of care.[13,14] Viewpoints and perspectives of various groups need to be considered for efficient, appropriate, and ethical use of the stretched resources.[15] A multidisciplinary approach embracing and involving groups such as local public, health care providers, volunteering organization, emergency medical services, public health experts, media people, local leaders, government, and international leaders can be the key to effective management during pandemics.[16]

THE HUMAN FACTOR, TRAININGS, AND SIMULATIONS

Mass casualty incidents are critical situations that require coordination, rapid response, and efficient decision-making.[9] Health care practitioners are frequently unprepared to anticipate and respond to an unexpected disaster.[17,18] Mass casualty incidents can be emotionally and physically challenging traumatic events, leading to post-traumatic stress disorder, anxiety, and depression.[19,20] First responders are those manifesting increased susceptibility to safety issues, such as infectious illnesses, adverse environmental exposures, and severe injuries, fear and difficult decisions, facing highly demanding situations for their well-being. Indeed, human factor and ethics play an essential role in decision-making process.[18]

Dealing with the human factors is critical for making fair and timely ethical choices.[19,20] Actions should always match with organizational values and the well-being of individuals should be prioritized by incorporating ethical principles into the management plans.[20]

Exercise and training are essential tools for ensuring readiness to face mass casualty incidents, including familiarization with triage protocol, understanding and incorporating ethical issues into decision-making and resource allocation, and understanding how to most effectively manage emergency medical needs.[9,18,19] Mock drill is a terminology used to depict a training exercise simulating a real-life scenario in which participants rehearse responding to a disaster. Simulation-based training provides health care practitioners to deal with challenges and failures and to evaluate an organization's preparedness to mass casualty incidents, with the unique chance to practice crisis resource management behaviors while handling high-fidelity clinical scenarios. Simulation allows providers to hone and advance their skills in resource allocation, leadership, and teamwork during triage procedures. Despite being a key component to training to ensure competence during emergencies, a small number of organizations provide a core curriculum or simulation opportunities to practice the skill set for triage during mass casualty incidents.[18]

By conducting mock drill regularly, health care practitioners can reinforce technical and nontechnical skills, including human factors, for the management of disasters and

Table 4
Perception and concerns of different populations and groups, their ethical implications, and possible solutions

Level	Perception and Concerns	Ethical Implications and Solutions for Triage
Marginalized and disabled population	Existing triage protocols and prognostication tools need to be modified to offer better justice for people with disability	Need to involve the human right experts and representatives from the people with disability while designing triage protocols to enhance justice, transparency, acceptability and to assure a personalized approach
Public	Anxiety, lack of preparedness, fear, feeling of uncertainty	Involvement of public is critical to maintain trust, transparency, and support for effective crisis management
Health care workers	Moral distress, failure to adapt to crisis situation and safety concerns	Support system from hospital for moral distress of the providers; transfer to non-critical role of the providers who are unable to adapt; best possible attempts from hospital to enhance safety of providers, especially prevention of infectious diseases
Researchers	Research during disasters and pandemics is challenging yet necessary	Research need to focus on improving treatment, patient safety and patient outcomes; formulation of national guidance for ethical approval of research works; the primary responsibility of providers to continue clinical care need to be ensured; autonomy, privacy, safety, and preferences of the patients need to be assured while conducting research works
Region or nation	Need of proper leadership, planning, collaboration and execution	Involvement of political leadership at national level; development of mechanism to acquire real-time data, provide situational awareness; collaboration with local leaders and international bodies to obtain synchronized efforts to deal with the situation; to ensure effective and best possible mobilization and allocation of available resources
International community	Lack of knowledge about local cultural, social and religious scenario; understanding the local needs, supporting which would benefit the community the most	International response groups need to coordinate with local authorities and need to get acquainted with local cultural and religious practices; to preferably consider support measures that not only addresses immediate needs, but would confer gains to the community that sustains after the disaster or pandemic

Adapted from refs[13–15,17]

educate themselves in how to make time-sensitive clinical judgments in a limited available resource setting.[18,20] Regular training, using high-fidelity simulation, procedural simulations, part-task trainers, simulated patients, screen-based simulations, serious games, and a full-scale maxi-simulation, demonstrated more successful acquisition and retention of skills in comparison to continual medical education based on self-learning static programs.[18] On the other hand, non-technical skills including social, cognitive, and personal resource skills can contribute to efficient and safe task performance in addition to achieving technical competence. Decision-making, situation awareness, leadership, and collaboration are examples of non-technical skills that, if not appropriately learned and reinforced, may lead to delays, mistakes, and accidents.[18,19] In addition to these skills, adequate training, triage protocols, and effective teamwork are crucial to foster health care practitioners who are able to make the most ethical decisions possible under challenging circumstances.[18–20]

LESSONS LEARNED FROM RECENT CATASTROPHES

Among the major recent natural disasters, numerous lessons have been learned. These lessons have revealed common themes and good practices gathered across various sectors. Some of these themes include the importance of planning since disasters will always be unexpected, if not unprecedented. Resilience is also seen as an interactive process that needs to be reinforced and sustained over time, especially before a disaster strikes. In addition, resilience is strengthened when it is shared, emphasizing the need for cooperation and collaboration. Every disaster is unique, presenting different triage challenges. **Table 5** shows the unique triage challenges in different type of catastrophes.

The recent mass disasters, such as the 2022 earthquake in Afghanistan, the 2023 earthquakes in Turkey and Syria, and the earthquakes in Japan over the last two decades, have taught us valuable lessons. One of the key lessons learned is the importance of effective disaster management planning and execution for both natural and man-made disasters. It is crucial to have a well-organized disaster team with clearly defined roles. An organizational model structured around five functional pavilions including preventive planning, immediate response, smooth coordinated functioning of the response team, and post-response phase long-term assistance and recovery, each running its own activities independently but in coordinated fashion make vital contributions to an overall emergency response.[21] Coordination at local, regional, national, or international level is imperative. Health systems play a vital role in disaster resilience, as timely delivery of health services is critical. An effective triage plan relies on medical personnel in charge of disaster situations having adequate knowledge of the plan and the ability to direct other personnel, including paramedics, armed forces, rescue personnel, and volunteers, who must work synergistically to ensure effective interventions and improve resilience. Beyond the medical assistance, the technical aspects of disaster preparedness include information dissemination, management of mass casualty incidents, triaging, assessment of damage, and humanitarian supply management. Operational synergy is challenging in the face of language disparities, shared, but limited resources, limited medical teams, law and order enforcement, and risk to volunteers. In addition to these time-sensitive issues, there is also a critical need to create public awareness of the associated risks of infectious disease post-disaster management.

A review of nine earthquakes in Japan in the twenty-first century recommends seven phase counter measures as a "Disaster Life Cycle," including three pre-event measures, including damage mitigation, preparedness and disaster prediction, and early

Table 5
Unique triage challenges in different types of mass casualty incidents

Incidents	Triage Challenges
Earthquake	• Large number of severely injured • Retrieving victims buried under debris • Triaging different types of physical trauma (orthotrauma, neurotrauma, abdominal injuries and thoracic trauma) • Airway management onsite (anticipated difficulty due to burns or inhalational injury) • Establishment of a medical transport corridor for safe fast transport to predefined medical facility • Secondary disaster post-earthquakes (outbreak of chemical contamination by industrial poisons, explosion or fires, catastrophic floods, tsunami in coastal areas, landslides, avalanches, volcanoes, traffic accidents, public sanitation and environmental concerns, biological contamination and infectious diseases)
Tsunami	• Drowning • Mostly lower limb injuries due to submerged water • Land usage plans due to limited land availability within defined coastal areas • Communication issues due to network breakdowns and power shutdowns • Debris clearance or waste management plans • Risk of infectious diseases
Terrorism	• High-energy injuries • Management of ballistic, blast, shrapnel injuries • Security issues among rescuers • Knowledge about biological and chemical weapons • Ethical controversy of prioritizing victims over terrorists
Air crash	• High-energy impact injury • Burns due to fires • Communication issues
Intrahospital emergencies (eg, fire)	• Complexity in evaluation of patients • Keeping safety of patients in mind • Communication issues • Hospital preparedness and logistics (medical equipment, fire-fighting devices, in-house evacuation plans, transport devices, manpower available for emergency management) • Hospital design (fire/mishap location, ventilation system, type of material burned)

warning, and four post–event measures, including damage assessment, emergency response, recovery, and reconstruction, with communication and information playing a central role.[22] Post-disaster, a critical review of the whole task accomplished, and a medical audit is mandatory.

Although the COVID-19 pandemic has demonstrated unprecedented initiatives at regional levels, leadership and global cooperation, triage plans need to function effectively in critical care and public health care systems both regionally and globally. Global emergencies require health care systems to shift to alternative operational states, so as to meet novel demands and overcome the resource constraints. Whether a pandemic occurs or not, the challenge for everyone in health care is to set egos aside and adhere to broader ethical principles.[9] International and multidisciplinary collaboration is required and an international task force should be created to adopt new resilience measures and draw up national networks from individual countries with a list of health care professionals and volunteers from different streams to be in the frontline in case of disasters. There should also be drafted plans to mobilize teams from one area and to deploy at the disaster site.

Managing casualties from flight crash accidents, especially during pandemics such as COVID-19 that require isolation, can be a challenging task. During air crashes, communication network may be in chaos due to post-crash fire, stormy bad weather or radio sets getting wet and thereby due to the technical snags, there may occur communication gap between onsite and medical centers. Mock disaster exercises must be performed at major airports based on evidence-based disaster planning guidelines with specified roles of disaster management performed at the mock exercise such as sending emergency response units to the scene, evacuation and fire-fighting drills, trained medical personnel carrying out triage, providing first aid services, and transportation of victims to different hospitals.[23] **Table 6** provides a comprehensive overview of emergency preparedness at airports.

The lessons learned from emerging terror attacks across the globe necessitate the development of stringent contingency plans and guidelines that should be continually revised, updated, and expanded to address terrorist acts and time-to-time review of intentional releases of newer chemical, biological, or nuclear agents and the weapons of mass destruction. Terror attacks usually do not have a geopolitically defined territory and can potentially threaten the entire nation, region or the world, so a "master plan" for coordinating the national government machinery, resources, and funding for related but geographically separate incidents should be there. From a meta-analysis of 68 terrorism acts with 616 lessons learnt, the data showed that despite the difference in nature of attacks, countries, and casualties involved, most of the lessons learned were similar.[24] They concluded that to save as many victims as possible, protect rescue forces from harm, and prepare hospitals at the best possible level, it is important to implement the lessons identified in training and preparation. The lack of knowledge on how to deal with injuries caused by firearms or explosive devices could

Table 6
Two-phase response model for disaster and casualty at airports

Responder	Primary Phase Response	Secondary Phase Response
First responding agency	Emergency medical services	Site medical teams from different hospitals of the region volunteers and NGOs
Subordinates	Fire brigade and fire department of the airports	Armed forces government agencies and law and order officials private ambulance companies
Personnel	Emergency medical technicians nurses	Physicians, nurses, and emergency medical technicians
Operations	Designate operation coordinator and key officers of medical incident Establish and operate command post, triage, treatment, and transportation area Establish vital communication to other agencies Ensure access and egress routes	Deploy optimal numbers of site medical teams according to level of incident Take over field command and medical works Dispatch patients and communicate with hospitals

Adapted from Lee WH, Chiu TF, Ng CJ, Chen JC. Emergency medical preparedness and response to a Singapore airliner crash. Acad Emerg Med 2002;9:194-8.

be remedied by consistent training and drills of emergency service staff. Consistent implementation of the "THREAT points" and implementation of the "3 Echo" interprofessional concept—enter, evaluate, and evacuate—in training and practice would be an important step toward further improving preparation for terror attacks.[25,26] After the 2017 German terror attacks, the Terror and Disaster Surgical Care course was developed by the German Trauma Society to enhance the preparation of hospitals to manage mass casualty incidents related to terror attacks, which might be extended to other nations for preparation.[27]

Given the potential uncertainties regarding health hazards to the public and rescue workers onsite, it is essential to have a structured plan to improve public health risk before, during, and after a disaster event.

SUMMARY

Medical triage protocols serve as invaluable tools in effective allocation of scarce resources during disasters and pandemics. At all times, resource allocation must be ethically justified. The basic principles of ethics such as justice, nonmaleficence, and autonomy need to be considered. Health care communities need to keep learning from the experiences during the disasters and pandemics and to adapt their patient-centered and multidisciplinary approaches.

CLINICS CARE POINTS

- In times of crises, catastrophes, and pandemics where resources are constrained, medical triage protocols serve as invaluable tools, directing health care workers to prioritize and allocate resources efficiently.
- Ethically navigating the fair allocation of resources presents considerable challenges as principles such as in the resource allocation process.
- Ethical resource allocation can be facilitated through patient-centered approaches, transparent processes for resource allocation, and the continuous refinement of existing protocols based on lessons learnt from disasters and pandemics.
- It is imperative to involve marginalized groups, ethicists, and policymakers in a multidisciplinary approach when formulating or revising triage protocols.

DISCLOSURE

The authors report no conflicts of interest. Funding source: No funding obtained.

REFERENCES

1. American College of Emergency Physicians. Advancing emergency care: policy compendium. Dallas: ACEP; 2008. p. 10.
2. Winslow GR. Triage. In: Post SG, editor. Encyclopedia of bioethics. 3rd edition, vol V. New York: Macmillan Reference—Thomson Gale; 2003. p. 2520–3.
3. Wynia MK. Oversimplifications II: public health ignores individual rights. Am J Bioeth 2005;5:6–8.
4. Moskop JC, Iserson KV. Triage in medicine, part II: Underlying values and principles. Ann Emerg Med 2007;49(3):282–7.
5. Holm S. Medical aid and disaster relief. In: Ashcroft RE, Dawson A, Draper H, et al, editors. Principles of healthcare ethics. Chichester: Wiley; 2007. p. 671–7.

6. Sztajnkrycer MD, Madsen BE, Báez AA. Unstable ethical plateaus and disaster triage. Emerg Med Clin 2006;24:749–68.
7. Gert HJ. How are emergencies different from other medical situations? Mt Sinai J Med 2005;72:216–20.
8. Elcigou O, Unluoglu I. Triage in terms of medicine and ethics. Saudi Med J 2004; 25:1815–9.
9. Zhu J, Brenna CT, McCoy LG, et al. An ethical analysis of clinical triage protocols and decision making frameworks: what do the principles of justice, freedom, and disability rights approach demand of us? BMC Med Ethics 2022 Feb;23:11.
10. Bazyar J, Farrokhi M, Khankeh H. Triage Systems in Mass Casualty Incidents and Disasters: A Review Study with A Worldwide Approach. Open Access Macedonian Journal of Medical Sciences 2019 Feb;7(3):482–94.
11. Garner A, Lee A, Harrison K, et al. Comparative analysis of multiple-casualty incident triage algorithms. Ann Emerg Med 2001 Nov;38(5):541–8.
12. Soola AH, Mehri S, Azizpour I. Evaluation of the factors affecting triage decision-making among emergency department nurses and emergency medical technicians in Iran: a study based on Benner's theory. BMC Emerg Med 2022 Oct; 22:174.
13. Biddison LD, Berkowitz KA, Courtney B, et al. Ethical considerations: care of the critically ill and injured during pandemics and disasters: CHEST consensus statement. Chest 2014;146(4 Suppl):e145S, 55S.
14. Christian MD, Sprung CL, King MA, et al. Triage: care of the critically ill and injured during pandemics and disasters: CHEST consensus statement. Chest 2014;146(4 Suppl):e61S–74S.
15. Devereaux AV, Tosh PK, Hick JL, et al. Engagement and education: care of the critically ill and injured during pandemics and disasters: CHEST consensus statement. Chest 2014;146(4 Suppl):e118S, 33S.
16. Braun BI, Wineman NV, Finn NL, et al. Integrating hospitals into community emergency preparedness planning. Ann Intern Med 2006;144:799–811.
17. Dichter JR, Kanter RK, Dries D, et al. System-level planning, coordination, and communication: care of the critically ill and injured during pandemic and disasters: CHEST consensus statement. Chest 2014;146(4 Suppl):e87S–102S.
18. Battaglini D, Ionescu Maddalena A, Caporusso R, et al. Acquisition of skills in critical emergency medicine: an experimental study on the SIAARTI Academy CREM experience. Minerva Anestesiol 2021;87:1174–82.
19. Pandit K, Healy E, Todman R, et al. Disaster Triage Skills Training: An Introductory Virtual Simulation for Medical Students. Cureus 2023;15:e39417.
20. Uddin H, Hasan MK, Castro-Delgado R. Effects of mass casualty incidents on anxiety, depression and PTSD among doctors and nurses: a systematic review protocol. BMJ Open 2023;13:e075478.
21. Scendoni R, Cingolani M, Tambone V, et al. Operational Health Pavilions in Mass Disasters: Lessons Learned from the 2023 Earthquake in Turkey and Syria. Healthcare (Basel) 2023;11(14):2052.
22. Meguro K. (2015) Lessons Learned from Past Big Earthquake Disasters and Comprehensive Disaster Management for Implementation of Disaster Resilient Society. Available at: https://sheltercluster.s3.eu-central-1.amazonaws.com/ public/docs/k.meguro-lessons_learned_from_past_big_earthquake_disasters_ and_comprehensive_disaster_management_for_implementation_of_disaster_ resilient_society.pdf. Accessed December 10, 2023.

23. Lee WH, Chiu TF, Ng CJ, et al. Emergency medical preparedness and response to a Singapore airliner crash. Acad Emerg Med 2002;9:194–8.

24. Schorscher N, Kippnich M, Meybohm P, et al. Lessons learned from terror attacks: thematic priorities and development since 2001-results from a systematic review. Eur J Trauma Emerg Surg 2022;48:2613–38.

25. Jacobs LM, Wade DS, McSwain NE, et al. The Hartford Consensus: THREAT, a medical disaster preparedness concept. J Am Coll Surg 2013;217:947–53.

26. Autrey AW, Hick JL, Bramer K, et al. 3 Echo: concept of operations for early care and evacuation of victims of mass violence. Prehospital Disaster Med 2014;29: 421–8.

27. Achatz G, Friemert B, Trentzsch H, et al. Terror and disaster surgical care: training experienced trauma surgeons in decision making for a MASCAL situation with a tabletop simulation game. Eur J Trauma Emerg Surg 2020;46: 717–24.

Ethics of Preanesthesia Mandatory Laboratory Testing

James Hunter, MD[a], Stephen H. Jackson, MD[b],
Gail A. Van Norman, MD[c],*

KEYWORDS

- Ethics • Preoperative testing • Pregnancy testing • COVID testing
- Mandatory testing

KEY POINTS

- Principles of informed consent for medical testing follow general principles of medical care that recognize respect for patient autonomy, beneficence, non-maleficence, and distributive justice.
- Mandatory medical testing without informed consent raises concerns about patient autonomy in medical decision-making.
- Mandatory medical testing may be allowable in scenarios where not testing would violate clearly established medical standards of care.
- In some circumstances, mandatory testing is not ethically justified; one example is mandatory pregnancy testing, which is not ethically justified in most cases.
- Mandatory preanesthesia testing for COVID infection was ethically justifiable on utilitarian principles early in the pandemic, but has become less ethically justifiable as the pandemic has evolved.

INTRODUCTION

Basic tenets of medical ethics—respect for patient autonomy, beneficence, non-maleficence, and justice—require that physicians respect and promote patient autonomy; intend and attempt whenever possible to provide care that is beneficial and avoids harm medically, psychologically, socially, and culturally; and treat patients fairly and equally with regard to care and access, without bias with regard to economic status, race, sex, religion, or other social or cultural characteristics.

[a] Department of Anesthesiology and Perioperative Medicine, University of Alabama at Birmingham, Birmingham, AL, USA; [b] Department of Anesthesiology, Good Samaritan Hospital, San Jose, CA, USA; [c] Department of Anesthesiology and Pain Medicine, University of Washington, Seattle, WA, USA
* Corresponding author.
E-mail address: gvn@uw.edu

Anesthesiology Clin 42 (2024) 473–490
https://doi.org/10.1016/j.anclin.2024.01.002
1932-2275/24/© 2024 Elsevier Inc. All rights reserved.

anesthesiology.theclinics.com

EVIDENCE BASED MEDICAL TESTS

Evidence-based medicine (EBM) relies on a traditional understanding of science and experimentation, and shares with medical ethics the goals of maximizing benefits and minimizing risks of medical tests and treatments, as well as engaging patients in shared informed decision-making. EBM practice rests on the concept that conscientious, judicious, and explicit use of the best available current information should be combined with clinical experience and systematic research in advising patients about medical tests and treatments. Importantly, this applies to preanesthesia testing, which should be based, whenever possible, on contemporaneous credible data and not arise out of the "habits" of personal clinical experience or historic and/or unsupported claims of collegial cohorts. Even long-accepted traditional practices and clinical protocols and policies mandating certain actions should, at some point in time, be placed under the scrutiny of systematic investigation because they may well not pass rigorous scientific examination. One aspect of preanesthesia care particularly deserving of periodic re-examination is the concept of recommended versus mandatory testing.

Appropriate preanesthesia medical testing guided by EBM can enable a better evaluation of the level of medical risks for particular patients, direct preoperative interventions designed to minimize risks, and better inform patients about the benefits and risks of anesthesia—thereby promoting their informed decisions and in so doing honoring the ethical principles of beneficence, non-maleficence, and respect for patient autonomy.[1] Preanesthesia testing should be applied only in appropriate clinical scenarios and to appropriate patient groups. For example, utilizing a test with only moderate sensitivity and specificity in a group of patients with a low prevalence of the condition of concern is counter to proper epidemiologic principles because this can result in higher false positive and/or false negative rates.

Inappropriate testing can be associated with significant harms and increased costs of care, for the individual patient as well as for society. It presents greater risks of a patient being falsely labeled as having a condition that causes patient distress and fear, and can lead to subsequent inappropriate tests and treatments with their potential attendant complications. Conversely, falsely labeling a patient as not having a serious condition that the patient actually does have can result in false reassurance and failure to perform further testing and treatments, thereby denying the patient early detection of disease and possible life-altering or life-saving intervention.

The prevalence of disease should play a significant role in determining whether to apply a test because the prevalence of a condition in the test population affects the positive predictive value of even highly sensitive and specific tests (**Table 1**).[2]

With both significant potential benefits and serious harms for patients at stake, principles of medical ethics together with adherence to EBM require us to consider

Table 1
Effect of prevalence of a condition on positive predictive value of a test with 90% sensitivity and 95% specificity

Prevalence of a Condition (%)	Positive Predictive Value[a] (%)
0.1	1.8
1.0	15.4
5.0	48.5
50	94.7

[a] PPV = portion of patients with a positive test who have the condition.
From Santini A, Man A, Voidazan S. Accuracy of diagnostic tests. J Crit Care Med 2020; 7:241-8.

whether testing is being appropriately applied to the right patients and leads to better medical and non-medical outcomes. The physician's challenge is to determine with reasonable certainty whether potential benefits outweigh the potential increase in harms and costs.

Tests need not be invasive to have ethically significant ramifications. A blood or urine test may carry little or no physical consequences, but increases healthcare costs, especially when over-testing occurs. Test results can also have significant non-medical, social consequences. Nonmedical harms are well-recognized by US courts and legislation, which have increasingly awarded damages for harms of even minor medical treatments and tests,[3,4] including privacy violations[4,5]; falsely labeling a patient as having a significant medical condition[6,7]; or falsely reassuring them of the absence of a significant medical condition[7–9]; social harms[6]; emotional and psychological harms[10]; complications, both physical and otherwise when further follow-up testing is undertaken; and financial impacts, both of the primary test and its follow-up.[11] Minimally invasive tests can have ethically significant considerations, but institutional and practice policies often do not address consent for routine laboratory tests, under the mistaken presumption that the patient provides "presumed consent" when they offer their arm for phlebotomy.[12,13] Presumed consent, however, is seldom informed consent, thus violating both legal and ethical standards for consent.

Not all medical tests are ethically "equal." A few of the tests widely recognized as falling into a category with special ethical concerns include genetic testing,[14] testing for illicit drugs,[15] and pregnancy screening.[16,17] Making such a test a condition of treatment, that is, *mandatory* screening tests, may not be ethically or legally justifiable.

INFORMED CONSENT AND LABORATORY TESTING

Mandatory preanesthesia testing (note that "routine" testing is often *de facto* mandatory testing) places a condition on access to surgical care, and it may be difficult or impossible for patients who desire or need anesthesia to freely refuse. This burden is particularly acute for patients who belong to vulnerable groups—for example, the poor or certain cultural, ethnic, religious, or gender-based groups—because these patients typically are at greater risk of lacking resources to become informed about, identify, find, and access alternative care from a provider who will honor their informed refusal. Mandatory testing therefore is potentially both coercive and discriminatory,[1] and a coerced consent is both ethically and legally invalid.

This does not mean that it is never ethically acceptable to require a medical test prior to anesthesia or surgery. Physicians are ethically not required to perform procedures that are (1) futile/non-beneficial (discussion of which is beyond the scope of this article), (2) of questionable scientific or rational basis, and/or few rational practitioners would offer, or (3) below the standard of care (that is in direct violation of written professional standards, or actually contrary to medical evidence, and not merely "less than ideal"). At the same time, there are circumstances in which performing an anesthetic (surgery/procedure) without a test would breech one of these conditions, and we accept that a patient's refusal to allow the test would, at times, justify denying the clinical service in order to practice within professional standards of medicine.

Informed Consent: A Brief Refresher

In the United States, the legal rights of patients to consent to or refuse medical care were established in 1914 in the case of *Schloendorff V. Society of New York Hospital*.[18] In that case, a woman consented to an anesthetic only for examination and diagnosis, but while under general anesthesia she was subjected to an unconsented surgery. Extended time on the operating room (OR) table caused an upper extremity injury, later requiring amputation of the fingers of one hand. Justice Benjamin Cardozo rendered his famous ruling:

> Every human being of adult years and sound mind has a right to determine what shall be done with his own body, and a surgeon who performs an operation without his patient's consent commits an assault.[18]

Later court rulings solidified that this condition applies to both tests and treatments. The legal obligation that consent be "informed" was established in 1957 in *Salgo v. Leland Stanford University Board of Trustees*, a case in which a patient suffered a devastating complication (paraplegia) resulting from a medical test (an aortogram) for which he had agreed, but had not been informed of the risks.[19] In 1972, a court ruled in *Canterbury v. Spence* that consent was "not worthy of the name" unless the patient was informed about options and risks, and that such consent was not legally valid if coerced.[20]

If a preanesthesia laboratory test is to be evidence-based and also fulfill our ethical obligations to inform patients about benefits and risks of testing, we must consider (1) what is known about medical harms from the anesthetic that can be elucidated and/or mitigated by the test, (2) what additional possible medical and nonmedical harms and benefits of the test itself present, and (3) whether testing avoids more net harms than it causes. In some cases, tests commonly mandated by anesthesiologists prior to surgery or anesthesia do not pass the scrutiny of any of these questions—and in others, substantial questions remain about their appropriateness even if the patient can benefit from them. In all cases, we are left with the crucial question of whether there are any circumstances in which we can, ethically or professionally, justify denying care when an autonomous, informed patient refuses a recommended test. We will examine 2 examples of preanesthesia testing with complex ethical and professional implications: mandatory preanesthesia pregnancy testing and mandatory preanesthesia COVID testing.

PREANESTHESIA PREGNANCY TESTING

Common arguments for mandating preanesthesia pregnancy testing generally fall into 2 categories: avoiding fetal harms and avoiding medico-legal liability when an abnormal infant is born to someone who was exposed to anesthesia during pregnancy.

Anesthesia Exposure In Utero

Concerns were raised in the mid 20th century by animal experiments demonstrating teratogenicity of some drugs used during anesthesia. Recent data now clearly demonstrate that there is a startling lack of inter-species translatability in pharmaceutical toxicology tests, even when the species are closely related. Approximately half of all drugs found to be safe in animals fail human trials due to toxicity, and potentially beneficial drugs never undergo human testing because animal toxicity tests prevent them from entering human trials.[21] There are many cases of drugs that are proven safe in animals that have had tragic human consequences, such as thalidomide and TGN1412.[22,23] Conversely, some drugs, such as penicillin (frequently fatal in guinea pigs[24]), are only available because their clinical use preceded US laws requiring safety trials in animals.

Complicating this issue is the high rate of spontaneous human fetal anomalies—occurring in about 3% of all live births—for which causes are largely unknown. Early loss of pregnancy or presence of an anomaly in a newborn after in utero exposure to anesthetic drugs is therefore not by itself sufficient evidence of causality.

Despite a multitude of studies, exposure to anesthetic drugs in clinical doses and duration in utero has not been shown to result in significant negative human fetal outcomes, including a significant increase in fetal loss after exposure to anesthetic agents. Multiple systematic reviews and medical professional society statements affirm that no anesthetic drug has been proven to be teratogenic to the human fetus at any gestational age, if used in standard concentrations and in a manner consistent with clinical anesthesia practice.[16,25–28] Three large, well-designed retrospective human studies failed to find a correlation between in utero exposure to anesthesia and early fetal loss.[28–32] A small but statistically insignificant increase in miscarriages in patients who underwent general anesthesia for abdominal or obstetrical-gynecologic procedures[28,29,31,32] suggested a relationship to the surgical procedure, rather than the anesthetic. Scientific evidence can never guarantee complete absence of risk of teratogenicity or miscarriage, but the risks appear to be too small to be indiscernible in large retrospective studies involving actual clinical practice. Arguments that retrospective studies can be scientifically weaker than randomized prospective trials are valid, but prospective, randomized controlled trials of "potential teratogens" in pregnant humans would not be ethically permissible.

Anesthesia and Fetal Neurocognitive Development

Research regarding adverse effects of anesthetics on human fetal brain development is concerning, but as yet inconclusive, despite a large number of studies.[33–35] Many cited studies involve animal models, which differ significantly among species in timing and brain location of synaptogenesis, and much longer and repetitive anesthetic exposures than generally used in clinical practice.[36,37] Extrapolation of human outcomes following general anesthesia in the first year of life to outcomes from fetal exposure in utero has never been scientifically validated. The necessity for surgery during the first year of life indicates something is unusual, and experts agree it is difficult to impute adverse outcomes to the anesthetic rather than the surgical procedure or the cause underlying the need for surgery.[35,36] The American College of Obstetricians and Gynecologists issued a joint statement with the American Society of Anesthesiologists (ASA) in 2021, stating:

> There is no evidence that in utero human exposure to anesthetic or sedative drugs has any effect on the developing fetal brain; and there are no animal data to support an effect with limited exposures less than 3 hours in duration.[38]

The US Food and Drug Administration (FDA) has issued a precautionary announcement that volatile anesthetics "might" be harmful to young and rapidly developing brains, but also stated that "recent human studies suggest that a single, relatively short exposure to general anesthetic and sedation drugs in infants or toddlers is unlikely to have negative effects on behavior or learning."[39]

There is not a current consensus regarding neurocognitive effects of anesthetics; however, the status of debate regarding fetal neurodevelopment and anesthetic exposure should be disclosed during any informed consent discussion with the potentially pregnant patient.

Accuracy of Pregnancy Tests versus Patient History—Are Pregnancy Tests Necessary?

A positive pregnancy test may not indicate pregnancy, and a negative test does not rule it out.

In small studies of adult female patients, positive preoperative pregnancy tests occurred in 0.15% to 2.2% of patients.[25] The true prevalence of early first trimester pregnancy in patients presenting for surgery is unknown, but the estimated low prevalence suggests that by epidemiologic principles, a screening test is problematic.

Human pregnancy tests need only be able to detect any form of human chorionic gonadotropin (hCG), including those not associated with pregnancy, to be FDA approved, and yield both false positive and false negative results.[40–42] Accuracy of a point of care (POC) pregnancy test depends on the day of pregnancy during which the test is performed, the test's ability to detect hyperglycosylated hCG (hCG-H), which controls pregnancy implantation and placental growth, and the day on which implantation occurs. Tests vary widely in sensitivity.[40,41] In an independent study of POC tests, all of which claimed 99% accuracy in detecting pregnancy 3 days after the first missed day of menses, the best performing product was accurate in detecting pregnancy only 77% of the time. Accuracy of tests from different manufacturers ranged from 43% to 67%.[41] As but one example, E.P.T. (Pfizer) tests detected pregnancy in 53% to 68% of patients on the first day of missed menses and in only 80% to 86% 3 days later.[41]

Positive pregnancy tests do not distinguish between current pregnancy, recent pregnancy or miscarriage, recent exogenous administration of hCG, elevated pituitary hCG, the presence of various cancers, trophoblastic disease,[43–45] other conditions such as familial hCG syndrome,[46] and the presence of antibodies against animal proteins commonly found in veterinarians and other animal workers.[44] Laboratory assays of total hCG are falsely positive in up to 5 out of 162 patients.[47]

In one clinical study using POC urine testing, false negative test result occurred in 11 out of 9447 tests,[48] usually in early pregnancy. Causes for falsely negative urine tests include very early pregnancy, the common inability of urine tests to detect hCG-H, dilution of hCG in high volumes of urine, and renal degradation of hCG. High levels of hCG degradation products can block hCG binding to the test device, causing a false negative test (the "hook" effect).[49] A large number of implantations occur after the first day of missed menses,[50] and hCG levels can be undetectable for several days during this time, even though the patient is pregnant.[51]

The "false negative" patient response rate to being asked if they could be pregnant in the emergency room or preoperative holding area is around 0.3%.[52] Several studies have failed to identify pregnancies among patients who were asked in a confidential setting if they could be pregnant.[53,54] One study found that only 11 of 8245 preoperative pregnancy tests were positive, but that over half were false positives.[55] A 2023 study found just one positive pregnancy test among 1195 subjects (0.02%).[56] In all of these studies, if a patient stated that they absolutely could not be pregnant, the error rate in the patient's self-assessment was lower than the error of any POC urine pregnancy test, thus raising doubt that performing a preoperative pregnancy test in an unselected group of patients is more accurate than simply asking an informed patient in a confidential setting whether they could be pregnant.[57]

Non-medical Harms of Pregnancy Testing

Financial costs
The "cost" of a POC urine pregnancy test is estimated to be about $35.[55,58] Because of the low prevalence of pregnancy in the preoperative setting, the total cost of detecting one pregnancy ranges from $1000 to $49,000—presenting concerns regarding cost containment and social and distributive justice in limited resource settings.[55,58–63]

Social harms
Studies demonstrate that many patients, particularly adolescents, will forgo even necessary medical care, if they believe that they will be pregnancy tested.[64] A positive

pregnancy test makes many women vulnerable to increased family and/or partner-based domestic violence, including homicide, which is doubled and tripled in adult and adolescent pregnant patients, respectively.[65] This risk is particularly severe in adolescent patients, possibly because pregnancy may be a marker for a serious crime—child sexual abuse within the home. Given that fetal harms from anesthesia exposure are unproven, it is difficult to justify exposing patients to the risk of such serious consequences if a breach of confidentiality occurs. In addition, maintaining confidentiality may be challenging. In many states, physicians are legally obliged to report possible cases of sexual assault in children (including adolescent pregnancy) to law enforcement authorities; in others, confidentiality for minors seeking reproductive care is mandatory.[66–70] Anesthesiologists may find themselves having to choose between ethical obligations of confidentiality and legal requirements to disclose.

Consent or assent of minors for pregnancy testing involves complex issues such as parental rights and shared decision-making. US legislation regarding minors' rights to health care without parental knowledge or consent varies considerably among the 50 states. Anesthesiologists have ethical obligations to involve patients in shared decision-making, including minors who have decisional capacity.[1,71–73] Additionally, the Federal Health Insurance Portability and Accountability Act protects the confidentiality of reproductive health care information for both adults and minors, thus often pitting federal law against that of individual states.[66] The ASA *Guidelines for the Ethical Practice of Anesthesiology* oblige anesthesiologists to obtain developmentally appropriate permission or assent for medical decisions involving minor patients.[71]

Standards of care

Mandatory preanesthesia pregnancy testing is not, and never has been, a standard of care. A single study found that one-third of US anesthesia practices mandated pregnancy testing, and only 1 of 5 anesthesiologists surveyed would refuse to provide anesthesia for a positive test.[74] The ASA Task force on Preoperative Evaluation, in partnership with the ASA Committee on Ethics, does not support mandatory pregnancy testing, recommending that pregnancy tests be *offered* to any "female" patient who may desire it, and informed consent or refusal be obtained.[75] We note that transgender men may have pregnancy concerns and that the language of the joint statement should be changed to reflect this.[76]

While there is no conclusive evidence that anesthetics harm fetuses, the same cannot be said for some surgeries. Procedures involving pelvic organ manipulation are associated with increases in fetal loss.[77] Fertility procedures may be rendered moot by a positive pregnancy test. Exposure to chemotherapy that may be given intraoperatively may increase fetal loss,[78] and intraoperative exposure of a fetus to ionizing radiation may approach doses known to cause fetal injury.[79] Professional standards of care for surgeons weigh in favor of pregnancy testing under specific circumstances where medical evidence does clearly support the possibility of fetal harm related to the procedure. In those cases, it is the ethical responsibility of the surgeon to disclose risks in order to facilitate shared decision-making with the patient. Anesthesiologists should be aware that patients might have undergone surgically indicated pregnancy testing and review the results of those tests for appropriate discussion with the patient of anesthesia considerations.

MEDICO-LEGAL LIABILITY CONCERNS

Medico-legal consequences to anesthesiologists for not performing pregnancy tests are practically nonexistent. The last acknowledged data from the Anesthesia Closed Claims Project in 2017 identified just 10 cases out of the 11,000 in the database in which a claim was pursued because anesthesia and surgery were performed in patients with an undiagnosed pregnancy (<0.1%).[16] Three of the oldest cases are irrelevant to modern medical practice. Four cases with 3 successful claims occurred in cases where a pregnancy test was obtained, but the results were not checked by the anesthesiologist. The remaining 3 cases occurred in patients who denied they could be pregnant, but it was discovered after surgery that they were. Only one of those cases led to an award. The ASA Committee on Quality Management and Departmental Administration concludes the following:

> Other than for surgical indications, routine pregnancy testing may pose greater medico-legal risk to anesthesiologists due to failure to check the result or failure to document informed consent of [perhaps minimal] risk of miscarriage prior to elective surgery.[16]

In summary, scientific evidence has not established that determining the pregnancy status of a patient prior to anesthesia care avoids fetal harms. Arguably, pregnancy testing in the preoperative holding area does not appear to be more accurate overall than simply asking the patient in confidence if they could be pregnant. Lack of mandatory pregnancy testing does not lead to a significant increase in medico-legal liability, and professional societies actually advise against it. Because a patient may decide to incorporate their pregnancy status in their decision-making regarding the anesthesia and procedure, ethical principles favor informing the patient about these facts and offering, but not requiring, pregnancy testing.[17]

MANDATORY COVID-19 TESTING: EXAMPLE OF A CHANGING LANDSCAPE AND CHANGING ETHICS
The Context

From our current vantage point, it is easy to forget the extreme devastation to human health and life that spread across the globe in 2020 during the global COVID pandemic. From the first suspected cases of COVID-19 infection in mid-November of 2019, the virus spread at astonishing speed, exceeding 57 million known cases worldwide 1 year later, with almost 1.4 million confirmed deaths.[80] By November of 2020, the United States had seen more total COVID-19 deaths than the pandemic's combined death toll for Australia, Canada, China, Japan, and Germany. US hospitalizations more than doubled in October 2020 alone.[81] Entire hospitals were converted to emergency wards for patients presenting with COVID. In January of 2021, approximately 180 US deaths occurred every hour.[82] The number of collateral deaths due to COVID (eg, deaths due to lack of ICU beds for patients suffering from non-COVID, life-threatening conditions) remains unknown.

The toll on hospital and health care systems nationwide was crippling. Health care workers were overworked, exhausted, and psychologically traumatized. And they, too, were becoming sick and dying from COVID, creating a shortage of physicians and other healthcare workers needed to manage the onslaught of critically ill patients. Shortages of personal protective equipment (PPE) occurred across the nation.[83] Maintaining a non-infected health care workforce became paramount, along with preserving dwindling supplies of PPE. Continuing elective surgeries was unjustifiable because it presented serious risks to physicians and other health care personnel. Mandatory preanesthesia testing of patients and symptomatic workers was instituted.[84,85] Suspension of elective surgeries brought the primary financial engine for many hospitals to a halt. Health care systems began to hemorrhage financially, and hospitals began to close, particularly in rural areas.[86]

Early on, policies and practices de-emphasized ethical principles that addressed the moral obligations of physicians to the interests and care of individual patients, in favor of those maximizing benefits to many patients with competing interests needing high intensity care.[a] Within this context, we can identify a few of the early perioperative measures enacted and their corresponding rationales and ethical principles[1,87,88] (**Table 2**):

Overall, these measures served as a stopgap early in the pandemic, aiming to achieve the ethical principle of distributive justice by maximizing utilitarian use of limited resources in order to take care of more of society's sickest patients.

As the pandemic evolved, several developments played key roles in shifting clinical and ethical considerations away from a pure approach of mandatory COVID testing to the gradual and still-ongoing return of the preeminence of principles focusing on the rights and autonomy of individual patients (**Table 3**). Examples included: (1) the development of safe and effective vaccines and the subsequent fall of infection rates and viral virulence, (2) increased supplies of PPE due to upscaling of manufacturing, (3) selective resumption of elective surgeries as infection rates fell, and (4) emergence of data showing that morbidity and mortality of anesthesia and surgery are significantly elevated for some period of time following COVID infection.

Today, fewer patients are suffering from COVID, and infections are less virulent, leading to less morbidity and mortality. Reducing the spread of disease continues to be maintained by isolation of active cases, but community COVID screening tests are no longer widespread.

It is less clear whether mandatory preanesthesia testing is still ethically warranted — active infection generally is less severe, and PPE is more readily available for use in "suspicious" cases. The exact point at which ethical principles weigh against mandatory screening tests depends on specific clinical contexts, such as a hospital's ability to absorb staff absences due to COVID, availability of sufficient supplies of PPE, and local community prevalence of disease.

Symptomatic patients or patients with known recent exposure are tested primarily in order to discuss risks and avoid elective surgery in a patient whose risks of morbidity and mortality are elevated and secondarily to keep the risk of in-hospital spread low. Instead of mandatory testing of all patients, testing at all of the authors' institutions is requested only of those patients prior to elective surgery who have suggestive symptoms or a known exposure. Patient refusal to be tested leads to a discussion among the surgeon, anesthesia team, and patient regarding risks and whether to delay surgery for at least 2 weeks since onset of symptoms — the timeframe in which postoperative pulmonary complications appear to be particularly elevated in patients who have had recent COVID infection.[89]

Thus, in the case of preoperative mandatory COVID testing, there has been an evolution of the balance of ethical principles. Early in the pandemic, principles that de-emphasize individual "rights" and autonomy were more justifiable than they are now, when the risks of infection and its consequences are reduced and the ability of health care workers to be protected from acquiring disease are heightened — and re-prioritizing patient autonomy becomes possible.

---

[a] Shifting between a focus on individual patients and entire patient populations can be understood broadly as shifting between a deontological framework and a utilitarian (consequentionalist) one. However, respecting individual patient autonomy versus maximizing the best outcomes for most patients need not correlate with a commitment to either deontology or utilitarianism, respectively.

Table 2
Examples of early-pandemic ethical considerations

Action	Rationale	Harms	Example Ethical Principle
Suspension of Elective Surgeries	• Decrease unnecessary exposure of health care workers and in-hospital patients to infection; preserve the health care workforce • Beds for elective surgical patients would reduce those available for medical patients	• Delay of beneficial but less urgent treatments, which may then progress to become more urgent or lead to prolonged suffering	• *Non-maleficence*—avoid creating more infected patients through COVID spread • *Beneficence*—maintain society's health care work force to take care of more COVID patients • *Justice*—utilization of available resources for those in most immediate need
Mandatory COVID Testing for Patients Needing Surgery and Symptomatic Providers	• Identify patients who might present infectious risks to both in-house patients (and would need isolation) and providers (who should use scarce PPE). • Identify infected health care workers, to be removed from clinical settings in order to prevent in-house spread of COVID	• Loss of patient/health care worker autonomy	• *Beneficence* (maximizing the ability to provide *necessary* operations) • *Non-maleficence*—avoiding further spread of infection to patients, loss of health care workers due to illness • *Non-maleficence* and *distributive justice*—preserving PPE for use only in appropriate cases

Table 3
Examples of ethical considerations in mid-late pandemic

Action	Rationale	Harms	Ethical Principle
Mandating Vaccination of Patient-Facing Health Care Workers	• Continue to reduce the spread of infection, now specifically targeted to COVID • Reduce patient exposure • Reduce health care worker infections and maintain the specialized workforce	• Loss of health care worker autonomy	• *Beneficence and non-maleficence*— reduce spread of infection, morbidity, and mortality
Selectively Resume Elective Surgeries	• As time passes, elective surgeries might become emergency surgeries; elective surgeries are more likely to be effective • Regain/preserve hospital financial solvency • Prevent hospital closures	• Risk of increased spread of COVID to in-patients and health care workers	• *Non-maleficence*: avoid preventable progression of disease • *Beneficence*: achieve a higher rate of successful surgical treatments by doing them earlier • *Beneficence*: support ability to meet community needs by preventing/reducing hospital closures • *Distributive justice*: smaller hospitals in underserved areas were more likely to close if elective surgeries could not resume
Mandatory Preanesthesia COVID Testing	• Identify patients who have current or recent COVID • For current COVID infection, continue to delay elective surgeries to protect health care workers, in-patients, and the patient themselves	• Loss of patient autonomy regarding testing • Loss of patient autonomy in weighing risks of proceeding with surgery in the setting of active COVID infection • Possible increased health risk due to delayed surgery	• *Non-maleficence*: avoid elective surgery during active infection when risks are highest and reduce risk of in-house spread of infection • *Beneficence*: allow surgeries to proceed before patient condition becomes emergent

(continued on next page)

Table 3
(continued)

Action	Rationale	Harms	Ethical Principle
	• For recent COVID or asymptomatic COVID patients: allow some surgeries that are "urgent" • Armed with data on surgical outcomes for patients with recent COVID infection, inform patients and surgeons about reducible risks		• *Respect for patient autonomy:* better able to inform patients of their individual risks of proceeding with non-emergent surgery

CLINICS CARE POINTS

- Preanesthesia testing should conform with principles of medical ethics and should be evidence-based whenever possible.
- Certain medical tests, such as preanesthesia pregnancy testing, have special medical implications due to potentially significant societal as well as medical harms; informed consent for such tests should be obtained and documented.
- Mandatory preanesthesia testing may be coercive and in most cases is not ethically warranted.
- Appropriate patients, including transgender men, should be informed of what is known about anesthesia and pregnancy and offered a pregnancy test if they want one.
- Mandatory COVID testing early in the pandemic was warranted under utilitarian principles; however, mandatory preanesthesia COVID screening may no longer be ethically justifiable.

ACKNOWLEDGMENTS

The authors wish to gratefully acknowledge the help of Gabrielle Jackson, PhD, from the Department of Philosophy, Stanford University, for her kind review of an early draft and recommended inserting the quote from the eminent philosopher Daniel Dennett (recently passed) that introduces the article, and in so doing, set the "focus and thrust" for the entire article. She has also served as a co-member of the Bioethics Committee of Boston Children's Hospital.

DISCLOSURES

All authors assert that they have no commercial or financial interests concerning this publication and have received no funding.

REFERENCES

1. Beauchamp T, Childress J. Principles of biomedical ethics. 8th edition. New York: Oxford University Press; 2019.
2. Santini A, Man A, Voidazan S. Accuracy of diagnostic tests. J Crit Care Med 2020;7:241–8.
3. Bazzano LA, Durant J, Brantley PR. A modern history of informed consent and the role of key information. Ochsner J 2021;21:81–5.
4. U.S. Department of Health and Human Services. Why is the HIPAA privacy rule needed? United States Department of Health and Human Services. 2006. Available at: https://www.hhs.gov/hipaa/for-professionals/faq/188/why-is-the-privacy-rule-needed/index.html. [Accessed 19 December 2023].
5. Showalter JS. Unintended consequence: patient privacy in the age of social media. Healthcare Financial Management Association (HFMA). 2018. Available at: https://www.hfma.org/legal-and-regulatory-compliance/privacy-and-hipaa/58918/. [Accessed 19 December 2023].
6. Wakefield JC. False positives in psychiatric diagnosis: implications for human freedom. Theor Med Bioeth 2010;31:5–17.
7. Troxel DB. Medicolegal aspects of errors in pathology. Arch Pathol Lab Med 2006;130:617–9.
8. Brenner RJ. False-negative mammograms. Medical, legal and risk management implications. Radiol Clin North Am 2000;38:741–5.

9. Wilson RM. Screening for breast and cervical cancer as a common cause for litigation. A false negative result may be one of an irreducible minimum of errors. BMJ 2000;320:1352–3.

10. Stein A. Medical malpractice and the middle-ground fallacy: should victims; families recover compensation for emotional harm? Bill of Health: Examining the Intersection of Health, Law, Biotechnology, and Bioethics. 2015. Available at: https://blog.petrieflom.law.harvard.edu/2015/05/20/medical-malpractice-and-middle-ground-fallacy-should-victims-families-recover-compensation-for-emotional-harm/. [Accessed 19 December 2023].

11. Korenstein D, Harris R, Elshaug AG, et al. To expand the evidence base about harms from tests and treatments. J Gen Intern Med 2021;36:2105–10.

12. Borovecki A, Mlinaric A, Horvat M, et al. Informed consent and ethics committee approval in laboratory medicine. Biochem Med 2018;28:030201.

13. Gronowski AM, Budelier MM, Campbell SM. Ethics for laboratory medicine. Clin Chem 2019;65:1497–507.

14. Rego S, Grove ME, Cho MK, et al. Informed consent in the genomics era. Cold Spring Harb Perspect Med 2020;10:a036582.

15. Warner EA, Walker RM, Friedmann PD. Should informed consent be required for laboratory testing for drugs of abuse in medical settings? Am J Med 2003; 115:54–8.

16. ASA Committee on Quality Management and Departmental Administration. Pregnancy testing prior to anesthesia and surgery. American Society of Anesthesiologists. 2021. Available at: https://www.asahq.org/standards-and-practice-parameters/statement-on-pregnancy-testing-prior-to-anesthesia-and-surgery. [Accessed 19 December 2023].

17. Jackson S, Hunter J, Van Norman GA. Ethical principles do not support mandatory preanesthesia pregnancy screening tests: a narrative review. Anesth Analg 2023. https://doi.org/10.1213/ANE0000000000006669.

18. Schloendorff v Society of New York Hospital. New York Court of Appeals. 211 N.Y. 125. 1914-04-14. Available at: https://opencasebook.org/documents/5974/. [Accessed 19 December 2023].

19. Salgo V. Leland Stanford University Board of Trustees 154 Cal.App.2d 560, 317 P.2d 170 (1957). Available at: https://casetext.com/case/salgo-v-leland-stanford-etc-bd-trustees. [Accessed 19 December 2023].

20. Canterbury V. Spence. Casetext.com. Available at: https://casetext.com/case/canterbury-v-spence. [Accessed 19 December 2023].

21. Van Norman GA. Limitations of animal studies for predicting toxicity in clinical trials: is it time ot rethink our current approach? JACC Basic Transl Sci 2019;4: 845–54.

22. Vargesson N. Thalidomide-induced teratogenesis: history and mechanisms. Birth Defect Res C Embryo Today 2015;105:140–56.

23. Suntharalingam G, Perry MR, Ward S, et al. Cytokine storm in phase 1 trial of the anti-CD28 monoclonal antibody TGN1312. N Engl J Med 2006;(355):1018–28.

24. Cormia FE, Lewis GM, Hopper ME. Toxicity of penicillin for the guinea pig. J Invest Dermatol 1947;9:261–7.

25. Bauchat JR, Van de Velde M. Nonobstetric surgery during pregnancy. In: Chestnut's obstetric anesthesia: principles and practice. 6th edition. Philadelphia PA: Elsevier Inc; 2020. p. 368–91.

26. Cheek T, Baird E. Anesthesia for nonobstetric surgery: maternal and fetal considerations. Clin Obstet Gynecol 2009;52:535–45.

27. Canadian Agency for Drugs and Technologies in Health. Anaesthetic agents in pregnant women undergoing non-obstetric surgical or endoscopic procedures: a systematic review of the safety and guidelines. 2015. Available at: https://www.cadth.ca/anaesthetic-agents-pregnant-women-undergoing-non-obstetric-surgical-or-endoscopic-procedures-review. [Accessed 19 December 2023].

28. Duncan P, Pope W, Cohen M, et al. Fetal risk of anesthesia and surgery during pregnancy. Anesthesiology 1986;64:790–4.

29. Cohen S. Risk of abortion following general anesthesia for surgery during pregnancy: anesthetic or surgical procedure? Anesthesiology 1986;65:706–7.

30. Mazze R, Kallen B. Reproductive outcome after anesthesia and operation during pregnancy: a registry study of 5405 cases. Am J Obstet Gynecol 1989;161:1178–85.

31. Balinskaite V, Bottle A, Sodhi V, et al. The risk of adverse pregnancy outcomes following nonobstetric surgery during pregnancy: estimates from a retrospective cohort study of 6.5 million pregnancies. Ann Surgery 2017;266:260–6.

32. Aylin P, Bennett P, Bottle A, et al. Estimating the risk of adverse birth outcomes in pregnant women undergoing non-obstetric surgery using routinely collected NHS data: an observational study. Southampton (UK): NIHR Journals Library; 2016.

33. Jevtovic-Todorovic V. Anaesthesia-induced developmental neurotoxicity: reality or fiction? Br J Anaesth 2017;119:455–7.

34. O'Leary J, Warner D. What do recent human studies tell us about the association between anaesthesia in young children and neurodevelopmental outcomes? Br J Anaesth 2017;119:458–64.

35. McCann M, Soriano S. Does general anesthesia affect neurodevelopment in infants and children? BMJ 2019;367:l6459. https://doi.org/10.1136/bmj.l645.

36. Useinovic N, Jevtovic-Todorovic V. Controversies in anesthesia-induced developmental neurotoxicity. Best Pract Res Clin Anaesthesiol 2023;37:28–39.

37. Bleeser T, Hubble TR, Van de Velde M, et al. Introduction and history of anesthesia-induced neurotoxicity and overview of animal models. Best Pract Res Clin Anaesthesiol 2023;37:3–15.

38. American College of Obstetricians and Gynecologists and American Society of Anesthesiologists. Committee on Obstetric Practice Opinion: Nonobstetric surgery during pregnancy. Committee Opinion Number 775. 2021. Available at: https://www.acog.org/clinical/clinical-guidance/committee-opinion/articles/2019/04/nonobstetric-surgery-during-pregnancy. [Accessed 19 December 2023].

39. United States Food and Drug Administration. FDA Drug Safety Communication: FDA review results in new warnings about using general anesthetics and sedation drugs in young children and pregnant women. Accessed Sept 8, 2023. Available at: https://www.fda.gov/drugs/drug-safety-and-availability/fda-drug-safety-communication-fda-review-results-new-warnings-about-using-general-anesthetics-and. [Accessed 19 December 2023].

40. Cole L. New discoveries on the biology and detection of human chorionic gonadotropin. Reprod Biol Endocrinol 2009;7:8. https://doi.org/10.1186/1477-7827-7-8.

41. Cole LA. The hCG assay or pregnancy test. Clin Chem Lab Med 2012;50:617–30.

42. Nerenz R, Song H, Gronowski A. Screening method to evaluate point-of-care human chorionic gonadotropin (hCG) devices for susceptibility to the hook effect by hCG beta core fragment: evaluation of 11 devices. Clin Chem 2014;60:667–74.

43. Braunstein G. False positive serum human chorionic gonadotropin test results: causes, characteristics and recognition. Am J Obstet Gynecol 2002;187:217–24.

44. Oyatogun O, Sandhu M, Barat-Kirby S, et al. A rational diagnostic approach to the "phantom hCG" and other clinical scenarios in which a patient is thought to be pregnant but is not. Ther Adv Reprod Healt 2021;15. 26334941211016412.

45. Bodin S, Edwards A, Roy R. False confidences in preoperative pregnancy testing. Anesth Analg 2010;110:256–7.

46. Cole L. Familial hCG syndrome. J Reprod Immunol 2012;93:52–7.

47. American College of Obstetrics and Gynecology Committee on Gynecologic Practice. Opinion No. 278. Avoiding inappropriate clinical decisions based on false-positive human chorionic gonadotropin test results. Obstet Gynecol 2002; 100:1057–9.

48. Cole L. hCG, the centerpiece of life and death. Int J Endocrinol Metabol 2012;9: 335–52.

49. Priyadarshini S, Manas F, Prabhu S. False negative urine pregnancy test: hook effect revealed. Cureus 2022;14:e2277.

50. Wilcox AJ, Baird DD, Dunson D, et al. Natural limits of pregnancy testing in relation to the expected menstrual period. JAMA 2001;286:1759–61.

51. Nepomnaschy PA, Weinberg CR, Wilcox A, et al. Urinary hCG patterns during the week following implantation. Hum Reprod 2008;23:271–7.

52. Manley S, De Kelaita G, Joseph NJ, et al. Preoperative pregnancy testing in ambulatory surgery. Incidence and impact of positive results. Anesthesiology 1995;83:690–3.

53. Minnerop M, Garra G, Chohan JK, et al. Patient history and physician suspicion accurately exclude pregnancy. Am J Emerg Med 2011;9:212–5.

54. Maliva S, D'Errico C, Reynolds P, et al. Should pregnancy testing be routine in adolescent patients prior to surgery? Anesth Analg 1996;83:854–7.

55. Gong X, Poterack K. Retrospective review of universal preoperative pregnancy testing. Results and perspectives. Anesth Analg 2018;127:e4–5.

56. Flanagan SG, Green MA. Is preoperative urine human chorionic gonadotropin (hCG) testing necessary for pediatric patients before oral and maxillofacial surgery procedures with sedation? J Oral Maxillofac Surg 2023;81:150–5.

57. Kerai S, Saxena K, Wadhwa B. Preoperative pregnancy testing in surgical populations: How useful is policy of routine testing. Indian J Anaesth 2019;63:786–90.

58. Hennrikus W, Shaw B, Geraldi JA. Prevalence of positive pregnancy testing in teenagers scheduled for orhtopedic surgery. J Pediatr Orthop 2001;21:677–9.

59. Wingfield RM, Mcmenamin M. Preoperative pregnancy testing. Br J Surg 2014; 101:1488–90.

60. Kahn RL, Stanton MA, Tong-Ngork S, et al. One-year experience with day-of-surgery pregnancy testing before elective orthopedic procedures. Anesth Analg 2008;106:1127–31.

61. Jackson S, Abbey K, Hunter J. Pre-anesthesia pregnancy testing in adolescents. In: Hunter JM, Caldwell JC, Mann DG, editors. Ethics handbook: an educational Resource for the Practice of Anesthesiology. American Society of anesthesiologists Committee on ethics. Schaumburg III: American Society of Anesthesiologists; 2021. p. 223–33.

62. Hutzler L, Kraemer K, Palmer N, et al. Cost benefit analysis of same day pregnancy tests in elective orthopaedic surgery. Bull Hosp Jt Dis 2014;72:164–6.

63. Mesrobian JR. Preop pregnancy testing revisited. Anesth Analg 1996;83:440–1.

64. English A, Ford C. The HIPAA privacy rule and adolescents: legal questions and clinical challenges. Perspect Sex Reprod Health 2004;36:80–6.

65. Krulewitch C, Roberts DW, Thompson LS. Adolescent pregnancy and homicide: findings from the Maryland office of the chief medical examiner, 1994-1998. Child Maltreat 2003;8:122–8.
66. English A, Guderman R. Understanding legal aspects of care. In: Neinstein LS, editor. *Neinstine's adolescent and young adult health care: a practical guide.* 7th edition. Philadelphia: Wolters Kluwer; 2023. p. 85–9.
67. Boostra HD, Nash E. Minors and rights to consent to health care. Guttmacher Institute. 2000. Available at: https://www.guttmacher.org/gpr/2000/08/minors-and-right-consent-health-care. [Accessed 19 December 2023].
68. Weiss C. Protecting minor's health information under the federal medical privacy regulations. American Civil Liberties Union. Available at: https://www.aclu.org/other/protecting-minors-health-information-under-federal-medical-privacy-regulations. [Accessed 19 December 2023].
69. State laws that enable a minor to provide informed consent to receive HIV and STD services. Centers for Disease Control and Prevention. 2021. Available at: https://www.cdc.gov/hiv/policies/law/states/minors.html. [Accessed 19 December 2023].
70. 45 CFR (Code of regulations) 164,502(g)(3). Legal Information Institute. Available at: https://www.law.cornell.edu/cfr/text/45/164.502. [Accessed 19 December 2023].
71. Guidelines for the Ethical Practice of Anesthesiology. American Society of Anesthesiologists. Last amended 12/13/20. 2022. Available at: https://www.asahq.org/standards-and-practice-parameters/guidelines-for-the-ethical-practice-of-anesthesiology. [Accessed 19 December 2023].
72. Homi H, Ahmed Z. Preoperative pregnancy testing: to test or not to test? (an anesthesiologist's dilemma). Society for Pediatric Anesthesia News 2012;15:1.
73. Katz A, Webb S. Committee on Bioethics. Informed consent in decision-making in pediatric practice. Pediatrics 2016;138. e20161485.
74. Kampen PM. Preoperative pregnancy testing: a survey of current practice. J Clin Anesth 1997;9:546–50.
75. American Society of Anesthesiologists Task force for Preoperative Evaluation. Practice advisory for preanesthesia evaluation. Anesthesiology 2012;116:1–17.
76. Brandt JS, Patel AJ, Marshall I, et al. Transgender men, pregnancy and the "new" advance paternal age: a review of the literature. Maturitas 2019;128:17–21.
77. Juhasz-Boss I, Solomayer E, Strik M, et al. Abdominal surgery in pregnancy—an interdisciplinary challenge. Dtsch Arzteble Int 2014;111:465–72.
78. Backes CH, Moorehead PA, Nelin LD. Cancer in pregnancy: fetal and neonatal outcomes. Clin Obstet Gynecol 2011;54:574–90.
79. American College of Radiology, Society for Pediatric Radiology ACR-SPR practice parameter for imaging pregnant or potentially pregnant adolescents and women with ionizing radiation. American College of Radiology 2008. 2018. Available at: https://www.acr.org/-/media/ACR/Files/Practice-Parameters/Pregnant-Pts.pdf. [Accessed 19 December 2023].
80. World Health Organization. Weekly operational update on Covid-19 20-November-2020. Available at: https://www.who.int/publications/m/item/weekly-operational-update-on-covid-19—20-november-2020. [Accessed 19 December 2023].
81. Maxouris C. Here's exactly how bad Covid-19 was in November. Available at: CNN 2020; https://www.cnn.com/2020/12/01/us/covid-november-numbers-records/index.html. [Accessed 19 December 2023].

82. Worldometer: Coronovirus. Daily new deaths in the United States. Available at: https://www.worldometers.info/coronavirus/country/us/. [Accessed 19 December 2023].

83. Querney J, Cubillos J, Ding Y, et al. Patient barrier acceptance during airway management among anesthesiologists: a simulation pilot study. Korean J Anesth 2021;74:254–61.

84. O'Connor K, McGee M, Gibson M, et al. Developing an outpatient pediatric pre-procedure COVID-19 testing model. J Perianesth Nurs 2021;36:367–71.

85. Huybens EM, Bus MPA, Massaad RA, et al. What is the preferred screening tool for COVID-19 in asymptomatic patients undergoing a surgical or diagnostic procedure? World J Surg 2020;44:3199–206.

86. Christensen J. How the pandemic killed a record number of rural hospitals. Available at: CNN Health 2021; https://www.cnn.com/2021/07/31/health/rural-hospital-closures-pandemic/index.html. [Accessed 19 December 2023].

87. Draper H. Introduction. In: Draper H, Scott W, editors. Ethics in anaesthesia and intensive care. Philadelphia Elsevier Inc; 2003. p. p1–16.

88. Johnson A. The birth of bioethics. Oxford. New York: Oxford University Press; 1998. p. 327–34.

89. El-Boghdadly K, Cook TM, Goodacre T, et al. Timing of elective surgery and risk assessment after SARS-CoV-2 infection: 2023 update: a multidisciplinary consensus statement on behalf of the Association of Anaesthetists, Federation of Surgical Specialty Associations, Royal College of Anaesthetists and Royal College of Surgeons of England. Anaethesia 2023;78:1147–52.

Maternal–Fetal Conflicts in Anesthesia Practice

Sebastian M. Seifert, MD[a],*, Leslie Matthews, MD, PharmD[b],
Lawrence C. Tsen, MD[a], Grace Lim, MD, MSc[c]

KEYWORDS

- Fetal • Patienthood • Maternal • Anesthesia • Obstetrics • Conflict resolution
- Ethics

KEY POINTS

- The *maternal–fetal conflict* arises when maternal interests or wishes are inconsistent with fetal benefit.
- The principle of maternal autonomy underpins most decisions regarding maternal–fetal surgery with informed decision-making in the framework of maternal–fetal dyad model.
- In obstetrics, maternal physical risks (conflict: non-maleficence) are often incurred for fetal benefit (beneficence) with or without direct maternal benefit.

INTRODUCTION

The *maternal–fetal conflict* is defined as: "any situation where maternal well-being or wishes contradict fetal benefit."[1] Anesthesiologists caring for obstetric patients frequently balance both maternal and fetal risks and benefits in the interest of patient safety. Occasionally, interventions conferring fetal benefits can impose maternal harms or risks, and mothers declining such interventions can pose an ethical challenge. Conversely, the standard care for emergency procedures during labor and delivery is often assumed for their direct fetal safety benefits, frequently with limited consideration to maternal physical and mental harms. In these situations, the ethical principles of nonmaleficence and beneficence can be in direct conflict, and the ethical principle of maternal autonomy underpins most decisions. For example, in fetal surgery, maternal physical risks (conflict: nonmaleficence) are incurred for fetal benefit (beneficence) without direct maternal benefit. Another example is emergent cesarean

[a] Department of Anesthesiology, Perioperative and Pain Medicine, Harvard Medical School, Brigham and Women's Hospital, 75 Francis Street, Boston, MA 02115, USA; [b] Department of Anesthesiology & Pain Medicine, Nationwide Children's Hospital, 700 Children's Drive, Columbus, OH 43205, USA; [c] Department of Anesthesiology and Perioperative Medicine, University of Pittsburgh School of Medicine, UPMC Magee Women's Hospital, 300 Halket Street Suite 3403, Pittsburgh, PA 15215, USA
* Corresponding author. 75 Francis Street, L1 Anesthesia Offices, Boston, MA 021115.
E-mail address: sseifert@bwh.harvard.edu

Anesthesiology Clin 42 (2024) 491–502
https://doi.org/10.1016/j.anclin.2023.12.007
1932-2275/24/© 2023 Elsevier Inc. All rights reserved.

delivery, where many urgent maternal physical interventions are inflicted with a distressed fetus in mind, but which may be simultaneously psychologically traumatic for the mother and increase risk for postpartum mental health complications.[2–4]

In this article, the authors review some common and uncommon clinical situations where the maternal–fetal conflict directly intersects with anesthesia care and management. The authors consider ethical frameworks to approach such situations and provide practical examples for how to apply these principles to clinical anesthesia practice.

CASE STUDY #1: NEURAXIAL VERSUS GENERAL ANESTHESIA
Key Consideration: Patient and Provider Conflicts on Anesthetic Selection

Case presentation
A 32-year-old gravida 1 para 0 (G1P0) at 36 weeks is scheduled for an urgent cesarean delivery. The patient had been laboring with nitrous oxide inhalation with the fetal heart rate monitor recording deep variable decelerations for the past 40 minutes. The patient has a body mass index of 42, diabetes, gestational hypertension, and gastroesophageal reflux disorder. She has a class 3 airway and her platelet count is 122K. The anesthesiologist desires to perform spinal anesthesia; however, the patient insists on receiving general anesthesia.

Clinical questions

1. What happens when the preferences of the patient and anesthesiologist are in conflict?
2. Does labor pain or the use of maternal analgesic agents affect the ability to consent?
3. Is there a role for other practitioners (eg, obstetrician/maternal fetal medicine specialist, neonatologist) in determining the route of anesthesia?
4. How can reflection, inquiry, and advocacy assist in the resolution of a difficult conversation?

Discussion
The optimal anesthetic management for a surgical intervention is based on myriad factors and relies on acceptance of the plan by the patient and all providers. Unique to surgery during pregnancy is the increased anesthetic risk profile due to pregnancy-related alterations in anatomy (eg, airway edema, friability), physiology (eg, increased metabolic demand, less functional residual capacity, faster desaturation), and pharmacology (eg, increased volume of distribution, less protein binding) as well as fetal concerns.[5]

General anesthesia for cesarean delivery has been associated with greater maternal mortality, mostly related to complications in airway management, aspiration, and ventilation when compared with neuraxial anesthesia.[6] Recent evidence from the Centers for Disease Control and Prevention, the Serious Complication Registry from the Society for Obstetric Anesthesia and Perinatology, the Multicenter Perioperative Outcomes Group, and the American Society of Anesthesiologists (ASA) Closed Claims Project has indicated that maternal airway management has become safer, at least in the United States and high-income countries. Improvements in equipment and training to manage expected and unexpected difficult airways, including video laryngoscopes and supraglottic airway devices, difficult airway algorithms and multidisciplinary simulation, and team training, have made a significant impact.[6] However, maternal mortality and morbidity from failed intubation, extubation difficulties, and postoperative respiratory and ventilation issues still occur.[7] When compared with neuraxial anesthesia, maternal general anesthesia has also been associated with intraoperative awareness, worse postoperative pain, delayed mobilization, and impaired breastfeeding success,[8] as well as lower fetal pH values, Apgar scores, and ventilatory independence.[9] Moreover, based on findings in rodent and nonhuman primate models, unresolved concerns exist on the effects of anesthetic agents, particularly halogenated gasses, on neurodevelopment: neuronal creation, migration, differentiation, synapsis formation, and reorganization. Of note, the clinical interpretation of these findings in humans remains elusive.[10]

General anesthesia is uncommon in modern obstetric practices; high rates of neuraxial anesthesia utilization allow for its avoidance, particularly in people at high risk for cesarean delivery or difficult airway management issues.[11] However, maternal morbidity related to neuraxial anesthesia (eg, headache, nerve injury) occurs, including pain and emotional distress resulting from sensations during surgery with the subsequent failure to provide sedation or induce general anesthesia.[8] As a result, each form of anesthesia offers risks that must be balanced with their potential benefits. General anesthesia provides an absence of all sensation but also an absence of the mother and partner in participating in delivery. Neuraxial anesthesia offers the opportunity to witness the birth, but with the possibility of feeling touch, pressure, and other sensations that may be assessed as unpleasant by some people.

Conversations between patients and providers should consider how specific benefits and risks related to general versus neuraxial anesthesia affect their own decision-making (**Table 1**). Courts and expert opinion indicate that "material risks," which are potential complications that a reasonable patient would consider important for decision-making, should be specifically discussed. Materials risks are most often interpreted as those that have high incidence, high morbidity, or a high probability of adverse fetal implications.[12]

When patient and provider decisions are not in alignment, optimal communication is essential. Four primary types of communication failure result from misunderstandings in the (1) occasion–situation or context; often a delay in test results, (2) audience–composition of group: key person missing from discussion, (3) purpose–reason unclear, not achieved or inappropriate: a disagreement on treatment plan, or (4) content–insufficient, inaccurate or no information: omission of needed information.[13] In our case example, improved communication and decisional unity could be fostered by greater sharing of content and purpose. Content and purpose account for 60% and 15%, respectively, of the communication failures that result in an anesthetic malpractice claim,[14] with 84% of these failures involving a patient or family members occurring before surgery. A place to start such discussions is with a common purpose (eg, "ensuring the most safe and optimal care and outcomes for mother and baby"); subsequently, decisional factors relevant to the current situation and practice environment can be shared (see **Table 1**).

Perceptions, interpretations, or values likely influence how decisional factors are interpreted. Providers known to the patient (eg, obstetricians) or those with novel information (eg, neonatologist, maternal fetal medicine obstetrician, and radiologist) can provide input into decisions. Racial and ethnic disparities regarding acceptability of various analgesia and anesthesia,[8] emotions, and identity issues (eg, what does this say about me?) may further influence a person's engagement in a discussion. Language or cultural barriers can be minimized with the use of translators or providers who speak the same language or are from similar backgrounds and the use of language-specific educational resources. Often used as a surrogate for comprehension, accurate recall does not seem to be influenced by labor discomfort, opioid premedication, age, education level, or previous epidural analgesia experience.[12]

Table 1
Decisional factors in considering neuraxial versus general anesthesia for cesarean delivery

Factor	Favoring Neuraxial	Favoring General
Maternal condition	Patient refusal of general anesthesia Aspiration risk Difficult airway Patient desires to witness the birth	Patient refusal of neuraxial anesthesia Uncorrected coagulopathy Hemodynamic instability Neurologic (brain/spinal cord) issues that preclude neuraxial Anticipated difficult neuraxial placement
Fetal conditions	Mitigates transplacental transfer of sedative agents	Facilitates rapid delivery in cases of severe fetal distress
Anesthesia concerns	Limited general anesthesia experience or equipment	Limited neuraxial anesthesia experience or equipment Greater maternal/mortality risk than with neuraxial anesthesia
Surgical concerns	History or risk for challenging postoperative pain management	Surgeries for which controlled ventilation, muscle relaxation, significant Trendelenburg positioning may be of value

In considering how these elements affect comprehension, consensus, and consent, three steps are helpful in reaching a mutual understanding: reflection, inquiry, and advocacy. Starting first with reflection (ie, assessing your own beliefs and biases and checking your emotions) and advancing to inquiry (ie, attempting to understand the other person's viewpoint, with nonjudgmental openness) will allow a good basis for acknowledgment and sensitivity to the issues and context surrounding each participant's viewpoint. Each subsequent cycle of inquiry and advocacy should be oriented toward gaining an agreement; agreements should not be a subordination of one viewpoint or a compromise between the two viewpoints, but rather the recognition of a third viewpoint as an optimal outcome in the particular situation. Summarizing the steps for comprehension and agreement then allows both parties to move forward.

Ultimately, patient autonomy is a dominant factor in medical decision-making and must be respected, with the mother accepting the possibility of positive or negative outcomes based on her decisions.[12] Improved communication, through the discussion of risks and benefits, and acknowledgment of how perceptions, interpretations, and values influence decisions can be augmented through a cycle(s) of reflection, inquiry, and advocacy (**Fig. 1**). These tools should be oriented toward gaining a perspective, which often represents a new third viewpoint, when this consensus has been made, consent and more definitive care can begin.

Summary: When deciding the optimal anesthetic management for surgical interventions during pregnancy, providers should prioritize shared decision-making. Although neuraxial anesthesia is generally preferred due to its safety profile, the potential risks and benefits of both neuraxial and general anesthesia should be thoroughly discussed with the patient. Effective communication, considering the specific risks and benefits of each option and acknowledging the influence of individual patient perceptions and values, is crucial in achieving patient autonomy and upholding informed consent.

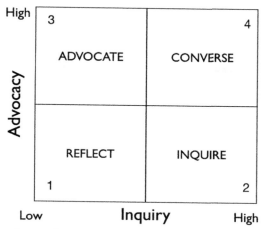

Fig. 1. Advocacy–inquiry two-by-two diagram.

Clinics care points

- An appreciation of the risks and benefits of selecting neuraxial versus general anesthesia includes maternal, fetal, anesthesia, and surgical issues.
- Difficult conversations are more than the known facts and include perceptions, emotions, and identity issues.
- Conflict resolution should begin with reflection, move to inquiry, and then finally advocacy in a desire to engage in a conversation that seeks resolution. An agreement, rather than compromise, should be sought and the plan articulated.

CASE STUDY #2: PAIN DURING CESAREAN DELIVERY
Key Consideration: Management of Pain During Cesarean Delivery and Long-Term Effects

Case presentation
A 27-year-old G1P1 patient presents to a follow-up appointment with her obstetrician, approximately 6 weeks following emergent cesarean delivery of a healthy female infant. She reports difficulty sleeping, irritability, and feelings of detachment from her newborn. She is unsure why she feels "nothing" when she holds her baby and feels unmotivated to continue breastfeeding. She attributes her feelings to being exhausted from having a new baby and considers this as being "normal" after a prolonged induction of labor and traumatic emergency delivery. She notes that her epidural pain relief "barely worked" and she felt tearing, stabbing pain followed by intense drowsiness with minimal recollection of the delivery. She is thankful that her baby did well without complications, but she is unsure whether she saw her baby until the day after delivery, and wonders if this is why she feels detached from the newborn bonding process.

Clinical questions

1. How do we balance the risks and benefits of anesthetic techniques in the management of intraoperative pain during cesarean delivery?
2. How do real-time clinical decisions impact patients in the immediate and future postoperative periods?

3. How best do we implement a shared decision-making model with patients while in a high acuity setting or in cases of patient distress?

Discussion

The anesthetic plan for cesarean delivery depends on many factors, including urgency of delivery and the patient's history with presence or absence of contraindications to neuraxial anesthesia. As discussed in Case #1, the patient's goals and priorities should be considered using a shared decision-making approach. Although most commonly performed under neuraxial anesthesia to reduce both maternal and fetal risks of general anesthesia, neuraxial anesthesia may be contraindicated or inadequate. In these circumstances, it is important to discuss the alternatives, whether it be supplemental intravenous medications or general anesthesia in the context of the potential benefits as well as risks. More data are becoming available regarding the incidence of patient-reported pain during cesarean delivery and the potential for long-term sequelae of uncontrolled pain related to inadequate neuraxial anesthesia.

A large systematic review reported the incidence of supplemental analgesia use to be 15% in elective cesarean deliveries with a similar incidence in a study including unplanned and intrapartum cesarean deliveries.[15,16] Several studies, and litigation against obstetric anesthesiologists, have highlighted the complication of poorly controlled pain during labor and cesarean delivery.[17] Not only is inadequate anesthesia distressing at the time of delivery but also the negative physical and psychological effects can persist for years. Failure or inadequacy of neuraxial anesthesia has been tied to postpartum depression and, in severe cases, post-traumatic stress disorder.[16,18]

One of the challenges with investigating failed neuraxial anesthesia is that pain is inherently subjective. An anesthesiologist may feel that a neuraxial anesthetic is functioning based on his or her assessment of the block, but ultimately the patient's perception of pain and experience in the operating room is the most important. For some patients, pressure and tugging sensations during cesarean delivery are quite uncomfortable and distressing and can lead to long-term emotional consequences. One of the common threads through cases in litigation, patient complaints, and discussion during debriefing conversations is that patients felt unheard or that their complaints of pain were not taken seriously.[19] Close communication with the patient during delivery, listening to concerns, respecting patient autonomy, and quickly acting on discomfort is just as critical in creating an environment of trust and promoting beneficence as is performing a neuraxial block itself. Part of being a skilled provider is recognizing the limitations of a procedure and having a plan to mitigate all outcomes.[20]

A unique feature of the labor and delivery setting is the frequency at which plans must adapt to dynamic conditions where rapid decision-making may be necessary in highly emotionally charged situations. True informed consent is often not feasible in these emergent scenarios. Therefore, it is important to consider two practice points. First, care systems can evolve such that advanced conversations with anesthesia providers are facilitated, before the onset of emergencies, so that clinicians can provide as much information as possible, patient preferences and attitudes can be explored, therapeutic alliances can be built, and a mutually agreed on plan can be developed and documented. Second, when advanced conversations are not possible, anesthesia clinicians must make every effort in a short period of time to engage such therapeutic conversations and to assist patients in establishing their goals for care.

In emergency cases where advanced conversations and care priorities could not be established, emergency consent or assent is invoked. Assent is the expression of approval or agreement with the care plans. If the patient cannot give assent in an emergency situation, presumed patient assent is invoked based on what is known about their preferences and the principle of beneficence. In an emergency situation, involving in which informed consent cannot be obtained because immediate treatment is required to preserve "life or limb" and to prevent serious health impairment. In these situations, patients (decision-makers) rely on the provider to provide care. It is assumed that medical and anesthesia providers act as agents for patient safety, and decisions are made based on existing care standards and reasonable practice. A decision to provide anxiolysis, sedation, repeat the neuraxial, or convert to general anesthesia, in cases of persistent discomfort with neuraxial anesthesia for cesarean delivery, depends on patient medical risk factors (airway examination, nil per os status), patient preferences, obstetric surgical considerations, and patient autonomy and assent.

Summary: Neuraxial anesthesia is usually preferred in cesarean delivery due to its safety profile for both the mother and fetus. However, recognizing instances where neuraxial anesthesia is contraindicated, inadequate, or not desired by the patient is crucial. Early conversations, before the eruption of an emergency, and ideally using a shared decision-making approach, are essential in the dynamic labor and delivery setting. Clinical care must emphasize the importance of providing comprehensive information efficiently to establish therapeutic alliances and ensure a safe and effective care plan. In cases where these plans could not be ascertained before the onset of an emergency, anesthesia providers are agents for patient safety, and the decision to adjust anesthesia care (eg, repeat neuraxial, anxiolysis, conversion to general anesthesia) is made based on existing care standards and reasonable practice given the specific care situation as well as patient assent.

Clinics care points

- Anesthetic plans should be tailored to the individual patient, taking into account the risks and benefits of each type of anesthetic to both the patient and the fetus, the clinical setting, as well as the patient's goals and preferences using a shared decision-making approach.

- Uncontrolled pain in labor and delivery is associated with long-term effects such as postpartum depression and post-traumatic stress disorder.

- In emergency situations, where shared decision-making and informed consent are not feasible due to the urgency of care, anesthesia providers make clinical decisions based on existing care standards and reasonable practice to safely conclude the essential procedures. Patient assent to treatment should also be considered in these situations.

CASE STUDY #3: FETAL SURGERY
Key Consideration: Ethical Dilemmas in Maternal–Fetal Surgery

Case presentation

A 21-year-old G1P0 with no significant past medical history presenting at 22 weeks 4 days with a fetus found to have an open neural tube defect at T9. The fetus has Chiari II hindbrain herniation with associated mild ventriculomegaly. She does not like the idea of having fetal surgery, but her partner and her family believe that an intrauterine repair is best for the fetus. The patient and her partner present for consultation.

Clinical questions

1. Who is the patient? Are there one or two patients in maternal–fetal surgery? Is there a primary patient?

2. Does the fetus have patienthood rights within an ethical framework? Does this pose a threat to a pregnant patient's autonomy?
3. How do you balance the risks and benefits between the pregnant patient and the fetus?
4. What components should be included in informed consent for these procedures?

Discussion

The practice of fetal surgery is rapidly evolving as technology and science advances. In part, this is due to improvements in antepartum diagnosis and the development of minimally invasive techniques. Historically, the only options people had when faced with a significant fetal diagnosis was to terminate the pregnancy or continue the pregnancy anticipating delivery of a child with a substantial medical condition. Initially, fetal intervention was only offered in severe cases that were expected to result in fetal or neonatal death because the risks to the fetus were so significant. Now, however, maternal–fetal surgery has advanced such that interventions are offered not as a means to ensure fetal survival, but rather as a mechanism to alleviate or eliminate childhood disability. In addition, anesthetic and surgical approaches are safer than before. Despite these advances in clinical options, there is often tension between maternal and fetal interests based on risk; inherently, maternal–fetal surgery is unique in that it involves varying degrees of risk to the pregnant patient depending on the invasiveness (percutaneous, fetoscopic, or open) without *direct* benefit but potential significant benefit for the fetal patient.[21–23] The progressing field of maternal–fetal surgery introduces critical ethical issues and it becomes necessary to consider the ethical framework for formal determination of conditions that meet ethical qualifications for intervention.[24–26]

In the case above, the historical standard treatment for spina bifida was postnatal surgical intervention such that there is no direct risk to the pregnant patient. The Management of Myelomeningocele Study, a randomized controlled trial comparing prenatal and postnatal repair, observed that prenatal surgery on fetuses up to 26 weeks improved the ability to walk independently with no differences in long-term need for CSF shunting or cognitive outcomes. Surgeries typically involve a laparotomy for the pregnant patient with either an open hysterotomy or a newer fetoscopic approach through the uterus. Neural tube defect surgeries have risks to both the pregnant patient and the fetal patient, including preterm labor or delivery (potentially emergently), chorioamnionitis, and placental abruption. Risks for the pregnant patient include allergic reactions, pulmonary edema, bleeding, risks associated with blood transfusions, hospital admission for 4 to 7 days, painful recovery, risks of neuraxial or nerve block procedures, risks of general anesthesia, increased risk for difficult airway in pregnancy, uterine rupture, and postoperative risks (urinary tract infection [UTI], deep vein thrombosis [DVT], and so forth). Risks for the fetus include preterm delivery (potentially emergently), chorioamniotic separation, further injury from the surgery itself, long exposure to general anesthesia, and oligohydramnios.[23] Other potential harms include psychological harm in addition to the costs of traveling to and staying near a center. However, pregnancy itself involves risks to the pregnant patient's health and well-being including pregnancy-related diseases and complications during birth and the postpartum period.[27]

In maternal–fetal surgery, a pregnant patient presents for care, and now, more than ever before, medical providers are able to provide treatment with fewer risks. Two important and controversial questions in thinking about the relationship between the pregnant patient and the fetal patient are "who is the patient" and "what are the potential fetal patienthood rights?" Pregnant people have autonomy and personhood status, but fetuses lack these key features as they exist within the maternal patient. The moral status of the fetus is largely considered dependent on a pregnant patient's autonomous control over her body. Autonomy is necessary for personhood, but may not be for patienthood. Because the pregnant patient is the one who presents for care, the fetus' patienthood status could be conceptualized as being conferred by the pregnant patient's decision to present for treatment.[27,28]

Three proposed models to describe patienthood status in maternal–fetal surgery include the following: (1) one-patient model with the fetus considered part of and dependent on the mother for the duration of the pregnancy; (2) two-patient model where both the pregnant patient and the fetal patient have equal patienthood rights; and (3) dyad models that acknowledge the interdependence of the pregnant patient and the fetus, such as a two-patient ecosystem model.[23,27]

In the one-patient model, the pregnant patient should be considered the sole patient to ensure her autonomous ability to make choices to undergo procedures with risk of bodily harm to her. In addition, this model allows us to not venture into legally regulating a pregnant patient's behavior based on the fetus. In a single-patient model, the fetal well-being is supported by ensuring the pregnant patient's autonomy. Generally, it is in the pregnant patient's best interest to optimize both her and her fetus' health and functional outcomes.[23,27]

Because the fetus has the potential to become a child, some would contend that this confers an independent value for the fetus. Conflict in the context of maternal–fetal surgery with a two-patient model could be a pregnant patient declining surgery despite potential benefit for the fetus. In this example, the medical provider may have a beneficence-based obligation to the fetus that would be in conflict with the provider's beneficence-based and autonomy-based obligations to the pregnant patient. There is also the principle of nonmaleficence of the pregnant person to the fetus and of the medical providers to their patients.[23,27]

The third model aligns with qualitative research into how pregnant patients and their families view the status of the fetus within the context of the pregnancy. Most of the patients surveyed in one study reported that it was morally acceptable for the pregnant patient to undergo surgery for the benefit of the fetus. Interestingly, if the first two models are too simplistic and the third model is accepted, fetal therapy can be conceptualized as benefiting the pregnant patient because she includes the fetus. Similarly, supporting the pregnant patient will support the fetus. Medical providers can then move forward working cooperatively with the pregnant patient for common linked goals of maternal, fetal, and family well-being. The issue may still remain that goals for each may be in conflict where medical providers have to balance their obligations. Of note, there is an ever evolving viability threshold that will be passed at some point, which further complicates these discussions.[23,27,28]

Informed consent is also a critical aspect of maternal–fetal surgery. Informed consent should be comprehensive and include prenatal and postnatal options as well as including discussions with maternal–fetal medicine, neonatologists, pediatric neurosurgeons, and anesthesiologists. A strong institutional support system with mental health providers is also an integral part of care.[21,22,29] Although the pregnant patient's partner will have their own views and interests, the American College of Obstetricians and Gynecologists Committee on Ethics and the American Academy of Pediatrics Committee on Bioethics have stated their support for the pregnant patient having ultimate autonomy over the decision to undergo maternal–fetal surgery. It should also be clear if the procedures in discussion are investigative rather than therapeutic. Last, many centers have an ethical oversight committee to review cases and assess risks and potential benefits. Similarly, the institutional review board can provide oversight and monitoring for investigative options and ongoing monitoring. As new maternal–fetal surgery centers are built and new interventions offer opportunities, equitable access to services should be a principal focus. Patients with a lower socio-economic status are more likely to have fetuses at risk for neural tube defects and lower engagement in care. The ethical principle of justice can be applied to ensure the accessibility of maternal–fetal interventions to all patients.[23]

Medical providers have beneficence-based ethical obligations to the pregnant patient to empower them to make informed decisions about the pregnancy and beneficence-based obligations to the fetal patients. In fetal surgery, it is easy to focus the fetus. Medical providers do, however, have autonomy-based ethical obligations only to the pregnancy patient. Therefore, many have advocated that pregnant patients should be centered so as not to jeopardize their autonomy. Instead of thinking about conflict, providers can think about ensuring informed decision-making and supporting autonomy in a dyad model. Any ethical framework should center the pregnant person's autonomy and prevent pregnant patients from being pressured into having a surgical procedure if they do not want it. In addition, the pregnant patient's view of the procedure, the risks, and the fetal status must be understood.[24,27]

Summary: Maternal–fetal surgery has evolved with technological advancements, shifting from survival-focused interventions to addressing childhood disability. Ethical complexities arise from tensions between maternal and fetal interests, influenced by the proposed patienthood models. Ensuring informed consent, oversight, and equitable access underscore the ethical considerations in this evolving field of health care.

SUMMARY

In conclusion, high-quality obstetric anesthesia practice often demands a delicate navigation through the complexities of maternal–fetal conflict, where the equilibrium between risks and benefits to both mother and fetus is paramount. The ethical principles of maternal autonomy, beneficence, and nonmaleficence serve as guiding posts in these challenging scenarios. Incorporating advocacy–inquiry into the informed consent process is a valuable tool to allow clinicians to explore and incorporate patient preferences, priorities, attitudes, and beliefs into clinical planning. By fostering a collaborative and informed decision-making process, obstetric anesthesia clinicians can strive for a balance that not only respects the autonomy of the mother but also prioritizes the well-being of both mother and fetus.

CLINICS CARE POINTS

- The principle of maternal autonomy underpins most decisions in maternal–fetal surgery with informed decision-making in the framework of maternal–fetal dyad model.
- When engaging in maternal–fetal surgery, it is imperative for medical providers to prioritize informed decision-making. Balancing beneficence toward the fetus with respect for the pregnant patient's autonomy ensures ethical and patient-centered care.

DISCLOSURE

G. Lim receives salary and research support from NIH UH3CA261067, NIH U01TR003719, and NIH R01MH134538 and receives research support, consulting honoraria, and chairs or is a member of advisory board from industry: Octapharma, Heron Pharmaceuticals, Edwards Lifesciences, Haemonetics, Werfen. Dr G. Lim receives stipends for medical expert testimony not related to this publication and receives royalties from Cambridge University Press for a textbook. Dr G. Lim is a consultant reviewer for ACOG and ASA liaison to the ACOG Alliance for Innovation on Maternal Health's (AIM) Clinical and Community Advisory Group.

REFERENCES

1. Fasouliotis SJ, Schenker JG. Maternal-fetal conflict. Eur J Obstet Gynecol Reprod Biol 2000;89(1):101–7.
2. Silverstein RG, Centore M, Pollack A, et al. Postpartum psychological distress after emergency team response during childbirth. J Psychosom Obstet Gynaecol 2019;40(4):304–10.
3. De Schepper S, Vercauteren T, Tersago J, et al. Post-traumatic stress disorder after childbirth and the influence of maternity team care during labour and birth: a cohort study. Midwifery 2016;32:87–92.
4. Chan SJ, Ein-Dor T, Mayopoulos PA, et al. Risk factors for developing posttraumatic stress disorder following childbirth. Psychiatr Res 2020;290:113090.
5. Bleeser T, Vally JC, Van de Velde M, et al. General anaesthesia for nonobstetric surgery during pregnancy: A narrative review. European Journal of Anaesthesiology Intensive Care 2022;1(2):e003.
6. Hawkins JL. Excess in moderation: general anesthesia for cesarean delivery. Anesth Analg 2015;120(6):1175–7.
7. Mhyre JM, Riesner MN, Polley LS, et al. A series of anesthesia-related maternal deaths in Michigan, 1985-2003. Anesthesiology 2007;106:1096–104.
8. Mhyre JM, Sultan P. General anesthesia for cesarean delivery: occasionally essential but best avoided. Anesthesiology 2019;130:864–6.
9. Palmer E, Ciechanowicz S, Reeve A, et al. Operating room-to-incision interval and neonatal outcome in emergency caesarean section: a retrospective 5-year cohort study. Anaesthesia 2018;73:825–31.
10. Ing C, Warner DO, Sun LS, et al. Anesthesia and developing brains: unanswered questions and proposed paths forward. Anesthesiology 2022;136:500–12.
11. Bauer ME, Kountanis JA, Tsen LC, et al. Risk factors for failed conversion of labor epidural analgesia to cesarean delivery anesthesia: a systematic review and meta-analysis of observational trials. Int J Obstet Anesth 2012;21:294–309.
12. Broaddus BM, Chandrasekhar S. Informed consent in obstetric anesthesia. Anesth Analg 2011;112:912–5.
13. Lingard L, Espin S, Whyte S, et al. Communication failures in the operating room: an observational classification of recurrent types and effects. Qual Saf Health Care 2004;13:330–4.
14. Douglas RN, Stephens LS, Posner KL, et al. Communication failures contributing to patient injury in anaesthesia malpractice claims. Br J Anaesth 2021;127:470–8.
15. Patel R, Kua J, Sharawi N, et al. Inadequate neuraxial anaesthesia in patients undergoing elective cesarean section: a systematic review. Anaesthesia 2022;77:598–604.
16. Sanchez J, Prabhu R, Guglielminotti J, et al. Pain during cesarean delivery: A patient-related prospective observational study assessing the incidence and risk factors for intraoperative pain and intravenous medication administration. Anaesth Crit Care Pain Med 2023;101310.
17. McCombe K, Bogod DG. Learning from the law. A review of 21 years of litigation for pain during cesarean section. Anaesthesia 2018;73:223–30.

18. Lim G, LaSorda K, Farrell L, et al. Obstetric pain correlates with postpartum depression symptoms: a pilot prospective observational study. BMC Pregnancy Childbirth 2020 Apr 22;20(1):240.

19. Stanford S. What is 'genuine' failure of neuraxial anaesthesia? Anaesthesia 2022; 77:523–6.

20. Ryan G, Brandi K. Informed consent and shared decision making in obstetrics and gynecology. Obstet Gynecol 2021 Feb 1;137(2):e34–41.

21. Austin MT, Cole TR, McCullough LB, et al. Ethical challenges in invasive maternal-fetal intervention. Semin Pediatr Surg 2019;28(4):150819.

22. Flake AW. Prenatal intervention: ethical considerations for life-threatening and non-life-threatening anomalies. Semin Pediatr Surg 2001;10(4):212–21.

23. Radic JAE, Illes J, McDonald PJ. Fetal repair of open neural tube defects: ethical, legal, and social issues. Camb Q Healthc Ethics 2019;28(3):476–87.

24. Antiel RM, Flake AW, Collura CA, et al. Weighing the social and ethical considerations of maternal-fetal surgery. Pediatrics 2017;140(6):e20170608.

25. Rousseau AC, Riggan KA, Schenone MH, et al. Ethical considerations of maternal-fetal surgery. J Perinat Med 2022;50(5):519–27. Published 2022 Jan 31.

26. Deprest JA, Flake AW, Gratacos E, et al. The making of fetal surgery. Prenat Diagn 2010;30(7):653–67.

27. Bartlett VL, Bliton MJ. Retrieving the moral in the ethics of maternal-fetal surgery. Camb Q Healthc Ethics 2020;29(3):480–93.

28. Begović D. Maternal-fetal surgery: does recognising fetal patienthood pose a threat to pregnant women's autonomy? Health Care Anal 2021;29(4):301–18.

29. Fry J, Antiel RM, Michelson K, et al. Ethics in prenatal consultation for surgically correctable anomalies and fetal intervention. Semin Pediatr Surg 2021;30(5): 151102.

Ethical Care of Pregnant Patients During Labor, Delivery, and Nonobstetric Surgery

Carlos Delgado, MD[a],*, Jo Davies, MB BS, FRCA[b]

KEYWORDS

- Pregnancy • Ethics • Nonobstetric surgery • Consent • Conflict

KEY POINTS

- The 4 basic ethical principles can conflict with each other when using them as a framework to guide difficult clinical decisions for the pregnant patient, so a careful assessment of the patient's goals of care, preferences, and social environment can inform and guide the consent and risks/benefits conversation.
- It is not uncommon to have dueling maternal and fetal interests at play, and the beneficence and autonomy-based obligations we have as providers to our 2 patients should be kept in mind in complex situations.
- Labor and mode of delivery (vaginal vs cesarean) should never be a barrier to have a thorough shared decision-making conversation with proper obtainment of consent.
- Nonobstetric surgery during pregnancy is not an uncommon scenario and a meticulous discussion of indications, risks, and benefits should be done ahead of the procedure, with special attention paid to defining necessity and extent of fetal monitoring and potential interventions.

INTRODUCTION

The care of pregnant women as they navigate labor and delivery, and when nonobstetric surgery is required, can be ethically fraught due to the potential conflicts between maternal and fetal interests. The vulnerability of both patients requires a unique understanding of ethical principles and concepts. This enables clear communication with pregnant patients, tailored to their individual needs and supportive of a trustworthy patient-provider relationship, while facilitating clinical decision-making. In this article, we will examine definitions and terminology from the foundations of medical ethics,

[a] Department of Anesthesiology and Pain Medicine, University of Washington, 1959 Northeast Pacific Street, Box 356540, Seattle WA 98195, USA; [b] Department of Anesthesiology and Pain Medicine, University of Washington, University of Washington Medical Center, 1959 Northeast Pacific Street, Box 356540, Seattle WA 98195, USA
* Corresponding author.
E-mail address: delgadou@uw.edu

Anesthesiology Clin 42 (2024) 503–514
https://doi.org/10.1016/j.anclin.2023.12.008
1932-2275/24/© 2024 Elsevier Inc. All rights reserved.

anesthesiology.theclinics.com

including consent, capacity, shared decision-making, and maternal-fetal conflict, framed in the setting of vaginal and cesarean delivery, and when nonobstetric surgery is indicated in a pregnant patient.

DEFINITIONS

Commonly, 4 basic ethics principles are used to guide medical decision-making. These principles should not be ordered in hierarchical order, and none is absolute or exceptionless.[1] Ethical conflict should be resolved by balancing and negotiating the impact each principle has on a specific clinical situation.

Beneficence

This concept can be understood as the obligation of a physician to act for the benefit of the patient. It includes defending individual's rights, preventing harm and removing conditions that endanger them. It also highlights the duty to benefit patients and promote their welfare.[2]

Nonmaleficence

Nonmaleficence compels physicians not to harm a patient, usually by balancing risks and benefits of interventions while understanding that both actions and omissions in care may affect the desired best outcome for the patient. It's important to recognize that most medical interventions are associated to some degree of harm.[3]

Autonomy

Allowing individuals to exercise the power to make rational decisions and moral choices constitutes the definition of autonomy. This principle does not extend to people that lack the capacity to act autonomously. A physician can make the determination of the presence or absence of decision-making capacities in a patient.[2] Disclosing information in a truthful and confidential manner, as well as obtaining appropriate informed consent, is essential to acknowledging autonomy.

Justice

This principle can be interpreted as the fair, equitable, and appropriate treatment of patients. In clinical situations, an important consideration relates to the appropriate distribution of health resources as well as the identification of financial, educational, or research conflicts of interest with the treating provider.[2] Ultimately, the implementation of fair practices geared toward eliminating social biases and disparities in access to health services allows for justice to be maintained when providing care.[3]

Commonly, these ethical principles can conflict with each other. There are useful questions a clinician can ask to evaluate the impact of each principle in patient care (**Table 1**). A balanced and systematic approach should include[4]

- A clinical assessment, identifying medical problems and treatment options
- Patient clarification of their preferences and goals of care
- An analysis of the effects of the medical problem and treatment plans on a patient's quality of life
- An awareness of the social, familiar, and cultural context surrounding the patient

TERMINOLOGY
Shared Decision-Making

Informed decision-making is the process by which a patient's autonomy can be exercised, demonstrated, and legally evaluated.[5] A physician provides pertinent

Table 1 Questions to address each ethical principle	
Autonomy	Is the patient empowered to give consent for interventions that align with their expressed values, beliefs, and preferences?
Beneficence	Is the proposed intervention consistent with what the patient says is in their best interest?
Nonmaleficence	Despite the risks associated with any intervention, is it doing a greater good than harm for this patient?
Justice	Is this patient being treated similarly to similarly situated patients? If not, what is the morally compelling explanation?

From Mann DG, Sutton CD. Ethics in the Labor and Delivery Unit. Anesthesiol Clin. 2021 Dec;39(4):839-849.

risks and benefits of a proposed course of action and then the patient analyses which choice may be the most beneficial for them in a specific situation. Both physician and patient decide on a mutually acceptable medical care choice,[6] after discussing the patient's values and emotional and social needs. It is important to note that when only 1 medically reasonable alternative is present, it should be strongly recommended.[7] A shared decision approach has been shown to improve patient satisfaction and reduce health care–related costs.[8] For anesthesia providers, the best location to adequately use a shared decision-making model is the preoperative clinic. Frequently, providers meet the patient right before their procedure or in an urgent/emergent setting, making these conversations challenging.[9] Anticipatory conversations in the preoperative clinic with not only the patient but also their social support system can make the shared decision model more successful. The use of decision aids, which are printed or audiovisual tools to facilitate counseling, can improve patient understanding of risks and benefits and lead to the provision of care that closely aligns with patient values.[10]

Informed Consent

Informed consent in modern medicine highlights the value of the ethical principle of autonomy and is a core element in the physician-patient relationship. Obtaining accurate and reliable consent in time-limited interactions can be a challenge for the anesthesiologist.[11] Physicians are required to provide their patients information that a reasonable individual would want to know when making a medical decision.[12] The process of obtaining consent requires patient capacity to understand and process the information provided, ask questions, and make a voluntary decision to accept or refuse what is being offered. This information exchange should be accurately documented.[13] It is important to highlight that consent is not simply a signed form; the form suggests a discussion took place, but it does not guarantee immunity if the delivered information was insufficient or if it was provided in the wrong setting.[14]

Capacity

Capacity can be understood as a patient's ability to understand, appreciate, and evaluate information to form a rational decision on how to proceed in a specific situation. Capacity is determined by the treating physician and can be impacted by situational stress, age, and mental status. It is important that the patient can communicate a decision after comparing risks and benefits of a treatment or intervention considering their own clinical situation.[11]

Maternal and Fetal Conflict

Many ethical conflicts in obstetrics revolve around the maternal-fetal relationship. Although most pregnant women aim to achieve a positive outcome for their pregnancy, which will likely result in a positive outcome for their unborn child, sometimes interests of the mother do not correspond with the interests of the fetus. In these situations, maternal-fetal conflict arises.[15] It is common to discuss which rights prevail in these situations. Rights-based reductionism is a concept in ethics where reasoning occurs solely based on the rights of the mother or the rights of the fetus. Unfortunately, this approach ignores the beneficence-based obligations to both mother and fetus. Complex clinical circumstances require the understanding of multiple complementing factors.[16] The professional responsibility model of ethics in obstetrics emphasizes the importance of scientific evidence and the offering of compassionate care to both mother and fetus.[7] A pregnant woman's autonomy is empowered by offering medically reasonable intervention and alternatives.[17]

The fetus as a patient

The fetus can be considered a patient in situations where it is presented as such to the clinician by the pregnant patient and there are interventions to be done that would do more good than harm to the child and the person it can later become.[18] Of note, beneficence-based care is the guiding principle in this scenario. The fetus, due to its immature nervous system at any gestational age, is incapable of asserting any autonomy-based requests for actual clinical practice.[7]

The viable fetus

For the viable fetus, depending on local and/or regional definitions, survival is expected in most cases. Since this survival can be expected to carry on into childhood, recommending care or alternatives that carry fetal benefit, that is, providing *directive counseling*, is appropriate. This aligns with the beneficence-based obligation a physician has to the fetus.[19]

The previable fetus

The previable fetus is not a patient independent from the pregnant woman's autonomy.[1] At the limits of viability, commonly 22 weeks of gestation but variable based on location and access to technological advances, current evidence indicates that survival of the fetus cannot be completely guaranteed. Therefore, nonaggressive obstetric and neonatal management strategies should be offered to the maternal-fetal dyad. These strategies could include, in some situations, avoidance of cesarean delivery or neonatal intubation/resuscitation.[16] *Non-directive counseling* is understood as offering women a choice between alternatives that may carry fetal benefit without causing harm to the pregnant patient.[19] The American Academy of Pediatrics and the American College of Obstetrics and Gynecology agree that when dealing with neonates of uncertain peri-viable state, parental wishes should guide the extent of care provided.[20,21]

ETHICAL ISSUES DURING LABOR AND DELIVERY
Labor

Birth plans

A birth plan is created with the goal of enhancing a patient's autonomy regarding decision-making during the birth process. It commonly outlines how the patient wishes her labor and delivery to progress and often contains a list of procedures and interventions which will or will not be tolerated. While all members of the obstetric team, including the anesthesiologist, attempt to honor the patient's choices described in their birth plan, it is important for patients to understand that unexpected events or unforeseen complications can occur during labor and delivery, and expectations may have to change to accommodate the situation.[22] Given the impact a birth plan can have on the patient's ultimate satisfaction with their labor and delivery experience, it would be highly beneficial to include the anesthesiology service when discussing a patient's birth plan antenatally.[23]

A "Ulysses directive" in obstetric care is used in a birth plan to describe a decision by the patient not to have epidural analgesia during labor even if, when the time comes, she changes her mind. However, this decision is often made prior to the patient experiencing the pain of labor, and possibly without adequate knowledge of the benefits and risks of the procedure. This brings into question if the decision is truly autonomous as opposed to a fully informed decision made during labor when the patient has true understanding of her labor experience and the procedure.[24] However, due to the unpredictability of labor, birth plans can have a profound impact on the ulterior consent process.

Capacity to consent

Many laboring women believe they have the capacity to consent and retain the information provided as readily as other groups of nonlaboring patients,[25] but there is regional variation. In the United States, studies have shown that a vast majority of patients and providers expressed they could give and obtain consent during labor, respectively, contrary to what other studies in Canada, Europe, and Australia have reported.[26,27] Interestingly, studies have shown that recall of risks does not vary based on the pain the patient was suffering at the time of consent.[28] A study on 206 patients in the postpartum period showed that those suffering from labor pain were more likely to be very satisfied with the communication of information than those without labor pain.[29]

Nevertheless, pregnant women prefer the discussion of interventions and their associated risks to take place before labor starts or a procedure is set to occur.[30] Limited language proficiency, level of education, and cultural and socioeconomic factors can impact the consent process as well. The latter becomes evident when assessing how voluntary a decision is made. It is well known that partner and family dynamics may influence the acceptance or refusal of a treatment. In these instances, taking the appropriate approach (ie, asking the family to step away for a while) may minimize the effect of these factors in the provision of consent.

Vaginal delivery and associated procedures

Obstetric patients are entitled to receive information regarding the degree of personal risk while attempting a vaginal delivery, as well as overall and relative risks of the interventions that might be derived from such an attempt.[31] While pregnant women may have differing views on how much information is presented to them during labor, frequent antenatal conversations can help provide realistic expectations and improve the care provided during vaginal delivery.[32]

Unconsented procedures during labor and delivery are a known issue. More than 30% of women were not consented for fetal monitoring during labor in a Dutch study,[33] and an Italian survey reported that close to 40% women in labor were not consented for an episiotomy.[34] Even when consent is obtained, it is frequently substandard. Women who have experienced operative vaginal deliveries report a higher level of dissatisfaction regarding the consent process compared to women undergoing both planned and nonscheduled cesarean deliveries.[35]

Cesarean Delivery

A cesarean delivery is the most common procedure in obstetric practice and requires a balance between the obstetrician's evidence-based clinical judgment (beneficence and nonmaleficence) and a patient's choice (autonomy), once fully informed of the risks and benefits of the procedure and possible alternatives.[17]

Patient-choice cesarean delivery

Patient-choice cesarean delivery is not without controversy, and there is currently insufficient evidence to fully support nonindicated cesarean delivery. Each case must be evaluated in isolation. It is the responsibility of the obstetrician to provide a deliberate and detailed explanation of the best available evidence discussing the benefits and risks of vaginal delivery versus cesarean delivery. The patient can only then truly make an informed decision. While it is important to acknowledge the patient's autonomy, this must be considered together with obstetrician's beneficence-based duty to the patient and the fetus.[17]

Trail of labor after cesarean delivery

In the event of trial of labor after cesarean delivery (TOLAC) after one prior low-transverse cesarean, both attempted vaginal delivery and repeat cesarean delivery are generally considered a safe course of action. Both these options can be offered to the patient with nondirective counseling. However, TOLAC after 2 previous low-transverse incisions is controversial and lacks substantive evidence. Deliberative shared decision-making is critical in this situation. In situations where a repeat cesarean delivery is clearly indicated (eg, previous classical incision) and supported by the evidence, a cesarean delivery should be recommended at the outset.[17]

Refusal of medically indicated cesarean delivery

There are scenarios where a cesarean delivery could maximize the well-being of the fetus, yet it is refused by the pregnant patient and/or their husband or family.[36,37] Providers will need to have a framework to navigate this scenario. The first step is to provide enhanced education, while trying to understand the patient's and the family's perspective. A history of past negative interactions, an unstable social support structure, or cultural and religious beliefs could be impacting her decision.[36] Assessing the degree of burden placed on the patient, as well as the understanding she has on the prospective outcome, is fundamental. Use of professional interpreters, when necessary, can be critical in these discussions. Seeking advice from ethical consultants is strongly encouraged in these challenging situations.[38]

When the goal to respect maternal autonomy conflicts with beneficence-based obligations to the viable fetal patient, persuasive counseling is often acceptable and may be warranted.[19] While coercion is ethically inadmissible, persuasive counseling involves removing biases the patient may have due to gaps in education or information. By providing the patient with an accurate interpretation of the information presented, they may be inclined to make a more rational decision. Persuasive counseling implies offering an impartial, evidence-driven medical opinion, as this is understood as the professional duty of a treating physician.[39]

If the patient refuses a strongly recommended cesarean section, the American College of Obstetricians and Gynecologists suggest that the following information be carefully documented:[38]

1. Verification that the need for the medical intervention has been fully explained, including the risks and benefits
2. The patient's refusal to consent to the medical intervention

3. The reasons (if any) stated by the patient for refusing
4. Confirmation that risks to the health and life of the patient, the fetus, or both, may be in jeopardy because of refusing, have been fully described.

Nonobstetric Surgery During Pregnancy

While the prevalence of nonobstetric surgery has decreased over time, it is still not an uncommon scenario that can bring stress to anesthesia providers. Recent estimates from a large meta-analysis reported a prevalence between 0.23% and 0.74%.[40] The most common types of procedures include abdominal surgery, followed by trauma and malignancy resection.[41] Commonly reported complications include reoperation, infection, wound morbidity, prolonged mechanical ventilation or reintubation, venous thromboembolism, and death, with the latter being reported at close to 0.25%.[42]

The maternal and fetal risks of nonobstetric surgery while pregnant have decreased over time; however, the risks of stillbirth and preterm birth and the need for unplanned cesarean delivery remain a possibility. Elucidating whether these risks are associated to the condition warranting a surgical procedure, the surgery itself, or a combination of both is complex.[40] There are no data to specifically address these concerns as conducting large population studies in these settings is difficult.

Timing and medical necessity

Whenever possible, surgery should be timed to minimize the potential risks to the pregnant patient and the fetus. Elective surgery should be delayed until after delivery. However, a pregnant woman should never be denied surgery that is medically indicated or have that surgery delayed which could negatively impact the patient and the fetus.[43]

Informed consent

The risks and benefits of surgery/procedure to the maternal-fetal dyad should be discussed preoperatively with the patient and, if possible, a member(s) of her support system. Ideally, both the surgeon and obstetric care provider should be involved in this discussion. An informed consent conversation respects the patient autonomy while maintaining the provider's beneficence-based duty to uphold fetal well-being, which can be at risk due to the primary condition requiring a surgical/procedural intervention.

In situations where emergency surgery is indicated, abbreviation of the consent discussion might be indicated.[44] In time-sensitive scenarios, medical decisions should be focused on beneficence and nonmaleficence.[25] Medical consent is based on a relationship of trust between the provider and patient. In emergencies, there is little time to develop this type of trust. The consenting provider should work to earn it by coming from a position of humility and open-mindedness.[45] If a patient is unable to give consent, and in the absence of an advanced directive, it is ethically acceptable for a physician to provide life-saving treatment using presumed consent.[46]

Maternal knowledge of the risks of general anesthesia in obstetrics is poor.[47] While risks such as occurrence of an allergic reaction or the presence of postoperative nausea and vomiting seems to be common, knowledge regarding difficult intubation, aspiration, dental damage, and malignant hyperthermia is quite limited. In addition, many anesthesia providers are reluctant to inform patients about the risks of general anesthesia.[48] It has been estimated that over 50% of pregnant women would like to be informed of the risks occurring in a proportion of 1:1000, with close to 30% wanting to know all the risks associated with general anesthesia (including difficult intubation, aspiration, teeth damage, awareness, allergy, and postoperative nausea and vomiting).[47]

When central neuraxial techniques are employed, risks that should frequently be discussed include those with high incidence, high morbidity, or adverse fetal effects, such as neurologic injury, postdural puncture headache, leg weakness, inadequate or failed block, hypotension, and fetal bradycardia.[11]

Fetal monitoring

The decision to perform fetal monitoring should be individualized and discussed with all team members (obstetricians, anesthesia providers, pediatricians, and perinatal nurses) in addition to the patient and her support system. The decision to do so and possible need for interventions should be clearly documented in the medical chart. This will allow for team members to be supported in their decision knowing that they are honoring the mother's wishes for her and on behalf of her child.

If the fetus is considered previable, documentation of fetal heart before and after the procedure is sufficient. In select circumstances, intraoperative fetal monitoring may be indicated for peri-viable fetuses to facilitate positioning or oxygenation interventions.[43] However, a clear course of action should be discussed with the patient and team members ahead of time, specifically when aggressive interventions (ie, delivery) are not to be employed in these circumstances.

For pregnancies with viable fetuses, intraoperative fetal heart rate monitoring is recommended to assess fetal well-being if it's feasible to perform, there should be an obstetric provider who can interpret and intervene, and the mother should be appropriately counseled about the risks and benefits of an emergent cesarean delivery. If none of these conditions apply, fetal heart rate and contraction monitoring should occur before and after the procedure. Due to the risk of preterm delivery, corticosteroid administration for fetal benefit should be considered for patients with fetuses at viable gestational ages, and evidence of preterm labor should be monitored in the perioperative period.[43]

Medication risks to fetus

Exposure to anesthetic agents causes concerns to providers due to the risk of teratogenicity. Luckily, multiple retrospectives studies in humans support the absence of teratogenic risks of commonly utilized anesthetic drugs for nonobstetric surgery, when used at standard clinical doses.[40,49] Another important concern regarding the use of anesthetic agents is the impact on neurodevelopment. Although conflicting results have been reported in the literature, there is insufficient evidence to recommend a specific technique or changes in current standards of practice.[41]

Medical maternal interventions include the administration of medications to the mother which can impact fetal physiology.[50] Commonly, these medications have the goal to improve fetal well-being. For example, administration of nitroglycerin to induce smooth uterine muscle relaxation will counteract tetanic contractions. Changes in positioning, optimization of oxygenation, and maintenance of systemic perfusion by using vasopressor medications can improve uteroplacental flow and revert intraoperative fetal bradycardia.

Fetal resuscitation

The issue of delivering the fetus and providing resuscitation is a nuanced and fraught ethical topic. A pregnant woman has autonomy over her body and the decisions that may impact the fetus. Ethically, as stated before, there are beneficence-based obligations to the fetus. In cases where severe prematurity or other coexisting fetal conditions may impact future quality of life or cause life-threatening multiorgan failure, parents are allowed to limit or withdraw potential care for the fetus.[51] A preoperative discussion addressing specifically resuscitation efforts should delivery be necessary is fundamental. Delivery is the choice of last resort, only used when in utero resuscitation therapies have failed.[52] Not only should the resuscitation process be explained but also what parents can expect regarding future quality of life if resuscitation is successful. It is also important to highlight that once delivery has occurred, the fetus becomes a newborn child, and they are deserving of all duties and considerations any child of any age is. This approach aligns with the ethical principle of justice, which attempts to provide equitable care to even the smallest newborn.[53] In many circumstances, an emergent delivery benefits both mother and fetus and does not imply compromising care of one over the other, given that the emergent situation is caused by maternal or uteroplacental deficits that can threaten the pregnant patient's life.[54]

SUMMARY

As anesthesia providers, we are uniquely positioned and expected to provide outstanding care to pregnant women. Our clinical decision-making for the patient undergoing labor and delivery or nonobstetric surgery can be guided by the 4 basic principles of ethics: beneficence, nonmaleficence, autonomy, and justice. Shared decision-making, supported by an adequate communication of evidence-based concepts, should facilitate conversations with the patients and facilitate obtaining informed consent, while promoting the principle of autonomy. When maternal-fetal conflict arises, beneficence-based obligations to both parties should be considered, in addition to autonomy-based duties to the mother.

Labor is not an impediment for women to provide consent for care, both for vaginal delivery and all interventions derived from this type of care. A careful balance between evidence-based clinical judgment and patient autonomy is necessary when addressing cesarean delivery, including both indicated and patient-requested cesarean, TOLAC, and refusal of a recommended cesarean delivery.

For nonobstetric surgery, discussion of anesthetic risks and the need for fetal monitoring and necessary interventions, especially emergent delivery, and fetal resuscitation, should be clearly documented. It is important to highlight that surgery that is medically indicated should never be denied to pregnant patients.

A structured and concept-based approach to complex ethical dilemmas should provide guidance to achieve resolution and provide our patients with the best possible and desired outcome.

CLINICS CARE POINTS

- Informed consent highlights the value of the ethical principle of autonomy. Capacity is necessary for adequate consent, and it is important to emphasize that being pregnant or in labor does not affect the ability to provide consent or retain risks/benefits information.
- Most pregnant women prefer discussion of interventions and their associated risks to take place before labor starts or a procedure is set to occur.
- While elective nonobstetric surgery should be delayed until after delivery, medically indicated interventions should not be withheld for pregnant patients.
- Over half of pregnant women would like to be informed of the risks of general anesthesia (including failed intubation and accidental awareness).
- For pregnancies with viable fetuses, intraoperative fetal heart rate monitoring is recommended during nonobstetric surgery if it's feasible to perform, there should be an obstetric provider who can interpret and intervene, and the mother should be appropriately counseled about the risks and benefits of an emergent cesarean delivery. For previable

fetuses, fetal heart rate monitoring should be obtained before and after the procedure. Intraprocedure monitoring should only occur in selected cases.

- A preoperative discussion specifically addressing resuscitation efforts for the fetus (should delivery be necessary) is critical.

DISCLOSURE

This research did not receive any specific grant from funding agencies in the public, commercial, or not-for-profit sectors. No conflicts of interest are disclosed.

REFERENCES

1. Digiovanni LM. Ethical issues in obstetrics. Obstet Gynecol Clin N Am 2010; 37(2):345–57.
2. Varkey B. Principles of clinical ethics and their application to practice. Med Princ Pract 2021;30(1):17–28.
3. Gallo L, Baxter C, Murphy J, et al. Ethics in plastic surgery: applying the four common principles to practice. Plast Reconstr Surg 2018;142(3):813–8.
4. Jonsen AR, Siegler M, Winslade WJ. Ethics: a practical approach to ethical decisions in clinical medicine. New York City, NY: McGraw Hill; 2015.
5. Schyns-van den Berg A, Claudot F, Baumann A. Anaesthesiology and ethics: autonomy in childbirth. Eur J Anaesthesiol 2018;35(8):553–5.
6. Legare F, Thompson-Leduc P. Twelve myths about shared decision making. Patient Educ Counsel 2014;96(3):281–6.
7. Chervenak FA, McCullough LB, Brent RL. The professional responsibility model of obstetrical ethics: avoiding the perils of clashing rights. Am J Obstet Gynecol 2011;205(4):315 e1–e5.
8. Oshima Lee E, Emanuel EJ. Shared decision making to improve care and reduce costs. N Engl J Med 2013;368(1):6–8.
9. Gustin AN Jr. Shared Decision-Making. Anesthesiol Clin 2019;37(3):573–80.
10. Poprzeczny AJ, Stocking K, Showell M, et al. Patient Decision Aids to Facilitate Shared Decision Making in Obstetrics and Gynecology: A Systematic Review and Meta-analysis. Obstet Gynecol 2020;135(2):444–51.
11. Wilson EH, Burkle CM. The Meaning of Consent and Its Implications for Anesthesiologists. Adv Anesth 2020;38:1–22.
12. Waisel DB, Truog RD. Informed consent. Anesthesiology 1997;87(4):968–78.
13. Green DS, MacKenzie CR. Nuances of informed consent: the paradigm of regional anesthesia. HSS J 2007;3(1):115–8.
14. Marco AP. Informed consent for surgical anesthesia care: has the time come for separate consent? Anesth Analg 2010;110(2):280–2.
15. van Bogaert LJ, Dhai A. Ethical challenges of treating the critically ill pregnant patient. Best Pract Res Clin Obstet Gynaecol 2008;22(5):983–96.
16. Chervenak FA, McCullough LB. Ethical issues in periviable birth. Semin Perinatol 2013;37(6):422–5.
17. Chervenak FA, McCullough LB. Ethical issues in cesarean delivery. Best Pract Res Clin Obstet Gynaecol 2017;43:68–75.
18. Chervenak FA, McCullough LB. Ethical dimensions of the fetus as a patient. Best Pract Res Clin Obstet Gynaecol 2017;43:2–9.
19. Mann DG, Sutton CD. Ethics in the labor and delivery unit. Anesthesiol Clin 2021; 39(4):839–49.

20. Obstetric Care Consensus No. 6 Summary: Periviable Birth. Obstet Gynecol 2017;130(4):926–8.
21. Cummings J, Committee On F, Newborn. Antenatal Counseling Regarding Resuscitation and Intensive Care Before 25 Weeks of Gestation. Pediatrics 2015;136(3):588–95.
22. ACOG. Sample Birth Plan Template. Accessed November 8, 2023. https://www.acog.org/womens-health/health-tools/sample-birth-plan.
23. Burcher P. The Ulysses contract in obstetrics: a woman's choices before and during labour. J Med Ethics 2013;39(1):27–30.
24. Ciliberto CG, Davies JM. Ulysses directives: should they take precedence over a laboring patient's request for labor analgesia? ASA Monitor. Aug 2014; 1(78):40–1.
25. Broaddus BM, Chandrasekhar S. Informed consent in obstetric anesthesia. Anesth Analg 2011;112(4):912–5.
26. Black JD, Cyna AM. Issues of consent for regional analgesia in labour: a survey of obstetric anaesthetists. Anaesth Intensive Care 2006;34(2):254–60.
27. Saunders TA, Stein DJ, Dilger JP. Informed consent for labor epidurals: a survey of Society for Obstetric Anesthesia and Perinatology anesthesiologists from the United States. Int J Obstet Anesth 2006;15(2):98–103.
28. Cheng WY, Cyna AM, Osborn KD. Risks of regional anaesthesia for caesarean section: women's recall and information sources. Anaesth Intensive Care 2007; 35(1):68–73.
29. Burkle CM, Olsen DA, Sviggum HP, et al. Parturient recall of neuraxial analgesia risks: Impact of labor pain vs no labor pain. J Clin Anesth 2017;36:158–63.
30. Beilin Y, Rosenblatt MA, Bodian CA, et al. Information and concerns about obstetric anesthesia: a survey of 320 obstetric patients. Int J Obstet Anesth 1996;5(3): 145–51.
31. Dietz HP, Callaghan S. Response to Vaginal delivery: An argument against requiring consent. Aust N Z J Obstet Gynaecol 2019;59(1):165.
32. Bringedal H, Aune I. Able to choose? Women's thoughts and experiences regarding informed choices during birth. Midwifery 2019;77:123–9.
33. van der Pijl MSG, Klein Essink M, van der Linden T, et al. Consent and refusal of procedures during labour and birth: a survey among 11 418 women in the Netherlands. BMJ Qual Saf 2023. https://doi.org/10.1136/bmjqs-2022-015538.
34. Valente EP, Mariani I, Covi B, et al. Quality of Informed Consent Practices around the Time of Childbirth: A Cross-Sectional Study in Italy. Int J Environ Res Publ Health 2022;(12):19. https://doi.org/10.3390/ijerph19127166.
35. Levy KS, Smith MK, Lacroix M, et al. Patient Satisfaction with Informed Consent for Cesarean and Operative Vaginal Delivery. J Obstet Gynaecol Can 2022; 44(7):785–90.
36. Deshpande NA, Oxford CM. Management of pregnant patients who refuse medically indicated cesarean delivery. Rev Obstet Gynecol 2012;5(3–4):e144–50.
37. Davies JM. Consent in laboring patients. In: Van Norman GJ S, Rosenbaum S, editors. Clinical ethics in anesthesiology: a case-based textbook. Cambridge, UK: Cambridge University Press; 2008. p. 44–8.
38. Committee Opinion No. 664 Summary: Refusal of Medically Recommended Treatment During Pregnancy. Obstet Gynecol 2016;127(6):1189–90. https://doi.org/10.1097/AOG.0000000000001479.
39. Shaw D, Elger B. Evidence-based persuasion: an ethical imperative. JAMA 2013; 309(16):1689–90.

40. Haataja A, Kokki H, Uimari O, et al. Non-obstetric surgery during pregnancy and the effects on maternal and fetal outcomes: A systematic review. Scand J Surg 2023;112(3):187–205.

41. Brakke BD, Sviggum HP. Anaesthesia for non-obstetric surgery during pregnancy. BJA Educ 2023;23(3):78–83.

42. Erekson EA, Brousseau EC, Dick-Biascoechea MA, et al. Maternal postoperative complications after nonobstetric antenatal surgery. J Matern Fetal Neonatal Med 2012;25(12):2639–44.

43. ACOG Committee Opinion No. Nonobstetric Surgery During Pregnancy. Obstet Gynecol 2019;133(4):e285–6. https://doi.org/10.1097/AOG.0000000000 003174, 775.

44. Bush DJ. A comparison of informed consent for obstetric anaesthesia in the USA and the UK. Int J Obstet Anesth 1995;4(1):1–6.

45. Blake J. Consent in Obstetrics. J Obstet Gynaecol Can 2020;42(4):391–3.

46. Informed Consent and Shared Decision Making in Obstetrics and Gynecology: ACOG Committee Opinion, Number 819. Obstet Gynecol 2021;137(2):e34–41. https://doi.org/10.1097/AOG.0000000000004247.

47. Jackson GN, Robinson PN, Lucas DN, et al. What mothers know, and want to know, about the complications of general anaesthesia. Acta Anaesthesiol Scand 2012;56(5):585–8.

48. Lanigan C, Reynolds F. Risk information supplied by obstetric anaesthetists in Britain and Ireland to mothers awaiting elective caesarean section. Int J Obstet Anesth 1995;4(1):7–13.

49. Cohen-Kerem R, Railton C, Oren D, et al. Pregnancy outcome following non-obstetric surgical intervention. Am J Surg 2005;190(3):467–73.

50. Chervenak FA, McCullough LB. The ethics of maternal-fetal surgery. Semin Fetal Neonatal Med 2018;23(1):64–7.

51. Perinatal Palliative Care: Acog committee opinion, Number 786. Obstet Gynecol 2019;134(3):e84–9.

52. Kukora SK, Fry JT. Resuscitation decisions in fetal myelomeningocele repair should center on parents' values: a counter analysis. J Perinatol 2022;42(7): 971–5.

53. Wolfe ID, Lillegard JB, Carter BS. Parental request for non-resuscitation in fetal myelomeningocele repair: an analysis of the novel ethical tensions in fetal intervention. J Perinatol 2022;42(7):856–9.

54. Sacco A, Van der Veeken L, Bagshaw E, et al. Maternal complications following open and fetoscopic fetal surgery: A systematic review and meta-analysis. Prenat Diagn 2019;39(4):251–68.

Ethical Issues in the Care of Patients Whose Personal, Religious, or Cultural Beliefs Impact Clinical Management Strategies

Lindsay K. Sween, MD, MPH[a], James M. West, MD, MA[b,*]

KEYWORDS

- Ethics • Autonomy • Informed consent • Personal beliefs • Jehovah's Witnesses

KEY POINTS

- Ethical principles regarding respect for patient autonomy in medical decision-making and the impact of religion, culture, and other issues on clinical care have been extensively reviewed in the medical literature.
- Each patient brings their own unique perspective to every clinical encounter informed by their life experiences, their religion, and their cultural upbringing.
- Ethical treatment of patients with specific personal, religious, or cultural beliefs that impact clinical decision-making includes not only respecting their autonomy, but also ensuring that in doing so they are able to comprehend the options and implications while balancing the protection of their privacy with the more communal nature of decision-making for some religious and cultural groups.

INTRODUCTION

Each patient brings their own unique perspective to every clinical encounter informed by their life experiences, their religion, and their cultural upbringing. Such personal beliefs may impact how an individual interacts with the health care system, including the providers from whom they will accept care, the persons to whom they are willing to have their medical information communicated, and which therapies they will and will not accept. Ethical treatment of patients with specific personal, religious, or cultural beliefs that impact clinical decision-making includes not only respecting their autonomy, but

[a] Northside Hospital, Northside Anesthesiology Clinicians, 1000 Johnson Ferry Road, Atlanta, GA 30342, USA; [b] Methodist Transplant Institute, Emeritus, Medical Anesthesia Group, Ret., 4th Floor Shorb Tower, 1265 Union Avenue, Memphis, TN 38104, USA
* Corresponding author. 5229 Cosgrove Cove, Memphis, TN 38117.
E-mail address: jwest1@comcast.net

Anesthesiology Clin 42 (2024) 515–528
https://doi.org/10.1016/j.anclin.2023.12.002
1932-2275/24/© 2023 Elsevier Inc. All rights reserved.

anesthesiology.theclinics.com

also ensuring that in doing so they are able to comprehend the options and implications while balancing the protection of their privacy with the more communal nature of decision-making for some religious and cultural groups. In addition, the decision-making and identification of treatment options requires thorough evaluation of how the physicians and hospital can most appropriately meet patient needs and goals of care given the constraints that certain beliefs may create.

In this review, the authors identify some of the health care-related beliefs of a few religious and cultural groups commonly encountered by health care providers in the United States and the ethical issues involved in providing care. Much of the discussion will focus on the care of Jehovah's Witnesses (JWs) and their refusal of blood products and a description of beliefs of other religious groups that impact clinical decision-making as examples of some of the ethical issues and challenges these beliefs have on delivery of evidence-based care in general and anesthesia care in particular. In our diverse society, the principles and approaches discussed are relevant to the ethical treatment of all patients and require that we exercise cultural sensitivity and knowledge of beliefs and customs of various faiths to understand how to manage challenging clinical situations appropriately.

RELIGIOUS AND CULTURAL OVERVIEW OF SELECT PATIENT POPULATIONS
Jehovah's Witnesses

The group now known as JWs was founded in the 1870s by Charles Taze Russell as a bible study group in Pittsburgh, Pennsylvania. The governing body of the JW church that determines official church doctrine is now called the Watch Tower Bible and Tract Society of Pennsylvania (colloquially known as the Watch Tower Society [WTS]) and is headquartered in Warwick, New York.[1] According to the 2020 US Religion Census, there are more than 3 million JWs in the United States.[2] JWs believe that the Bible is the divinely inspired word of God, and therefore, it should be interpreted literally except for passages that are clearly allegorical.[3,4] WTS banned followers' acceptance of blood transfusions in 1945 based on several biblical passages[5,6]:

Genesis 9:3: "Only flesh with its life – with its blood – you must not eat."

Leviticus 17:10-16: "If any man of the house of Israel or any foreigner who is residing in your midst eats any sort of blood, I will certainly set my face against the one who is eating the blood, and I will cut him off from among his people. For the life of the flesh is in the blood, and I myself have given it on the altar for you to make atonement for yourselves, because it is the blood that makes atonement by means of the life in it. That is why I have said to the Israelites: 'None of you should eat blood, and no foreigner who is residing in your midst should eat blood.'"

Deuteronomy 15:23: "But you must not eat its blood; you should pour it out on the ground like water."

Acts 15:28-29: "...to keep abstaining from things sacrificed to idols and from blood..."

A July 1951 *Watchtower* article explained WTSs reasoning for the blood transfusion ban based on the biblical proscriptions against eating blood: "When sugar solutions are given intravenously, it is called intravenous feeding...The transfusion is feeding the patient blood and...[the patient] is eating [blood] through his veins."[7] (See **Table 1**, for a list of which blood products are prohibited and which therapies are considered the personal decision of each JW.)

Since 1961, WTS has enforced its prohibition of blood transfusion by "disfellowshipping" (ie, expelling) any member who voices disapproval of the ban or accepts a banned blood component without appropriately repenting afterward.[8] The church

Table 1
Blood product guidelines for Jehovah's Witness patients[a]

Types of Blood Product or Procedure	Accepts/Refuse/ Personal Decision (PD)[b]	Specific Concerns
Whole blood	Refuse	
PRBCs	Refuse	
Plasma	Refuse	
Platelets	Refuse	
White blood cells	Refuse	
Cryoprecipitate	PD	
Cryo-poor plasma (cryosupernatant)	PD	
Platelet gel	PD	
Fractionated factors	PD	Most will accept
Albumin	PD	Most will accept
Erythropoietin	PD	Most erythropoietin is albumin coated and is PD; darbepoetin contains no albumin
Recombinant factor VII, VIII, and IX	PD	Not made from blood, although some may still object
Cell saver	PD	Continuous circuit
Acute normovolemic hemodilution	PD	Continuous circuit
Cardiopulmonary or veno-venous bypass	PD	Continuous circuit
Renal hemodialysis	PD	Continuous circuit
Stored autologous blood	Refuse	Completely separated from body
Organ and bone marrow transplant	PD	
Donation of blood	Refuse	
Organ donation	Refuse	

[a] The worksheet that many Jehovah's Witnesses have does not include all of these products and/or techniques but those not on the worksheet have been verified by their lead office.
[b] The term "personal decision" is used here to denote actions that the Jehovah's Witness governing body has said are optional. In reality, these are all personal decisions for each patient.
Abbreviations: PD, personal decision; PRBC, packed red blood cells.
From West JM. Ethical issues in the care of Jehovah's Witnesses. Current Opin Anesthesiol. 2014;27(2):170 to 176. Used with permission.

instructs members to discontinue any spiritual fellowship, such as Bible study, prayer, or discussing matters of church doctrine, with a disfellowshipped person, although marital and familial ties can theoretically remain intact.[3,8] In practice, disfellowshipped individuals are often completely ostracized by their JW social groups, and the church may grant an exception to its usual proscription against marital separation when one spouse is disfellowshipped due to "absolute endangerment of spirituality."[8,9] In June 2000, WTS issued a policy change from disfellowshipping, in which a committee revokes a JWs membership if he/she is found to have received a blood transfusion and is considered by that committee to be unrepentant, to disassociation, in which an individual voluntarily excuses him/herself from the church through the action of accepting a blood transfusion. The church's official statement read: "If a baptized member of the faith willfully and without regret accepts blood transfusions, he indicates by his own actions that he no longer wishes to be one of JWs."[10] Although the social implications of disassociation are equivalent to disfellowshipping, because disassociation is initiated by self-disclosure, an individual could choose to keep a blood transfusion confidential and remain a JW member.[10]

Furthermore, it is a common misconception that if a JW is transfused blood against their will, then the church believes that the individual is still subject to eternal damnation. Another misconception is that if a JW patient accepts blood, he/she would be subject to eternal damnation with no chance of redemption. Neither of these misunderstandings is true. According to James Pellechia, past associate editor of the Watch Tower:

A forced blood transfusion would not be viewed as a sin. Also, if under extreme pressure and while experiencing undue stress a JW were to compromise their belief and accept a blood transfusion, in other words, if they caved in at a moment of spiritual weakness yet still held to their beliefs, that individual would not be ostracized by the JW community. Rather, kindness would be shown and pastoral help offered. Nevertheless, a forced transfusion or a compromise with one's conscience may leave the patient with deep emotional scars.[11]

Despite this clarification, many JW patients and their families still believe in dire implications should they receive blood or blood products either based on prior consent or against their will.

Arab Americans and Muslims

There are more than 3 million Arab Americans in the United States, about 10% to 30% of whom are Muslim.[12] The 2020 US Religion Census estimated that there are more than 4.4 million American Muslims.[2] Although Western health care and medical ethics tend to emphasize the individual, the family plays an important role in making health care decisions in Arab and Muslim cultures. Observant Muslims may adhere to strict gender roles, and a woman may defer to her husband in making medical decisions for her.[11]

Both Muslim men and women are encouraged to dress modestly, and women may wear a hijab that covers the head and sometimes the body. In keeping with modesty, women who observe the hijab may desire that a health care provider announce him/herself before entering a room to allow time for her to cover herself (of course common courtesy requires we do this with all patients). Arabs and Muslims prefer health care providers of the same sex, although Islam does permit cross-gender providers to treat a patient in life-threatening situations or when an alternative provider is not available. Some Muslims may not shake hands or make eye contact with health care providers of the opposite sex.[11]

The desire for privacy may impact decision-making regarding particular forms of medical care particularly for female Muslims. For example, although standard reproductive system examinations, such as Papanicolaou tests and pelvic examinations, are acceptable for married and formerly married women, such examinations are typically not accepted by never-married female patients unless there is a serious medical situation requiring them. Muslim women may avoid talking with their health care providers about sexual education, sexual health and dysfunction, sexually transmitted diseases, and domestic violence.[11] Most married Muslim women will accept reversible forms of preconception birth control, such as birth control pills, but many will not accept methods that prevent implantation of a fertilized egg, such as an intrauterine device. Permanent sterilization with tubal ligation or vasectomy is generally refused.[11]

Certain Arabic cultural and religious traditions conflict with Western medical practices. For example, Arabs traditionally believe that complete bed rest hastens recovery for most ailments, whereas current Western medical opinion tends to favor activity as tolerated to prevent deconditioning and thromboembolic complications. Muslims that follow *halal*, Islamic dietary laws, may require a pork-free or vegetarian diet while in the hospital and may refuse any medical therapeutics derived from pigs. Although not necessarily a tenet of Islam, for many Arabs and Muslims mental illness is a culturally and religiously taboo subject and is frequently viewed as shameful, a sign of weakness, or an indication that an individual is not following the Islamic tenets. Because many Muslims believe that one cannot become mentally ill if appropriately adhering to Islamic law, they may not view pharmacologic or other interventions to treat mental illness as legitimate therapies. During the holy month of Ramadan, some Muslim patients may wish to fast during daylight hours, although they could otherwise be exempted by illness. Such a fast includes oral, intramuscular, and intravenous medications, intravenous fluids, enteric and total parenteral nutrition, and transfusion of blood and blood components.[11]

Orthodox Jews

According to the 2020 US Religion Census, there are approximately 940,000 Orthodox Jews living in the United States.[2] Orthodox Jews believe that God gave the Torah (the first five books of the Old Testament) to Moses on Mount Sinai, and *halacha,* the laws contained in the Torah that govern every aspect of life, should be strictly observed.[12,13] Similar to Muslims, Orthodox Jews adhere to modesty laws, called *tzniut*. These laws are observed by avoiding any physical contact with a member of the opposite sex, including handshakes, dressing modestly (including covering the hair, knees, elbows, and collarbones for women), and making minimal eye contact with individuals outside of the immediate family. Orthodox Jews are typically more comfortable with same-sex clinicians.[12]

Orthodox Jews are prohibited from using electrical devices or driving a car on the Sabbath (from Friday at sundown until Saturday at nightfall) and Jewish holidays. Therefore, they may be non-adherent with medical devices that require electricity, such as continuous positive airway pressure (CPAP) machines, on these occasions and may delay clinic appointments, elective surgeries, or presenting to the emergency room until after the Sabbath or holiday.[12]

Pikuach nefesh, the preservation of life, represents a fundamental concept in health care decision-making for Orthodox Jews. This principle does not mean that life must be prolonged at all cost regardless of life duration or amount of suffering, but it means that individuals must sustain their health and take action to restore it in times of illness whenever feasible.[13] Because Jews believe that human beings are created in the image of God, every life has inherent value and dignity, and illness, infirmity, or disability remove that dignity. It is seen as meritorious and necessary for extended family and even the community to care for those in need.[13] As opposed to the Western focus on the individual, Judaism is a collectivistic culture. Orthodox Jews recognize the right of autonomy, but patients may exercise their autonomy by asking health care providers to consult with their rabbi regarding medical treatment decisions to confirm observance of *pikuach nefesh* and other *halacha* laws.[12,13] At the end of life, an Orthodox Jewish family may request that a prayer group consisting of at least 10 men, called a *minyan*, be at the patient's bedside to recite particular prayers as the patient dies. Such a large group may be in conflict with a hospital's visitation policy in the intensive care unit (ICU), and health care providers must have cultural awareness to know to accommodate such a request.[13]

Amish

The Amish are a population of approximately 320,000 Anabaptist-Christian people of Swiss-German descent living in rural areas of the United States and Canada.[2,14,15] The Amish community consists of closely associated kinship and congregational networks that are led by male bishops and community elders. The Amish avoid technology, do not drive cars, and usually do not have their homes hooked up to phone lines or electricity grids. Because Amish transportation to hospitals or medical appointments is limited to taxis, drivers' services, horse-and-buggy, or bicycle, bundling appointments or providing home-based services can improve health care access by reducing the time and expense involved in seeking medical care. Some more progressive Amish may have cell phones for work purposes and may use generators or propane tanks to power lights and household appliances. Others rely on written letters or phones at non-Amish neighbors' homes for communication. Health care providers should ensure that communications to patients remain private. Leaving voicemail messages should be carefully considered unless the provider can ensure that the message is not received by someone other than the patient. If not, health information may have to be provided through traditional paper mail or after leaving a message for a patient to return a nondescript phone message. When patients are provided medical devices requiring electricity, equipment should be battery-powered, and batteries may need to be charged at doctors' offices or at non-Amish homes.[14,15]

Although Amish people will accept most traditional medical care, they are also more likely than non-Amish individuals to explore complementary and alternative medical care options, including chiropractic services, natural remedies and dietary supplements, massage therapy, and prayer. The Amish usually do not have any commercial health insurance, so payment for medical services either comes from direct payment or from an Amish church's hospital aid program that is funded by contributions from members. Providers can help alleviate the cost of out-of-pocket medical care by limiting the number of tests ordered, minimizing the duration of hospital stays, using homecare whenever possible, and offering payment plans.[14]

Members of the Amish community believe in early withdrawal of care in severely or terminally ill patients, including children, preferring to care for community members at home to reduce suffering as well as to minimize costs. Physicians should be aware of and sensitive to these perspectives, understanding the underlying guiding principles, both religious and cultural. To do so may require the physician and hospital to understand why an Amish parent might refuse treatment for a child and provide culturally sensitive education about the options for care, assist in identifying potential sources of funding for care as well as engaging with ethics committees to clarify the issues rather than reporting concerns about child neglect to the county or state patient protection offices.[14]

Abortion is prohibited, and contraception is discouraged in the Amish community, although enforcement differs by church. Similarly, members of some Amish churches may reject mental health counseling due to the belief that mental health professionals may usurp the role of ministers and impart outside ideas that contradict church teachings.[14]

Church of Christ Scientist (Christian Science)

Church of Christ Scientist is a Christian sect that was started by Mary Baker Eddy in 1879. Members of the church believe in spiritual healing, and the most fervent of them will not seek medical help for anything. This sect reached its peak in the United States in 1939 when it had about 270,000 members. By 2009, membership had dwindled to about 50,000.[16]

Although generally thought that members of the church actively avoid all medical care, the church does not absolutely require that Christian Scientists avoid medical care. Many members of the church will receive care from dentists, optometrists, obstetricians, and physicians for selected clinical problems such as bone fractures and will accept vaccination when required by law. At the same time, they believe that Christian Science prayer is most effective when not combined with medicine.[17]

According to their Web site "Christian Scientists are always free to choose for themselves and their families the kind of health care that meets their needs. However, by practicing Christian Science, many have lived happy and healthy lives free of drugs and other systems of physical care."[18]

Therefore, if a Christian Scientist does seek medical care, good communication will be required to ensure their autonomy is protected. In some cases, they might have a surrogate who is not a believer and encourages care the individual patient may decline. Extensive discussion may be required to understand what care is acceptable to the patient and what is not—often discussed with the patient alone without a surrogate, assuming the patient is competent to make personal health care decisions. Most important for the physicians to understand, when a Christian Scientist provides informed consent for surgery and anesthesia, the patient is unlikely to put any restrictions on specific techniques or treatments.

ETHICAL PRINCIPLES

Ethical dilemmas can be examined in the context of the four basic principles of medical ethics defined by Beauchamp and Childress: (1) respect for autonomy—recognizing a patient's decision-making capacity, (2) beneficence—balancing benefits against risks, (3) non-maleficence—avoiding harm, and (4) justice—a group of norms for distributing benefits, risk, and costs fairly.[19] In the United States, the principle of respect for patient autonomy is usually the most heavily weighted of the four, whereas in many European countries, the principle of beneficence may weigh more heavily than respecting individual autonomy.

Physicians demonstrate respect for the autonomy of competent patients by accepting their informed decisions, whether or not they consent to medical treatment. It seems self-evident that without respect for informed refusal, the concept of informed consent is invalidated. "Consent" would then merely be acquiescence of the patient to the physician's recommendations. A physician does not have to agree with a patient's decision, nor be compelled to give inappropriate, bizarre, or substandard care. The physician should, however, clarify how the disagreement about the plan for care will be managed and when clinically appropriate can recommend transfer of care to another provider who may be willing and able to fulfill the patient's goals.

One of the keys to ensuring support for patient autonomy is to provide sufficient information to a patient to allow the patient to give informed consent. To do so requires that the patient has appropriate decision-making capacity, is able to understand the nature of the procedure, the risks, benefits, and alternatives, including the option to do nothing and the probable outcomes of both acceptance and refusal of the proposed procedure. Perhaps most important, the decision must be made free of coercion. Because some patients are intimidated by the health care system and the "language" of health care, it is critical to ensure that the patient does not feel threatened, bullied, or subjected to irresistible pressure, such as the fear of ostracization, to make a decision they would otherwise not make.

LEGAL PRECEDENTS

Although legal decisions are not always synonymous with ethical ones, a review of some legal precedents related to medical decision-making is helpful in putting the ethical constructs guiding practice into perspective. As one example, the legal challenges related to refusal to accept blood or blood products by JWs provides important background to guide decision-making by anesthesiologists and other providers caring for this patient population, both adults and minors. The experience related to refusal of blood products has evolved over time and provides some insight into how medical ethics, at least in the United States has shifted from a paternalistic and/or beneficence-based emphasis to one of respect for autonomy.

In the early 1960s, the courts would often allow involuntary transfusion of JW patients based on the idea that their faith did not forbid a forced transfusion only a consensual one.[20] Over the last 40 years, however, US courts have rejected these older decisions and consistently upheld the rights of adult JWs to refuse blood, even when a transfusion would be life-saving and when others, such as dependent children, may be affected. The decisions related to transfusion of minors have taken a different position. When a minor child has required blood products and the JW parents refused to consent, hospitals have sought and received court orders to give blood believed to be necessary to preserve life. In some cases, court orders have been denied when a JW adolescent who is able to fully understand the consequences declines transfusion.[21–25]

ISSUES TO CONSIDER WHEN PATIENTS HAVE PERSONAL OR RELIGIOUS BELIEFS IMPACTING CLINICAL MANAGEMENT

Several key questions arise when confronted with a patient who has religious, cultural, or other beliefs that impact clinical management, whether in the operating room or any other health care environment.

1. Does the patient have appropriate decision-making capacity?
2. Have all appropriate risks, benefits, and alternatives been explained?
3. Does the patient truly practice the relevant faith and are they free of coercion?
4. What is the proper role of surrogate decision makers?
5. What therapies and blood products will the patient accept?
6. What are the relevant medical issues?
7. Does the surgical team, including anesthesia, have the experience and capabilities necessary to work under restrictive circumstances?
8. Will the constraints placed by the patient make them an inappropriate candidate for a limited resource, such as giving a JW a donated organ?
9. Is an anesthesiologist obligated to care for a patient whose personal beliefs may lead them to make medical decisions that said anesthesiologist may consider substandard care?

Does the Patient Have Decision-Making Capacity?

When caring for any patient, the providers should ensure that each patient has the capacity to understand the plan of care, the risks, benefits, and alternatives of care and is able to consent. Although most patients are able to do so, ensuring that the patient understands what is being proposed and their alternative options can be challenging. The health care environment is intimidating to patients and their families. The environment in which discussions take place is often hectic and, in many cases, distracting. Providers should clarify the level of understanding of the options and when appropriate have patient-approved family members or other surrogates present to assist in the discussions. At the same time, when planning care for a patient who has religious or cultural beliefs that restrict options, it is critically important to have an understanding of the patient's wishes, not the wishes of others. After a discussion with the patient and family/surrogates, the provider should have a separate discussion with the patient alone, assuming the patient has capacity to understand the discussion, plans, and alternatives. The outcome of the discussion should be clearly documented in the medical record. If there are concerns about patient's capacity to understand and the provider does not think the family or surrogate is representing the patient's wishes, alternative approaches including requests for appointment of a conservator may be necessary.

Have All Appropriate Risks, Benefits, and Alternatives Been Explained?

Aside from the usual explanation of anesthesia and surgical risks, there are often other important issues that must be addressed. In the case of JWs, these topics include but are not limited to explaining the specifics of blood conservation techniques, clarifying the risks of not accepting blood in the face of massive hemorrhage, and in the case of organ transplants, assuring that the patient understands that there are some residual blood cells in solid organs. In addition, some JWs will accept some blood products, but not others; some will accept cardiopulmonary bypass in which blood leaves the body in the circuit, whereas others refuse to accept any blood once it has left the circulation. The key ethical principle is that the anesthesiologist should have a detailed discussion with every patient about whether there are any restrictions to care that will impact anesthesia and perioperative management. If so, the provider should clarify what is and what is not acceptable, review the options for management, and determine whether proceeding with the surgical plan is appropriate or not. In some cases, although the anesthesia preoperative assessment is completed within minutes of the planned case start time, delay or cancellation may be necessary to ensure all clinical and ethical concerns have been identified and a plan is in place to address them.

Is the Patient Truly a Practitioner of Their Faith and Free of Coercion?

Patients often indicate that they have religious or other beliefs that impact clinical care and decision-making. One of the most challenging aspects encountered by the providers is ensuring that the decisions related to restrictions in care are being made by the patient rather than by family members, "advocates," or religious leaders. For example, in the case of a JW patient, patients may be reported as JWs by family members who are believers without input from the patient. Alternatively, patients who consider themselves JWs, but have not been baptized into the faith may not have the same strong beliefs about blood transfusions as those who are baptized JWs. It is important to verify with patients themselves what their beliefs truly are. This is true of a member of any faith who may refuse any therapies that impact clinical decision-making.

A most important part of the patient–provider relationship, particularly from an ethical perspective is that all patients should be free of coercion from family clergy, advocates, or health care providers. They must be assured that, regardless of their personal choices, their doctors will not abandon them. Providers must strive to ensure that the choices a patient makes are *truly* their own.

As noted previously, sometimes the decisions that JW patients express in the presence of family and church members are different from those they later express in private. It is, therefore, important that at some point before surgery and anesthesia, the patient have an opportunity to express their transfusion preferences to the anesthesiologist in private.[8] This might be done in a preoperative holding area or even in the OR after the family and/or church members have gone to the waiting room. The intent should *not* be to talk the patient into receiving blood, which would itself be coercive, but to ensure that their true wishes are known and followed. If the patient does recant, it is then important to determine what, if anything, should be communicated to family members, particularly in the case of the JW patient and decisions regarding administration of blood products. JW members who accept blood transfusion are subject to the church's communal shunning policy. The principles of patient confidentiality demand that specifics of treatment only be discussed with the patient unless they have authorized release of information to specific individuals or entities.

What Is the Proper Role of Surrogate Decision Makers?

While not the case for most religions, all JWs are encouraged to carry a special durable power of attorney that explains in detail their beliefs regarding blood and blood products. This document becomes important if the patient loses decision-making capacity before their wishes can be expressed. If a power of attorney for health care is not available and a provider cannot otherwise verify that a patient is a practicing JW, the providers generally err on the side of transfusion in emergent situations. Consultation with the ethics committee and hospital counsel may be helpful in clarifying management options, if time permits.

In some cases, the patient expressed their intentions preoperatively, but while under anesthesia, the need for blood becomes more critical. It is important to remember that the principle of substituted judgment dictates that surrogates make the decision that a patient would make if they were able to do so. The challenge for the providers is to confirm that the decisions of the surrogate accurately represent the *patient's wishes* and not the wishes of the surrogate. Once the patient's wishes are clarified, whether physicians agree or not, those decisions should stand unless new information becomes available that brings the previous determination into question. Respecting a patient's wishes can be particularly difficult if they have refused a treatment that the physician believes is life-saving, and the physician knows, believes, or even hopes that the surrogate would capitulate and allow the prohibited treatment. Continued badgering of the surrogate to change that decision is not appropriate and can be considered coercion.

What Therapies and Blood Products Will the Patient Accept?

Although decisions related to administration of blood products are relevant primarily to the care provided to JWs, the examples of some of the considerations that must be taken into account for this population of patients have relevance to the care and decision-making for other patients with strong beliefs about what care to accept and what care to decline, including decisions regarding reproductive health and other issues. For the JW patient, although the issues regarding restrictions on the administration of blood and blood products are critically important, it is also important to determine what each individual patient is willing to accept and what is restricted. Some JW patients will accept some blood products and not others. In one study, for example, up to 10% of pregnant JW patients indicated they would accept blood in an emergency.[26] There is also a sect known as "Advocates for Jehovah's Witness Reform on Blood (AJWRB)" that will accept blood products in many situations.[27,28] Nevertheless, in general, few practicing JWs will accept whole blood, packed red blood cells, plasma, platelet concentrates, or white blood cell transfusions.[4] Stored autologous blood is also not acceptable, because it is out of contact with the body for a significant period of time. Fractionated products such as albumin, cryoprecipitate, cryo-poor plasma, and individual factors are left to the "discretion of the practicing Christian," as is organ and bone marrow transplantation.[29]

Other "gray areas" include but are not limited to cell saver, acute normovolemic hemodilution (ANH), cardiopulmonary bypass, and renal dialysis. In these situations, *The Watchtower* has stated that if the blood is kept in continuous circuit with the body and not stored for any length of time, then accepting it is a personal decision. Cardiopulmonary bypass and dialysis would almost always involve a continuous circuit. Cell saver and ANH do not necessarily involve a continuous circuit, but one can easily be created (**Table 1**).[29]

What Are the Relevant Medical Issues?

A discussion of the ethical treatment of patients cannot help but overlap with a discussion of proper medical treatment. Although this article is not a treatise on the medical treatment of JW or other patients whose personal beliefs inform their medical decisions, it is important to remember that the principles of beneficence and non-maleficence dictate that we make use of every available tool to manage each patient in a way that optimizes their care, even in the face of restrictions to what can be provided. Blood-sparing surgical techniques can be used for patients who refuse to receive blood products. Other approaches to care can be used to minimize the likelihood of an undesired outcome or need for therapies a patient is rejecting. When encountering these challenging ethical and clinical issues, it is important for all providers to have a clearly defined plan of care to minimize the need for unwanted therapies or procedures. If the techniques or approaches are not available at a particular institution or providers do not have experience with them, identifying alternative providers or facilities to perform the procedures might be appropriate. In addition, if the clinical ramifications of the restrictions on care have not been adequately addressed preoperatively, it might be necessary and appropriate to delay the procedure until the patient is optimized or until the best operating room (OR) team is available.

What Are the Capabilities of the Surgical Team?

Patients whose personal beliefs lead them to refuse specific medical treatments or request certain accommodations, such as same-gender health care providers, and require advanced planning and preparation in non-emergent situations. In the case of JWs as well as any other cases, when procedures that may involve significant hemorrhage or other interventions that the patient refuses to undergo, the principle of non-maleficence dictates that we assess whether the surgical and anesthesia team have the skills, experience, and resources necessary to perform the procedure. It could become necessary to refuse to do the surgery, modify the surgical plan, or refer the patient to another center as has become more common in the care of JW patients who can be referred to institutions with experience in using "bloodless" surgical techniques. There are centers in the United States, for example, that have created a niche in caring for high-risk JW patients. They can be found by contacting the official JW Web site[a]. Consultation with or referral to such centers may be useful.

Surgeries Involving Extremely Limited Resources, Such as Solid Organ Transplant

In most routine surgical and anesthesia cases, distributive justice (fair allocation of scarce resources) is not a large consideration in the decision-making process.

---

[a] https://www.jw.org.

However, solid organ transplantation involves use of a very limited resource. Even centers that specialize in organ transplants in JWs have strict criteria for selecting the proper candidates for organ transplantation. If there is relative certainty that the preoperative status of the patient will mandate the use of blood products during the transplantation, then a JW patient probably should not be a candidate if they would refuse such transfusions. However, if the team feels that the transplant could reasonably be performed without the need for blood products, then we believe that the surgery can proceed.[30]

What Are the Health Care Provider's Rights and Obligations?

Many anesthesia providers feel that the refusal of standard care in the operating room, such as blood transfusions, places them in the untenable position of not being able to fulfill their professional duties. The American Society of Anesthesiologists has developed the Statement on Ethical Guidelines for the Anesthesia Care of Patients with Do-Not-Resuscitate Orders,[31] which is also applicable to other directives that limit treatment, which specify the following:

When an anesthesiologist finds the patient's or surgeon's limitations of intervention decisions to be irreconcilable with one's own moral views, then the anesthesiologist should withdraw in a nonjudgmental fashion, providing an alternative for care in a timely fashion. If such alternatives are not feasible within the time frame necessary to prevent further morbidity or suffering, then in accordance with the American Medical Association's Principles of Medical Ethics, care should proceed with reasonable adherence to the patient's directives, being mindful of the patient's goals and values.

In non-emergent situations, anesthesiologists have the right to recuse themselves from a patient's care, as long as they are willing to refer the patient to another provider who is capable and available to assume responsibility for care. In some cases, the referral is most appropriately made to another medical center that has expertise in caring for a certain group of patients, including, but not limited to JWs.[31]

If the clinical situation is a life-or-death emergency with no time to make a referral, the anesthesiologist is obligated to care for the patient, trying as much as possible to adhere to the patient's wishes. However, if the anesthesiologist is concerned that they will not be able to comply, then the patient or surrogate should be so informed.[31,32]

DISCUSSION

Some patients with religious, cultural, or other beliefs will refuse medical treatments, surgery, and administration of blood or blood products that the physician considers standard of care and, in some cases, life-sustaining. Other beliefs or life experiences can cause challenges for providers and health systems when patients have very specific needs that may be challenging to address. For example, some patients or their surrogates will require same-sex health care providers, access to alternative therapies (nutraceuticals, herbs, and other nontraditional therapies) that though maybe not refusing specific evidence-based treatments, may cause logistical problems and other challenges. The principle of respect for autonomy requires that health care providers honor a patient's right to refuse treatment or attempt to accommodate a request for alteration of standard practice, assuming a given situation is non-emergent, there is time to do so, and to the extent possible the providers can confirm that these alternatives do not interfere with standard practices nor have significant side effects or risk. In making decisions believed to be in the patient's best interest, the principles of beneficence and autonomy require that you ascertain that the patient has proper decision-making capacity and is free of coercion from health care providers and from family, friends, and religious advocates. The principle of non-maleficence requires that you limit or refer these patients to other providers capable of fulfilling the patient's requests. In those situations in which there is doubt about the patient's decision-making ability or to understand the consequences of the requests, about your obligations to the patient, or other issues, the hospital's ethics committee and/or legal counsel should be consulted. In addition and critically important, as our society has become increasingly diverse, it is extremely important for health care providers to develop cultural sensitivity skills. This can be accomplished by continuing education, through consultation with proper institutional departments, or most important by listening to patients.

CLINICS CARE POINTS

- Owing to strongly held beliefs, many patients will refuse certain medical interventions. These beliefs can be personal, religious, or cultural. Providers should identify whether these beliefs will impact clinical care and how to reconcile differences of opinion regarding medical management options.

- Respect for patient autonomy is the primary ethical principle applied in the United States, whereas the principle of beneficence is more strongly held in other countries.

- Respect for autonomy supports the concept that adult, competent patients have the right to refuse any medical therapy.

- Commitment to the principles of beneficence and non-maleficence requires anesthesiologists to offer the best care available within and consistent with the constraints of the patient's wishes—including appropriate preoperative planning to identify alternative therapies or management options and, in some cases, referring patients to alternative providers.

DISCLOSURE

Neither author has any conflicts of interest to disclose.

REFERENCES

1. Melton JG. Jehovah's Witness. Britannica; 1999. Updated June 30, 2023. Available at: https://www.britannica.com/topic/Jehovahs-Witnesses. Accessed July 31, 2023.
2. 2020 U.S. Religion Census Available at: https://www.usreligioncensus.org/index.php. Accessed August 1, 2023.
3. Ridley DT. Jehovah's Witnesses' refusal of blood: obedience to scripture and religious conscience. J Med Ethics 1999;25:469–72.
4. What Do Jehovah's Witnesses Believe? JW.ORG Available at: https://www.jw.org/en/jehovahs-witnesses/faq/jehovah-witness-beliefs/. Accessed July 31, 2023.
5. How Can Blood Save Your Life? JW.ORG Available at: https://www.jw.org/en/library/books/How-Can-Blood-Save-Your-Life/. Accessed July 31, 2023.
6. Bible. New World Translation; 2013. Genesis 9:3, Leviticus 17:10-16, Deuteronomy 15:23, Acts 15:28-29.
7. Questions from Readers. The Watchtower. July 1, 1951: 415 Available at: https://wol.jw.org/en/wol/d/r1/lp-e/1951487. Accessed July 31, 2023.
8. Muramoto O. Medical confidentiality and the protection of Jehovah's Witnesses' autonomous refusal of blood. J Med Ethics 2000;26:381–6.
9. When marital peace is threatened. The Watchtower. November 1, 1988: 20-25 Available at: https://wol.jw.org/en/wol/d/r1/lp-e/1988807. Accessed July 31, 2023.

10. Muramoto O. Bioethical aspects of the recent changes in the policy of refusal of blood by Jehovah's Witnesses. BMJ 2001;322:37–9.
11. Personal correspondence between the J. West and Mr. Pellechia; 2009.
12. Hammoud MM, White CB, Fetters MD. Opening cultural doors: Providing culturally sensitive healthcare to Arab American and American Muslim patients. AJOG 2005;193:1307–11.
13. Wecker L. Increasing cultural competence with Orthodox Jews: A primer for mental health clinicians. The Los Angeles Psychologist. Spring 2018: 6-7 Available at: https://www.lacpa.org/assets/LAP/Wecker%20LACPA%20Spring%2018.pdf. Accessed August 1, 2023.
14. Bressler T, Popp B. Ethical challenges when caring for Orthodox Jewish patients at the end of life. J Hospice Palliat Nurs 2018;20(1):36–44.
15. Anderson C, Potts L. The Amish health culture and culturally sensitive health services: An exhaustive narrative review. Soc Sci Med 2020;265:113466.
16. Anderson C, Potts L. Research trends in Amish population health, a growing literature about a growing rural population. J Rural Soc Sci 2021;36(1):6.
17. Prothero D, Callahan TD. UFOs, chemtrails, and aliens: what science says. Indiana University Press; 2017. p. 165.
18. Christian Science. Wikipedia Foundation. Updated July 2023 Available at: https://en.wikipedia.org/wiki/Christian_Science#Governance. Accessed September 4, 2023.
19. How Can I Be Healed. Christian Science Available at: https://www.christianscience.com/christian-healing-today/how-can-i-be-healed. Accessed September 4, 2023.
20. Beauchamp TL, Childress JF. Principles of biomedical ethics. 5th edition. Oxford University Press; 2001.
21. Georgetown College v Jones. 118 U.S. App. D.C. 80 (1964).
22. Re T. Adult: Refusal of Medical Treatment). Great Britain Court of Appeal, Civil Division. All Engl Law Rep 1992;30(4):649–70.
23. de Cruz P. Comparative health care law. Cavendish Publishing Ltd; 2001. p. 295.
24. Loriau J, Manaoulli C, Montpellier D, et al. Surgery and transfusion in Jehovah's Witness patient. Medical legal review. Ann Chir 2004;129(5):263–8.
25. Honig JF, Lilie H, Merten HA, et al. The refusal to consent to blood transfusion. Legal and medical aspects using Jehovah's Witnesses as an example. Anaesthetist 1992;41(7):396–8.
26. Furrow BR, Greaney TL, Johnson SH, et al. Health law: cases, materials and problems. 4th edition. West Group; 2001.
27. Gyamfi C, Berkowitz RL. Responses by pregnant Jehovah's Witnesses on healthcare proxies. Obstet Gynecol 2004;104:541–4.
28. Advocates for Jehovah's Witness Reform on Blood Available at: https://www.ajwrb.org/physicians. Accessed August 27, 2023.
29. Elder L. Why some Jehovah's Witnesses accept blood and conscientiously reject official Watchtower Society policy. J Med Ethics 2000;26:375–80.
30. Lin ES, Kaye AD, Baluch AR. Preanesthetic assessment of the Jehovah's Witness patient. Ochsner J 2012;12:61–9.
31. Stoye A, Chapin JW, Botha J, et al. Bloodless liver transplantation in a Jehovah's Witness. Int Anesthesiol Clin 2011;49:108–15.
32. Statement on Ethical Guidelines for the Anesthesia Care of Patients with Do-Not-Resuscitate Orders. Schaumburg, IL: American Society of Anesthesiologists; 2001. Updated 2018 https://www.asahq.orgstandards-and-practice-parameters/statement-on-ethical-guidelines-for-the-anesthesia-care-of-patients-with-do-not-resuscitate-orders. Accessed August 27, 2023.

Disclosure of Adverse Events and Medical Errors
A Framework for Anesthesiologists

Katherine O. Heller, MD*, Karen J. Souter, MB, BS, FRCA, MACM, PCC

KEYWORDS

- Medical error • Adverse events • Disclosure • Medical ethics • Training • Apology
- Malpractice

KEY POINTS

- Adverse events and medical errors remain an intrinsic part of the practice of medicine, including anesthesiology.
- Anesthesiologists face unique challenges in providing timely disclosure of adverse events and medical errors to their patients.
- Disclosure of adverse events and medical errors is strongly supported by patients, providers, national medical societies, and regulatory organizations.
- Training in disclosure techniques and communication strategies is an important component in supporting physicians in carrying out competent and ethical disclosure of adverse events and medical errors.
- The disclosure of adverse events and medical errors supports patient safety and allows for properly informed quality improvement practices.

INTRODUCTION

Adverse events and medical errors are an unfortunate but intrinsic part of the practice of medicine. Despite our best efforts, bad outcomes, including illness, injury, and death, occur as a result of these events. There has been an increased focus on the recognition and prevention of medical errors since the landmark report *To Err is Human* in 1999,[1] but medical error remains common in the practice of modern medicine. Adverse events are estimated to occur in up to one-quarter of hospital admissions,[2] and there are an estimated 200,000–400,000 deaths associated with preventable harm in hospitals each year in the United States.[3,4]

Department of Anesthesiology and Pain Medicine, University of Washington Medical Center, Seattle, WA, USA
* Corresponding author. Department of Anesthesiology & Pain Medicine University of Washington, Box 356540, 1959 NE Pacific Street, Seattle, WA 98195-6540.
E-mail address: oldenk@uw.edu

Anesthesiology Clin 42 (2024) 529–538
https://doi.org/10.1016/j.anclin.2023.12.003
1932-2275/24/© 2024 Elsevier Inc. All rights reserved.
anesthesiology.theclinics.com

Ethically and competently managing the disclosure of adverse events and medical errors to patients and their families is both a challenge and an opportunity for the practicing anesthesiologist. Prompt, honest disclosure is recommended by most professional societies and regulatory bodies, including the AMA[5] and the Joint Commission (formerly known as the Joint Commission on Accreditation of Healthcare Organizations).[6] There are many potential advantages to this approach, including improved doctor–patient relationships, better understanding and tracking of the causes of medical error, increased morale for medical providers, and potential prevention or reduction in malpractice claims. The disclosure of adverse events and medical errors ensures ethical, patient-centered care in supporting the need for patients to be fully appraised of all the facts to make informed decisions regarding their care. However, implementing appropriate disclosure policies remains difficult because of concerns over litigation, provider embarrassment and shame around adverse events, and medical errors as well as lack of experience and comfort in describing the adverse event and its consequences. Such conversations are challenging to manage in a calm and tactful manner. Anesthesiologists face the specific additional challenge as a result of brief initial patient contacts, events related to care of the anesthetized or sedated patient, multispecialty practice in complex care environments with many stakeholders, and often the need to provide ongoing patient care when an initial family disclosure conversation is occurring.

Although human error may be inevitable, better safety systems can help mitigate potential error and prevent patient harm. Willingness to promptly and honestly disclosure an adverse event or medical error is essential to maintaining a culture of safety and allowing root cause analysis (RCA) for sentinel events. Institutional training in communication strategies and the involvement of risk management and patient relations personnel can help encourage the disclosure of adverse events and medical errors in a way that benefits patients, their families, and the medical system.

HISTORICAL CONTEXT

Historically, anesthesiologists have been on the leading edge of patient safety work. The creation of the Anesthesia Patient Safety Foundation (APSF) in 1985 was an important milestone in establishing patient safety as a priority and framing it as something that can be improved with study and effort. The APSF vision, that *"no patient shall be harmed by anesthesia care"* preceded the 1999 *To Err is Human* report by nearly 15 years. Nonetheless, the turn of the century also marked a turning point in medicine; medical errors are viewed as potentially preventable events that should be addressed and mitigated by the larger medical system, rather than hidden or blamed on individual providers.

The frequency of adverse events and medical errors in anesthesia is hard to estimate, as many minor errors in medication dosing or patient management go unreported or in some cases even unrecognized. Perioperative medication administration is particularly prone to human error, as it necessarily bypasses checks that are standard in other parts of the hospital, including physician order entry, pharmacy verification, and multiple nursing confirmations. Self-reported rates of error are likely underestimates. The incidence of medication errors was estimated to be approximately 1 in 133 cases when anonymously reported[7] and most practicing anesthesiologists report involvement in at least one medical error.[8] More recently a prospective observational study reported that 1 in 20 perioperative medication administrations included a medical error and/or adverse drug event. Of these, 33% led to an observed adverse drug event and an additional 45.8% had the potential for patient harm.[9]

Thankfully, most errors do not result in lasting patient harm, but, in rare instances, more serious or even devastating errors do occur.

The Institute of Medicine[1] report changed the way health care professionals approach adverse events and medical errors and stimulated the redesign of health care systems to promote safety. Part of this transition has been a focus on transparency and disclosure. Since 2001, the Joint Commission has required disclosure of unanticipated outcomes of care and in 2006, the National Quality Forum recommended patients and families receive a *"timely, transparent, and clear communication about what is known about the event."* It is also recommended that an explicit, empathetic expression of regret be included with an apology in cases of clear error or system failure.[10]

THE ADVANTAGES AND OPPORTUNITIES ASSOCIATED WITH DISCLOSURE OF ADVERSE EVENTS AND MEDICAL ERRORS

The disclosure of adverse events and medical errors to patients and their families is grounded in ethical principles and has several clear advantages. First and foremost, it respects patient autonomy and empowers the patient to make fully informed decisions about their care at the time and in the future. Disclosure is consistent with our ethical obligation to be truthful and supports the ethical principle of justice, especially in cases of significant patient harm. For patients injured by adverse events or medical error, the first step toward accessing legal compensation is receiving proper notification that an error or system failure occurred.

Patients themselves report a strong preference for honesty and disclosure,[11-13] and a study of marginalized populations confirmed that population's general preference for disclosure of adverse events and medical errors.[14] When patients and their families participated in adverse event review, they reported timely communication, closing the loop on follow up, and centering the patient and family experience as specific priorities.[15] The majority of physicians supports disclosure[16]; recognition and disclosure of adverse events and medical errors is not only consistent with our obligations to patients, but also an essential part of professional obligations to ourselves and the community. Disclosing adverse events and medical errors within a supportive system can minimize secondary trauma to providers that can occur after serious harm events.

CHALLENGES OF DISCLOSURE AND THE *"DISCLOSURE GAP"*

Although providers, patients, and most medical societies support prompt and honest disclosure of adverse events and medical errors, there is still a gap between these recommendations and the reality of error disclosure. Providers may support error disclosure in theory but fail to provide that disclosure in practice. There are several reasons for this "disclosure gap,"[17] These reasons include fear of the patient's response and a loss of trust between physician and patient, a lack of knowledge of best practices for approaching a potentially difficult conversation, and the provider's own emotional response to the adverse event. The provider may fear loss of reputation or professional consequences, including liability, malpractice proceedings, and a loss of licensure to practice. Additionally, many physicians lack training and experience in potentially difficult conversations and may be concerned they will not be able to balance the patient's needs with their own concerns. Providers also experience a range of negative emotions when an error occurs and may feel shame and guilt around the time of disclosure.[18] Formally disclosing unexpected adverse events and medical errors implies a public admission of error, opening the door to perceived negative outcomes. Assumption about the patient's pre-existing knowledge and presumed preferences can also affect the likelihood of disclosure,[11] with physicians being less likely to disclosure adverse events and medical errors to patients they think might not want or understand the information.

ERROR DISCLOSURE IN THE CONTEXT OF ANESTHESIOLOGY PRACTICE

Anesthesiologists face additional specific challenges to adequate disclosure of adverse events and medical errors.[19] Anesthesiologists often have only brief contact with a patient before caring for them in a high-stakes environment. Anesthesiologists function as part of a multispecialty team in the operating room, along with other providers and medical staff, all of whom have a stake in any potential error or adverse event. For intra-operative events, the attending anesthesiologist is often responsible for the ongoing care and stabilization of the patient at the time when the first, and often critical, conversation with a patient's family member is likely to take place, usually led by the surgical team. The operating room is a complex environment, with multiple systems functioning in tandem. In the case of an adverse event, it may not initially be clear where the system failure and/or error occurred and this can add additional complexity to any patient or family discussions.

MALPRACTICE LEGISLATION

As disclosure of medical error becomes the expected standard of care in the opinion of patients and their care providers, there is increasing concern about the effect of error disclosure on potential liability and litigation outcomes. Two opposing opinions are prevalent; on one hand patients report an increased likelihood of pursuing legal action where there is perceived dishonesty, secrecy, or less than a complete explanation and apology.[20] With an increasing societal emphasis on disclosure, it was hoped that increased honesty and transparency around adverse events and medical errors, along with the opportunity for providers to express empathy and apologize, would reduce malpractice claims. On the other hand, disclosure also calls attention to the adverse event or medical error and allows the patient to avail themselves of the legal system, armed with knowledge gained during that disclosure conversation.[21] To encourage full, prompt, and honest disclosure, many of the United States have implemented "*apology laws*" that fully or partially protect the medical care provider from liability as a result of statements made during admissions of adverse events and medical errors. Currently, 39 states and the District of Colombia have provisions regarding medical professionals apologizing or making sympathetic gestures.[22] These laws offer varying protection. Some protect general admissions of sympathy from being admissible but preserve the admissibility of apologies that admit fault. In contrast, 9 states have more complete apology laws that protect not only expressions of sympathy and regret, but also admissions of fault or failure from being admissible in malpractice litigation, often for a set time after the event.[23] However, even these laws vary in exactly what types of apologies and admissions are covered.

Outcomes of institutional programs that focus on systematic disclosure of medical error have been mixed with some single institution studies reporting no increase in malpractice suits or costs after implementing error disclosure programs.[24] However, the overall malpractice claim frequency has not been reduced.[25,26] and the implementation of apology laws alone has not been shown to reduce the frequency or cost of malpractice claims in the United States.[23,27,28] Partial apology laws may limit the positive effects of disclosure, as a partial apology or expression of sympathy without full disclosure can be perceived as dishonest by patients and families.[23] In the absence of a comprehensive health system program around disclosure and compensation, apologies and disclosure may not reduce malpractice claims. In states such as Pennsylvania that mandate disclosure of medical error, one review found no increase in the total frequency of lawsuits but did find an association between disclosure and higher payout amount.[24]

COMMUNICATION AND RESOLUTION PROGRAMS

Communication and resolution programs (CRPs) have recently become more popular in large health care systems. These programs are one example of alternative dispute resolution models, which allow providers and health systems in which they operate to openly acknowledge when errors have occurred and offer compensation to the injured parties. The programs attempt to balance the needs of health care systems to ethically disclosure adverse events and medical errors and participate in rigorous quality improvement with the need for patients to receive compensation for error-related harm.[24] The University of Michigan Health System was an early adopter of a CRP, implementing an early settlement model in 2001. This model has 4 components: (1) acknowledging when patients are injured due to adverse events and medical errors; (2) compensating fairly (commensurate with degree of harm) and quickly when there is a deviation from the standard of care; (3) aggressively defending against meritless cases; and (4) studying all adverse events and medical errors to determine how health care delivery can be improved.[24] This model showed significant reduction in the frequency of malpractice claims and in total malpractice costs after implementation of the CRP.[29] CRPs are rapidly becoming popular and are now in use in at least 200 hospitals.[30] Similar programs have also shown reduced malpractice claims and costs, with one program showing 43% of events with medical error resolved by apology alone, even though 60% of these patients had legal representation.[26]

A toolkit for communication and optimal resolution containing implementation guidance for CRPs was released by the Agency for Healthcare Research and Quality in May 2016. Although the evidence for cost improvement (or at least cost neutrality) seems strong, the potential patient safety benefit remains to be seen.[31] CRPs are a logical next step in an ethical disclosure policy that supports both patients and providers, but their implementation remains challenging. Some centers have chosen an alternative CRP model focused on limited reimbursement. In these programs, there is less focus on error disclosure and events that result in serious harm or are otherwise likely to involve litigation are usually excluded. Rather, if upon review, a patient's medical care is deemed to be less than standard of care, patients and their families are proactively offered compensation and reimbursement for medical costs up to a limited amount. For government entities, the ability to proactively offer compensation for iatrogenic harm can be limited by both available funds and the laws governing disbursement of state or federal funding.

RISK MANAGEMENT BEST PRACTICES

One concern around the standardization of adverse event and medical error disclosure is increased exposure to liability. Many hospitals and health systems have risk management departments that aim to both improve patient safety and prevent or minimize adverse events and medical errors.[32] The strategies of risk management departments can be reactive to adverse events and medical errors or more proactive in terms of identifying and minimizing potential risks, often with the use of facility specific data. Risk management department professionals as well as patient relations staff can be essential in aiding providers after an adverse event or and medical error occurs, both in terms of advising on disclosure and apology, and in assuring later follow-up with the injured parties. A tracking system for reporting adverse events, medical errors, patient harm, and near misses is essential to enable risk management departments to improve patient care over time. It is in providers' best interest to understand the specific laws in their state that address adverse event and medical error disclosure, and to be aware of specifically what kinds of statements are covered under any applicable apology laws. Although honest disclosure of adverse events and medical errors is both ethically and professionally recommended, in initial discussions, it is best to avoid apologizing or placing blame if events are not fully understood. The risk management department in some institutions is available on call to advise on initial disclosure conversations. They are, however, most useful in subsequent contacts with an affected patient and/or their family. Some sentinel events, medication errors, and medical device malfunctions are mandated reportable events, and risk management can aid in ensuring compliance with necessary reporting.[33]

COMMUNICATION STRATEGIES AND TRAINING

Increasingly, the culture of medicine is shifting to encourage disclosure of adverse events and medical errors. With this shift comes a number of challenges around training current and new providers to responsibly engage in challenging conversations while disclosing an adverse event or medical error. Many hospital and graduate medical training programs have begun to incorporate training in error disclosure into their curriculums. These are most often brief didactic or small group role playing sessions.[34] Medical residents report increasing willingness to disclosure errors over historical cohorts,[35] and a formal curriculum and structured workshops have increased disclosure skills in standardized patient discussions.[36] In a large survey of residents, the presence of a formal curriculum had the largest positive affect on willingness to disclose error, while exposure to negative role-modeling was independently associated with an increased likelihood of trainees' nontransparent behavior in response to an error.[37] Outside a formal curriculum, the importance of role-modeling was demonstrated in a survey where physicians who witnessed their mentor's disclosing errors to patients were compared with those who did not. The results indicated that the physicians who witnessed error disclosure practices were more likely to do the same in front of their students and residents than those who did not (71.0% vs 29.0%, respectively, P-value = .008).[18] Practice atmosphere and climate in surgical versus medical settings may also affect anesthesiologists; a survey of surgical versus nonsurgical residents found that surgical residents were more concerned about potential negative feedback around error and less likely than nonsurgical residents to feel free to express concerns to other members of the team about medical errors.[38]

Although skill at adverse event and medical error disclosure increases with experience, even experienced providers have less than ideal error disclosure conversations in the absence of previous training.[39] Outside of training programs, just-in-time resources or coaching can be used to enable better error disclosure discussions at the time of the event. Depending on the institution, risk management resources may also be available for consultation. An additional positive outcome of routine adverse event and medical error disclosure is the ability to identify providers who may need additional support and counseling after significant patient harm events, with the hope of avoiding burnout. Most educational programs focus on maintaining a patient-centered and family-centered approach, allowing time for the affected patient or family to express emotion and ask questions, and ensuring a review and follow up of the event.

CULTURE OF SAFETY, AND ROOT CAUSE ANALYSIS

A root cause is defined as a deficiency or decision that, if corrected or avoided, will eliminate the undesirable consequence. RCA is a structured method used to analyze serious adverse events. Initially developed to analyze industrial accidents, RCA is now widely deployed as an error analysis tool in health care.[40] RCA seeks to identify the underlying systemic issues that allow errors to happen, rather than blaming individual providers. The RCA process has been mandated in response to sentinel events by the Joint Commission since 1997.[40] The first step of the RCA is to assemble a multidisciplinary team to identify and define the problem. The RCA team investigates and attempts to determines the root cause (or causes) of the adverse event or medical error. In the detailed phase of identifying what occurred, the full disclosure of adverse events and medical errors is a critical part. The need for creating a culture of support for the medical team members involved in the event and their ability to fully disclose what happened cannot be overestimated. Once the RCA team has identified all the system issues and missteps that led to the adverse event or medical error, it will propose changes to various hospital systems with the intention of avoiding or mitigating future risk.[41] When this system works well, it creates a feedback loop that ideally reduces future sentinel events, adverse events, and medical errors. However, implementing sustainable change can prove challenging, even in the face of serious adverse events. One large review of RCAs found that only 35% resulted in clear proposed corrective measures. The most common solution types were training, process change, and policy reinforcement. The disclosure of adverse events and medical errors and a strong culture of safety that supports transparency is therefore essential to the success of any RCA process.

SUMMARY

Patients, major medical societies, government entities, and providers all agree that the prompt, honest disclosure of adverse events and medical errors is standard practice. This disclosure fulfills our ethical obligations to patients and, in the right setting, may help the medical system to improve and reduce errors in the future. However, significant barriers still exist to the disclosure of adverse events and medical errors. All providers may experience worry over professional consequences, patient responses, and the potential for increased liability or loss of licensure. Anesthesiologists have the additional challenges of short preoperative patient contact, practice in a multispecialty environment with multiple stakeholders, and the need to continue care for affected patients at the time of initial disclosure conversations. Apology laws, and measures to protect physicians expressing empathy or in some cases admitting fault have had mixed results. CRPs that combine adverse event and medical error disclosure with patient follow up and the offer of compensation when appropriate are a promising way forward. Formal training in adverse event and medical error disclosure may help providers feel more comfortable with these challenging conversations. One predictor of the willingness to disclose error is having seen mentors or colleague model appropriate error disclosure, it is hopeful that the current progress in willingness to disclose adverse events and medical errors will continue. Risk management departments and analysis of error in a continuing quality improvement cycle to minimize preventable adverse events and medical errors are essential parts of an institution's commitment to their patients. Root cause analysis is an important tool where the focus should be held on developing specific, system level changes to aid in preventing future adverse events and medical errors. Anesthesiologists face a challenging landscape around adverse event and medical error disclosure that can be ameliorated by a strong culture of safety and transparency in the workplace, role modeling of error disclosure by colleagues, and risk management departments support after an adverse event or medical error has occurred.

CLINICS CARE POINTS

- Prompt, honest disclosure of medical adverse events and errors to patients and their families is a difficult but necessary part of the ethical practice of medicine
- Error disclosure and apologies for medical errors are legally protected in some, but not all, states and the degree of protection varies from state to state
- Disclosure conversations with patients and their families are best approached in a calm environment, focusing on discussion of the known facts and expressions of empathy, with assurances of further follow up and communication
- Health care systems should consider instituting provider training in disclosure conversations, risk management systems, and potentially communication and resolution programs to improve both the patient and provider experience around adverse medical events.

DISCLOSURE

K.O. Heller and K.J. Souter have no relevant commercial or financial conflicts of interest and no funding sources to disclose.

REFERENCES

1. Bates DW, Levine DM, Salmasian H, et al. The safety of inpatient health care. N Engl J Med 2023;388:142–53.
2. James JT. A new, evidence-based estimate of patient harms associated with hospital care. J Patient Saf 2013;9:122–8.
3. Kavanagh KT, Saman DM, Bartel R, et al. Estimating hospital-related deaths due to medical error: a perspective from patient advocates. J Patient Saf 2017;13:1–5.
4. American Medical Association. Promoting Patient Safety: Code of Medical Ethics Opinion 8.6. Accessed Oct 18, 2023. https://www.ama-assn.org/delivering-care/ethics/promoting-patient-safety.
5. LeGros N, Pinkall JD. The new JCAHO patient safety standards and the disclosure of unanticipated outcomes. Joint Commission on Accreditation of Healthcare Organizations. J Health Law 2002;35:189–210.
6. Webster CS, Merry AF, Larsson L, et al. The frequency and nature of drug administration error during anaesthesia. Anaesth Intensive Care 2001;29:494–500.
7. Orser BA, Chen RJ, Yee DA. Medication errors in anesthetic practice: a survey of 687 practitioners. Can J Anaesth 2001;48:139–46.
8. Nanji KC, Patel A, Shaikh S, et al. Evaluation of perioperative medication errors and adverse drug events. Anesthesiology 2016;124:25–34.
9. National Quality Forum. Safe practices for better healthcare - 2010 Update: A Consensus Report. Washington, DC: 20010.
10. O'Connor E, Coates HM, Yardley IE, et al. Disclosure of patient safety incidents: a comprehensive review. Int J Qual Health Care 2010;22:371–9.
11. Gallagher TH, Waterman AD, Ebers AG, et al. Patients' and physicians' attitudes regarding the disclosure of medical errors. JAMA 2023;289:1001–7.
12. Moore M, Mello MM. Patients' experiences with communication-and-resolution programs after medical injury. JAMA Intern Med 2017;177:1595–603.

13. Olazo K, Wang K, Sierra M, et al. Preferences and Perceptions of Medical Error Disclosure Among Marginalized Populations: A Narrative Review. Joint Comm J Qual Patient Saf 2022;48:539–48.

14. McQueen JM, Gibson KR, Manson M, et al. Adverse event reviews in healthcare: what matters to patients and their family? A qualitative study exploring the perspective of patients and family. BMJ Open 2022;12:e060158.

15. Gallagher TH, Waterman AD, Garbutt JM, et al. US and Canadian physicians' attitudes and experiences regarding disclosing errors to patients. Arch Intern Med 2006;166:1605–11.

16. Ghalandarpoorattar SM, Kaviani A, Asghari F. Medical error disclosure: the gap between attitude and practice. Postgrad Med 2012;88:130–3.

17. Mansour R, Ammar K, Al-Tabba A, et al. Disclosure of medical errors: physicians' knowledge, attitudes and practices (KAP) in an oncology center. BMC Med Ethics 2020;21:74.

18. Souter KJ, Gallagher TH. The disclosure of unanticipated outcomes of care and medical errors: what does this mean for anesthesiologists? Anesth Analg 2012; 114:615–21.

19. Vincent C, Young M, Phillips A. Why do people sue doctors? A study of patients and relatives taking legal action. Lancet 1994;343:1609–13.

20. Kachalia A, Shojania KG, Hofer TP, et al. Does full disclosure of medical errors affect malpractice liability? The jury is still out. Joint Comm J Qual Saf 2003;29: 503–11.

21. Morton H. Medical Professional Apologies Statutes 2021. Available at: https:// www.ncsl.org/financial-services/medical-professional-apologies-statutes. Accessed November 9, 2023.

22. Ross NE, Newman WJ. The role of apology laws in medical malpractice. J Am Acad Psychiatr Law 2021;JAAPL:200107–20.

23. Painter LM, Kidwell KM, Kidwell RP, et al. Do written disclosures of serious events increase risk of malpractice claims? one health care system's experience. J Patient Saf 2018;14:87–94.

24. Kachalia A, Kaufman SR, Boothman R, et al. Liability claims and costs before and after implementation of a medical error disclosure program. Ann Intern Med 2010;153:213–21.

25. LeCraw FR, Montanera D, Jackson JP, et al. Changes in liability claims, costs, and resolution times following the introduction of a communication-and-resolution program in Tennessee. J Patient Saf Risk Manag 2018;23:13–8.

26. Fields AC, Mello MM, Kachalia A. Apology laws and malpractice liability: what have we learned? BMJ Qual Saf 2020;30.

27. McMichael BJ, Van Horn RL, Viscusi WK. "Sorry" is never enough: how state apology laws fail to reduce medical malpractice liability risk. Stanford Law Rev 2019; 71:341–409.

28. Kass JS, Rose RV. Medical malpractice reform - historical approaches, alternative models, and communication and resolution programs. AMA J Ethics 2016;18: 299–310.

29. McDonald TB, Van Niel M, Gocke H, et al. Implementing communication and resolution programs: lessons learned from the first 200 hospitals. J Patient Safety Risk Manage 2018;23:73–8.

30. Gallagher TH, Mello MM, Sage WM, et al. Can communication-and-resolution programs achieve their potential? five key questions. Health Aff 2018;37: 1845–52.

31. McGowan J, Wojahn A, Nicolini JR. Risk Management Event Evaluation and Responsibilities. [Updated 2023 Aug 23]. In: StatPearls [Internet]. Treasure Island (FL): StatPearls Publishing; 2023. Available at: https://www.ncbi.nlm.nih.gov/books/NBK559326/

32. What Is Risk Management in Healthcare? NEJM Catalyst. 2018. Available at: https://catalyst.nejm.org/doi/full/10.1056/CAT.18.0197. Accessed November 10, 2023.

33. Stroud L, Wong BM, Hollenberg E, et al. Teaching medical error disclosure to physicians-in-training: a scoping review. Acad Med 2013;88:884–92.

34. Varjavand N, Bachegowda LS, Gracely E, et al. Changes in intern attitudes toward medical error and disclosure. Med Educ 2012;46:668–77.

35. Wong BM, Coffey M, Nousiainen MT, et al. Learning through experience: influence of formal and informal training on medical error disclosure skills in residents. J Grad Med Educ 2017;9:66–72.

36. Martinez W, Hickson GB, Miller BM, et al. Role-modeling and medical error disclosure: a national survey of trainees. Acad Med 2014;89:482–9.

37. Martinez W, Lehmann LS. The "hidden curriculum" and residents' attitudes about medical error disclosure: comparison of surgical and nonsurgical residents. J Am Coll Surg 2013;217:1145–50.

38. Crimmins AC, Wong AH, Bonz JW, et al. To Err is human' but disclosure must be taught. Simulat Healthc J Soc Med Simulat 2018;13:107–16.

39. AHRQ. Root Cause analysis. patient safety primer. 2014. Available at: https://psnet.ahrq.gov/primers/primer/10/root-cause-analysis. Accessed November 10, 2023.

40. Singh G, Patel RH, Boster J. Root cause analysis and medical error prevention. In: StatPearls [internet]. Treasure Island (FL): StatPearls Publishing; 2023. Available at: https://www.ncbi.nlm.nih.gov/books/NBK570638/. Accessed November 10, 2023.

41. Kellogg KM, Hettinger Z, Shah M, et al. Our current approach to root cause analysis: is it contributing to our failure to improve patient safety? BMJ Qual Saf 2017; 26:381–7.

Conscientious Objection

Gail A. Van Norman, MD*

KEYWORDS

- Physician conscientious objection • Moral distress • Accommodation
- Conscience clause

KEY POINTS

- Conscientious objection occurs when a physician objects to or refuses to provide patient care that is within medical standards due to a deeply held moral belief that to do so would be morally wrong.
- In the United States, conscientious objection in medicine is protected by the federal and state laws, but raises concerns regarding discrimination and limitations in healthcare access for vulnerable patients.
- Accommodation of conscientious objections also increases burdens on colleagues and institutions.
- Benefits of accommodation are greater ethical and moral diversity among health care providers and encouragement for morally passionate and committed physicians to enter the medical profession.
- Most ethicists and professional society statements agree that physician conscientious objection should be accommodated, when possible, but should be limited in ways to avoid discrimination and other patient harms, such as loss of access to medically valid care that meets professional standards.

INTRODUCTION

A core precept of medical ethics sets the patient's interest generally above that of the physician. However, it is not rare for physicians to confront personal moral conflicts in clinical care situations. Solving such conflicts, when patient desires or needs for medical treatments, are legal and within the standard of care can be a deeply challenging problem for physicians and practices. When surveyed, 27% of intensive care clinicians and nurses reported that they had acted in a manner contrary to personal or professional beliefs.[1] Forty-two percent of physicians overall and 58% of physicians rated as having "high religiosity" stated in a separate survey that they believed they are never obliged to do what they personally believe to be wrong.[2]

Professor Emeritus, Anesthesiology and Pain Medicine, Past Adjunct Professor Bioethics, University of Washington, Seattle, WA, USA
* Corresponding author.
E-mail address: gvn@uw.edu

Anesthesiology Clin 42 (2024) 539–554
https://doi.org/10.1016/j.anclin.2023.11.004
1932-2275/24/© 2023 Elsevier Inc. All rights reserved.

As modern medical ethics and legal decisions have increasingly enforced the primacy of patient rights and the requirement of respect for patient autonomy, it is to be expected that physicians will face more moral conflicts in a world that now affords them less paternalistic power to simply do what they personally believe is right. Physician "conscientious objection" to providing legal and accepted medical care when they feel morally conflicted has drawn increasing debate and legislative protection, placing it squarely in confrontation with burgeoning patient rights. Debates about conscientious objection often focus on special obligations and restrictions placed on the objector, but there are also important reasons for the medical community to accommodate objections when such accommodations do not create greater harms for patients or communities.

Although the origin of conscientious objection in medicine in the United States is often claimed to have started with the legalization of abortion protections afforded by the US Supreme Court decision in Roe v. Wade,[3] many other medical advances of the mid- and late-twentieth century were equally important, for example, the development of mechanical ventilation, the growth of organ transplantation, the legalization in some states of physician aid-dying, and the advocacy of religious groups such as the Jehovah's Witness Church to refuse blood transfusions. Such developments fostered "moral disagreements" between patients and physicians and raised questions of whether physicians can be required to provide care when they feel it violates their moral integrity.[4]

Many aspects of practice within the specialty of anesthesiology confront conscientious objections. These include refusals to honor patients' directives to forego certain treatments in the operating room and intensive care unit, including implementing advance directives requesting withdrawal of artificial nutrition and hydration or mechanical ventilation and patient refusals to receive blood transfusions and initiation of cardiopulmonary resuscitation in the operative room. It also includes objections to the provision of valid treatments that are requested by patients, including palliative sedation at end of life or physician aid-in-dying. Finally, anesthesiologist objections to participating in certain operating room procedures include providing anesthesia for pregnancy terminations, contraceptive procedures, and gender reassignment surgery,[5,6] among others.

CONSCIENCE AND OBJECTION

Conscientious objection in medicine is defined as a refusal by a physician or institution to provide medical care that is legal, valid, accepted, and within the standard of care due to a deep moral, ethical, cultural, or religious belief that to do so would violate their moral integrity and lead to a crisis of conscience. Physicians are never ethically obliged to provide futile, bizarre, or substandard care under principles of beneficence, non-maleficence, and in keeping with standards of professionalism. But their rights to raise a conscientious objection to other care, even though legally protected, are ethically limited.

The Conscience

Understanding what constitutes conscientious objection and what motivates conscientious objectors requires considering the very concept that lies at its heart: the conscience. The concept of conscience has long occupied a prominent place in philosophy and religion, but even now there is no general consensus on its meaning.[7-12] Various concepts of the conscience proffered by ethicists and philosophers are often sorted into one of two main categories: that of the "internal voice" versus that of a rational, externally validated moral framework.[9,13,14]

The concept of conscience as an internal voice expressing a person's sense of truth, and of right and wrong, asserts that the truth is absolute and immutable. Many philosophers, ethicists, and theologians express conscience as an "inner light" or even a gift bestowed by God. Rousseau called conscience the "voice of the soul,"[9,13] claiming that reason often deceives, but the conscience "never does."[13] Conversely, other ethicists have argued that such an "inner voice" can lead persons astray[15] and that the true conscience is instead a rational aspect of morality in which moral rules are reached via reason together with the external validation of observation and experience.[16,17] The rational concept of conscience holds that the inner voice is not necessarily a conduit to God but may be based in personal psychology and biases. The inner voice may sometimes merely be giving sway to undesirable, even despicable, internal personal judgments, and discrimination, and many medical ethicists argue that it cannot justify swerving from the principle of putting the patient first. There exists no test by which an objector can prove that their objection is sincere and not based in other subliminal or undisclosed motives, irrespective of what concept of conscience they hold.[16,17] These two concepts of conscience are nearly impossible to reconcile with one another, because one relies on "belief" and the other on "reason," and yet both may be in play in a conscientious objection.

Most ethicists' discussions of conscience do not include additional perspectives that are rooted in psychiatry and neurobiology, such as conscience, as a function of self-assessment that is developed from exposure to parents, family, and culture and regulates one's own behavior and identity.[18,19] Ethics discussions also do not usually address a malfunctioning conscience that may be the result of mental health conditions such as depression and obsessive compulsive disorder, both of which involve actions seated in deep feelings of shame and guilt,[20] and some of which may even have a physical basis in neurotransmitter physiology.

The lack of consensus regarding the concept of "the conscience" in any philosophic, historical, psychological, or neurobiological context, presents serious problems when we try to have a reasonable dialogue with one another about conscience, freedom of conscience, conscientious objection, and accommodation of beliefs. Despite a lack of consensus as to what conscience is, and regardless of the concepts out of which it arises, conscience clearly gives birth to deep moral conflicts in physicians. Nearly all ethical and philosophic concepts of conscience agree that conscience binds us to our actions in several critical ways: "moral" persons must avoid "immoral" acts, and once a moral obligation is accepted, there is a duty, or promise, to fulfill it that cannot be dismissed in the face of mere discomfort or difficulties.[7]

Conscientious Objections

There are many situations in which a physician may object to providing medical care. A physician may raise an objection that the requested treatment is futile or bizarre (ie, does not conform to acknowledged medical principles) or does not meet the standard of care, for example. A provider may raise legitimate doubts about the scientific merit of a treatment even if it is accepted or about the appropriateness of a treatment in a specific clinical context. A provider may argue that providing the care would violate other medical ethical principles that outweigh obligations to treat: one example is a violation of a principle of distributive justice if the care of one person in a mass casualty situation would divert critical resources from multiple other patients who might otherwise survive. However, although all of these objections can certainly be valid in some circumstances, none of them is a *conscientious* objection.[21]

A refusal to act due to personal threat is also not a conscientious objection, but a surrender to coercion—indeed, examples abound of conscientious objections in nonmedical contexts that have *created* significant, even extreme personal risks for the objector. One example is that of Desmond Doss, who served as a medic in World War II, and refused to carry a firearm due to his religious beliefs. Yet he went repeatedly unarmed and under fire onto the battlefield to retrieve wounded soldiers at the Battle of Hacksaw Ridge in Okinawa and personally saved the lives of more than 75 men.[22] In another more recent example, many US government employees refused to separate children from their families at the US-Mexico border in 2018 despite federal government policies requiring them to do so and under personal threat of job loss, prosecution, and incarceration.[23]

A conscientious objection in medicine usually involves a refusal to act based on a specific personal moral belief that is in tension with accepted medical standards of care. For a conscientious objection to be valid, it has to be morally substantial, such that to perform the act would seriously damage the moral integrity of the individual, and not merely cause personal discomfort, inconvenience, or even a small degree of personal risk.[24] Conscientious objection lies in the premise that physicians as individuals have personal core moral values that contribute to that person's understanding of *who they are*,[25] and violating such values would challenge the very core of that physician's moral identity.

Many people associate conscientious objection with religious proscripts, but conscientious objection need not be based in a religious doctrine.[26] If those were required, then physicians who are atheists or who do not practice a specific religion would not be able to raise moral objections, even when acting would cause them extreme moral distress. Furthermore, when the objector is citing a religious basis, their personal interpretation and exercise of that religion does not need to conform to formal doctrine: few physicians are religious scholars, and faith-based beliefs of all individuals often diverge from strict theological creeds. The only "test" of whether an objection is conscientious, is whether the objector holds a deep personal belief, the violation of which would be soul-crushing.

Conscientious objection should also be distinguished from political activism and civil disobedience—which can also arise out of physicians' moral or religious beliefs. Civil disobedience is defined as a willful unlawful and public act with political or moral principles at stake that is motivated by a will to affect political, legal, or social change.[7,27] Conscientious objection, in contrast, is a private, and (usually) legal refusal to act in response to a personal moral conviction. Note that in this context, "private" does not mean "confidential," but rather that the act's *primary* intention is not to effect a public, societal change.

ACCOMMODATING CONSCIENTIOUS OBJECTIONS

Perspectives regarding accommodation of conscientious objections take the form of several common assertions: (1) conscientious absolutism, (2) the "incompatibility thesis," and (3) the "moderate view."

Absolutists

An absolutist point of view insists that a practitioner who has a moral obligation to a legal and professionally accepted medical treatment has no obligation to participate or to refer the patient to a willing provider, lest such aid make the provider morally complicit in the objectionable care.[28] The simplest definition of moral complicity is "abetting" an act that is immoral, either by directly participating in the act itself or facilitating its occurrence in a meaningful way. Absolutists argue that referring a patient to another provider who will perform anesthesia for what is in their view an "immoral" procedure, such as gender-affirming surgery, for example, would be as immoral as performing the anesthetic themself, because the "objectionable" outcome (in this example gender reassignment) is the same. Surveys show that close to half of physicians, whether conscientious objectors or not, agree with this assertion.[29] But this argument assumes a very broad and overly simplistic view of what makes one morally complicit. Most ethicists agree that moral complicity involves more complex questions[11,30] and many assert that required referrals are morally permissible.[31]

Whether an act of one person is morally complicit with the act of another depends on a number of factors and nuances. Lipora and Goodin proposed that an argument for moral complicity is stronger if (1) the degree of "wrong doing" is significant—that is, the act would clearly be considered wrong in most contexts and cultures, (2) the objector knows the act is wrong in most contexts and cultures, (3) the wrong doing could or would not occur without their referral or other aid, and (4) there is "shared purpose" between the referring doctor with the principle "wrong-doer"—that is, *the objector both approves of and shares the same goal with the principle actor*.[30] Note that in such a case the objector's claim of conscientious objection is "insincere," because they tacitly approve of the action and are facilitating it, but simply do not want to bear blame for it.

The Incompatibility Thesis

The incompatibility thesis asserts that joining the medical profession is voluntary and that by doing so the physician has committed themselves to take on specific and well-publicized moral obligations to promote the health of patients, to respect patient autonomy and to place patient interests above their own.[32] If the person cannot keep these commitments, they should not become doctors in the first place.[33] Problems with this assertion are (1) it assumes that all potential objections are known to the person before they become a physician and (2) it does not take into account the possibility that the physician as a moral entity will experience personal change and may adopt new faith-based beliefs or receive other moral revelations as time goes by, such that their initial "commitment" no longer makes sense to them.

Some proponents of the incompatibility thesis point out that within the medical profession, there is broad latitude within which practitioners can make choices of specialty and practice locations to minimize confronting obligations that conflict with their moral integrity. An abortion objector, for example, could choose to work solely in Catholic institutions.[34] One problem with such practice restriction is the question of whether it is fair to require confinement to a less inspiring or less lucrative career as the price of moral integrity.

Proponents of the incompatibility thesis often demand that conscientious objectors leave the medical profession or specialty entirely when a repeated conscientious objection occurs.[33] In other contexts, this has also been proposed as a way for conscientious objectors to solve their dilemmas. The Jehovah's Witness Church, for example, exhorts conscientious objectors in their congregations to "carry their own load of responsibility," not push burdens off onto others—and to seek employment of another kind, "even though it may not be as rewarding from a financial standpoint."[35] But forcing out of the medical profession those individuals who develop moral beliefs that occasionally conflict with practice is wasteful of the physician as a resource and in the long run may serve the profession poorly by excluding thoughtful, committed, passionate, and moral providers from practicing at all and by failing to develop understanding and respect for diverse beliefs among medical colleagues.

Some ethicists argue against accommodation, asking the question of whether an objection can truly be a conscientious objection if the objector demands to be able to deflect the costs their beliefs place on them, rather than bear the costs themselves.[8] They posit that accommodation of conscientious objection is always a gift and not an obligation. But in so doing, they fail to recognize ethical obligations that we also bear toward our professional community and colleagues to respect and support each other in a meaningful professional life. The American Society of Anesthesiologists (ASA) Guidelines on the Ethical Practice of Anesthesiology refer to the obligation to foster a cooperative and respectful relationship with colleagues,[36] and we should find it difficult to simply ignore the moral distress of a colleague or dismiss them from our professional company.

Absolutism and the incompatibility thesis, though nearly polar opposites, share in common an intolerance for morally diverse points of view and are thus difficult to unswervingly support in a society that now consists of many different cultural, moral, and religious perspectives. As the United States has become less monolithic in culture and beliefs, both absolutism and the incompatibility thesis not only become harder and harder to support, but they reflect less and less the diverse beliefs of our profession's own members, as well as that of our patients.

Arguments Against Accommodation

Accommodating conscientious objection in medicine creates some formidable problems. At times, accommodation can and does end up erecting barriers to desired and/ or necessary medical treatments[37] — compromising health care and causing direct patient harm as a result.[38] Many patients will not be able to overcome the impediments created by a conscientious objector, whether the objector is an individual or an institution. Such barriers are unlikely to hinder those who are financially well-off, for example, but place burdens disproportionately on vulnerable patient groups—such as women, adolescents, the elderly, the poor, members of the LBTQ community, and patients of non-"mainstream" cultures, and ethnicity—who are more likely to already experience compromised health care access and are comparatively more likely to suffer from illness that is also due to societal disparities. When a conscientious objector is the sole provider or one of a limited number of providers in a region that can provide the service, accommodating conscientious objection could have devastating consequences for these groups of patients.

Conscientious objection can be asserted by institutions as well as individuals, and a high density of "conscience-protected beds" could make it impossible for an individual patient to find a place to receive desired care, even when there are sufficient numbers of providers. Such instances have real-world consequences. In 2020, for example, more than 41% of hospital beds in the state of Washington were run by Catholic Health Initiatives (CHI) Franciscan, a Catholic institution that prohibits pregnancy terminations, contraception services, aid-in-dying, and transgender care, all of which are legal services in the state.[39] A merger between CHI Franciscan and the Virginia Mason health system threatened to deprive large areas of the state of *all* of these services. The state was already familiar with the problems that would result: a merger between another Catholic health care organization and local hospitals in 2012 had led to a complete cessation of abortion services for a large swath of the Seattle area, and the entire city of Bellingham saw complete loss of those services under similar mergers. Catholic institutions currently account for one in six of all hospital beds in the United States,[39] and as such mergers continue, worries about the scope of service denials due to institutional and physician conscientious objections across the nation are not overblown.

Conscientious objection also presents hardships to non-objecting medical systems and to individual clinicians. Non-objecting institutions face challenges in taking on the burden of care other institutions are denying patients, and thus take on potentially an unfair share of patients whose care is less well reimbursed, for example.[26] Institutions must develop policies and hire staffing that permit conscientious objections among their own staff. Colleagues may be required to take on more work, and more stressful cases—many conscientious objections relate to refusals to treat patients for whom an emergency termination of pregnancy may be life-saving (eg, ectopic pregnancy, spontaneous miscarriage, and during cardiopulmonary resuscitation of a pregnant patient), as well as many other objections related to intensive care and end-of-life care, presenting significant psychological and emotional stresses to physicians who much step in and shoulder a larger burden of emergency and ICU cases. A recent study from Quebec confirms that burdens related to aid-in-dying are distributed unevenly as a result of conscientious objection and that patient access also suffers.[40] Such issues also can potentially create significant friction over pay equity and workload disparities. All of this poses problematic questions for institutional and public policies and professional standards, particularly when they occur in communities that are medically underserved to begin with.

Arguments for Accommodation

Despite concerns regarding accommodation of conscientious objection, there are powerful reasons to respect many, if not most of them. Certainly, at times, threats occur to the moral integrity of many doctors that would interfere with them being able to lead what, in their view, would be a moral and meaningful life if they were not allowed to recuse themselves from certain aspects of patient care. Not allowing conscientious objection could negatively impact what type of person wants to enter the medical profession—discouraging those with a strong moral identity and moral commitment, for example.[41] Disrespecting conscious objection also breeds intolerance for diverse moral beliefs among physicians and, by extension, patients.

The "moderate" view and reasonable accommodation

The moderate view toward conscientious objections holds that understanding and respecting practitioner's moral objections is an important part of our medical community. It supports a diversity of cultural, philosophic, and political ideals in medicine and promotes empathy of practitioners with patients who experience diverse beliefs and customs. Respect for conscientious objection draws our attention to practices and philosophies that may have become outdated or irrelevant. It promotes sensitivity and empathy among providers and fulfills an ethical obligation to promote the moral, philosophic, and ethical "health" of colleagues.[36]

However, this point of view also recognizes that not all conscientious objections are equal. Providing an accommodation for some circumstances is easier and far less burdensome than others, for example. Allowing a provider to wear a personal religious symbol at work presents a lower threat to the quality of care of individual and groups of patients, compared with someone refusing to provide anesthesia for an emergency treatment of ectopic pregnancy, for example–it can hardly be ethically distinguished from other personal ornaments with significant moral meaning that are commonly accepted, such as wedding rings.

Reasonable accommodation requires that both parties accept that a diversity of opinions exist and work to resolve disagreements respectfully while also recognizing the primacy of the responsibility that physicians have toward patient well-being. Thus, the moderate view favors accommodation, but sets limits. There is widespread agreement among ethicists that accommodations that would violate certain foundational concepts in medicine, or that would endanger patients, should not be allowed (**Box 1**)[7,11,12,26,42–44] and also the objector must, whenever possible, raise conscientious objections in advance if they know that they have them.

Some objectors argue that requiring advance notice raises physician privacy concerns. However, this argument is difficult to sustain when the objecting physician is indicating that they are going to act out their beliefs publicly if the patient care issue arises. Furthermore, employers have rights to know limited private information about their employees, if it affects the employee's ability to perform specific tasks that are explicitly detailed in their employment contract.[42,45]

American Society of Anesthesiologists and American Medical Association Guidelines

The ASA Guidelines for the Ethical Practice of Anesthesiology recognizes also the American Medical Association's (AMAs) Principles of Medical Ethics.[36,46] Both acknowledge physician rights to conscientious objection but also include the concept of required referral. The ASA Committee Ethics Committee's Statement on Ethical Guidelines for the Anesthesia Care of Patients with Do-Not-Resuscitate Orders[47] also requires that anesthesiologists who morally object to providing care should withdraw "in a nonjudgmental fashion, providing an alternative for care in a timely fashion." The AMA Code of Ethics[46] states that physicians "are expected to uphold the ethical

---

Box 1
Commonly recognized characteristics of an unallowable conscientious objection (moderate view of accommodation)

- The objection permits, promotes, or results in discrimination against a class or group of persons.

- The objection is based on a false clinical belief, that is, inaccurate factual understanding of a treatment—for example, an anesthesiologist who refuses to perform anesthesia in a possibly pregnant patient asserting that anesthetic agents are teratogenic, when studies demonstrate that this is not true.

- The objection harms patients or burdens them to an unacceptable degree. For example, a refusal to provide care that would result in a patient having to travel one mile in a nonemergency situation to obtain alternate care is ethically less problematic than one with a requirement to travel to a different city, state, or country, for the same care for a patient who could not shoulder the expense of the travel, or has limited ability to accomplish it.

- The objector refuses to provide critical patient information, that is, to disclose relevant legal and standard clinical options, including those that might be morally objectionable to the practitioner.

- The objector refuses to refer a patient to a "willing provider."

- The objector fails to give appropriate advance notice of limitations in service. An objection that is likely to occur more than once, such as when an anesthesiologist refuses to provide anesthesia for pregnancy terminations, should be disclosed to a practice before hire, with an understanding that the size of the practice may not allow accommodation of such an objection.

- The objection is being exercised in an emergency situation in which access to alternative care will be compromised and/or would cause a grievous delay in life-saving or life-altering medical care.

From Refs.[7,11,12,26,42–44]

norms of their profession, including fidelity to patients and respect for patient self-determination" but also asserts that the physician's freedom to act or refrain from acting according to conscience is limited and generally agree with many of the limits suggested by ethicists (see Box 1). They also state that if a physician refuses to refer, they still must help the patient identify how to obtain access to the desired services. This last requirement is unlikely to satisfy absolutists, because it still provides "aid" to the patient in obtaining the objected care.

LEGISLATIVE ISSUES

Not all countries or agencies recognize the same rights to conscientious objections for physicians. There is no legal right to conscientious objection for any profession in Sweden due to overriding cultural commitment to public service and ideals about nondiscrimination.[48] In Ontario, a court recently ruled that a referral requirement for a conscientious objector was a reasonable limitation on physicians' religious freedoms, to prevent patient harm and inequitable health care access.[49] In Australia, institutional conscientious objection to aid-in-dying (which is legalized) is not explicitly legally protected in Victoria, Tasmania, or other states of Western Australia, but regulations in South Australia, Queensland, and New South Wales strike a balance between patient access and institutional perspectives.[50] Many countries include referral obligations in conscience legislation regarding abortion, including Argentina, some Australian states, Chile, Colombia, China, Portugal, South Africa, and Zambia; however, multiple studies have found that refusal to refer is common among objecting practitioners despite the legal requirement to do so.[37] The rights of physicians and health care institutions to refuse to provide health care that conflicts with deeply held beliefs is well ensconced in both US federal and state laws, in what are referred to as "conscience clauses."

US Federal Law

In 2019, a politically conservative administration issued a final rule[a] that broadened federal protections for health care providers exercising a conscientious objection and expanded enforcement for existing conscience laws protecting the religious rights of health care workers and institutions.[51–53] Although a primary focus of the many of the protections in question related to abortion, they also included sterilization, transgender care, assisted suicide, advance directives, and vaccinations and included language that suggested it could be used to expand the scope of federal laws to apply to additional procedures and treatments. The new rule was vacated almost immediately by three federal courts, but a revision proposed in January 2023 retained many of the aspects of the original 2019 rule.[54,55] A summary of the progression of major federal legislation protecting conscientious objection can be found in **Table 1**.[56–60]

US State Laws

As of late 2019, 46 states had adopted conscience protections relating to abortion, many of which regarded sterilization and contraception. Twenty-six states imposed no conditions on the rights to refuse to treat. Only 13 states limited conscience

---

[a] Final rules are administrative rules issued to implement a new regulation, modify and existing one, or rescind a previous one for federal agencies. The rules are issued, usually after a period of public comment, when the federal agency has reached a conclusion that the rule will solve a previously identified problem in a regulation or better accomplish the goals behind the regulation. Rules are not legislation that is voted-on by elected officials. Objections to rules are made through the judicial system or by introduction of laws countermanding them. See Refs.[52,53]

Table 1
Examples of US federal laws addressing conscientious objection

The First Amendment of the US Constitution	The "Free Exercise" Clause Prohibits Government Interference with a person's Exercise of Their Religious Beliefs.
The Church Amendment (named for Frank Church, senator from Idaho)—a part of the Health Programs Extension Act of 1973	A response to the Supreme Court's ruling in Roe v. Wade (providing certain federal protections for obtaining abortion services) prohibited entities that receive federal funds from requiring providers or health care facilities to perform or assist in sterilizations or abortions
The Federal Religious Freedom Restoration Act (1993)	Augmented the First Amendment by requiring that laws of "general applicability" (ie, they applied to all individuals without regard for religion) at the federal, state, and local level could only interfere with free exercise of religion if there was a compelling government interest and could only do so in the least restrictive way. This law was expanded later to include corporations. Legally, health care institutions were not required to disclose religious or conscience-related restrictions on medical services in advance and do not require referrals to "willing providers"
The Coates-Snow Amendment (1996)	Prohibited discrimination against any health care entities, including physicians or postgraduate training programs (or their participants) that refuse to undergo training in pregnancy termination or refuse to make referrals to "willing providers"
The Affordable Care Act (2010)	Does not require health insurance to cover abortion as an essential health benefit, and does not permit insurance plans to discriminate against institutions or providers who refuse to provide, pay for, cover, or refer for abortions. It also explicitly protects conscientious objection to participating in physician-assisted suicide.

From[56–60]

objection during emergencies, 4 for miscarriages, and 3 for ectopic pregnancy.[61] There is evidence that patients have been injured as a result of denial of abortion under conscience laws, even when it seems to be in violation of the standard of care,[38] but 37 states provide immunity from civil liability in such cases, and legal remedies are limited when harm occurs.[61,62] Only five states require advance notice to patients of care refusals (Nebraska, Illinois, New York, Oregon, and Pennsylvania).[61] Two states require referral to a willing provider (Georgia and Illinois), and two states require that information be given to patients regarding alternative access to the care (Illinois and New York).[61]

Conscience clauses apply to individuals and health care institutions and to other aspects of health care management as well. In 2020, the Department of Health and Human Services Office for Civil Rights sanctioned the state of California, which had mandated that all insurance plans provide abortion coverage since 2014.[63]

Concerns about broad conscience protections in medicine are that they are one-sided, and "privilege the doctor over vulnerable patients, deny patients care that conforms with nationally and professionally accepted guidelines, contradict long-standing principles relating to informed consent, and leave the patient or their family without means of redress for harm resulting from the refusal,"[64] and not all conscience protections make exceptions for when violations of professional standards of care occur. Many ethicists worry that religious, ethical, or moral objections may be used merely as pretexts for discrimination in the US health care system, in which implicit and explicit discrimination is already well established.[64]

SUMMARY

In the course of medical practice, physicians regularly encounter ethical questions and dilemmas, some of which challenge them to choose between providing standard and acceptable medical treatments and following their own deeply personal, moral beliefs that oppose such treatments. The law protects, and ethical principles support the rights of physicians to conscientiously object to providing care that would cause them severe moral distress. However, those rights are ethically limited, and protecting patient interests remains the single, central moral obligation of medical practice. Conscientious objections sometimes present risks of patient harm, reduced patient access to care, denial of emergency services, or promotion of intolerable societal consequences, such as systematic discrimination against classes of people. On the other hand, conscientious objectors are important to the profession; their presence promotes ethical diversity, alternative perspectives, reconsideration of outdated principles, and commitment to the moral integrity of the practitioner. Moreover, ethical obligations of physicians to each other include a commitment to find respectful resolutions when a physician faces an intolerable moral threat.

Whenever possible, physicians and institutions on each side of the objection should seek to resolve moral threats and find accommodations for their colleagues that respect the concept of moral integrity while acknowledging and mitigating as far as possible the burdens the accommodation imposes. Not all conscientious objections can be anticipated in advance, but whenever an objection can be anticipated, objectors are obliged to notify patients and institutions, so that all can work together to find reasonable solutions. Solutions may include allowing practitioners to avoid specific care situations that present such threats or encouraging conscientious objectors to seek out practices that do not present known objections.

Not all objections can be accommodated, and in all cases, patient interests remain the central, most important ethical obligation of physicians. When it is not possible to provide an accommodation and a conscientious objector refuses to provide care, they have an ethical obligation to refer the patient to another willing provider in a timely manner—or even to proceed with the care if the result of a refusal would result in irreversible patient harm.[42,65]

CLINICS CARE POINTS

- Conscientious objection in medicine creates ethical obligations for the objector, their colleagues/institution as well as patients.

- Before raising a conscientious objection, an objector should consider whether their discomfort with providing care arises out of a deep moral belief or is based on some other principle, for example, a concern that the care is not medically appropriate for this particular patient in this particular clinical situation. Other types of objections call for different solutions than conscientious objection. In some situations, it might be appropriate to obtain consultation with colleagues about medical decision-making and have further discussions with the patient before declaring a conscientious objection.
- An objector should consider whether the conscientious objection they are contemplating violates important medical ethical principles—does the objection discriminate against a certain class of patients—create insurmountable barriers for the patient to obtain the care elsewhere, or increase risk to the patient in an emergency situation? In such cases, most ethicists believe that an objection should not be accommodated.
- An objector should consider the burdens that their objection imposes on colleagues and institutions and to the best of their ability offers mitigation to the burdens. Can they pick up other cases of equal stress to balance the additional burden their colleagues will assume?
- An objector should supply advance notice to colleagues about concerns related to the care requested by the patient and their implications, when they are identified. By doing so, there is the opportunity to make accommodations that are mutually acceptable to all parties.
- Finally, an objector should consider whether adjustments in an individual's practice focus or location will allow them to avoid situations that raise moral distress.
- Colleagues of conscientious objectors should be aware that accommodation of conscientious objection is not only required by law but also offers benefits to the profession a whole.
- Colleagues also have ethical obligations to support colleagues with allowable conscientious objections because supporting moral health is important in maintaining integrity in the profession and professional satisfaction.
- Conscientious objectors deserve—and physician colleagues are ethically obliged to provide—respectful acknowledgment of the objection and sincere efforts to attain an acceptable accommodation for all, provided the objection does not create unacceptable discrimination, unacceptable barriers to patients who want to obtain care, or other unacceptable violation of norms of ethical norms of the medical profession.

DISCLOSURE

The author serves as an Editorial Board member for Clinical Reviews and update reviewer for Procedures Videos for Elsevier Inc, Philadelphia PA. The author has no other financial interests or funding relevant to this publication.

REFERENCES

1. Piers RD, Azoulay E, Ricou B, et al. Perceptions of appropriateness of care among European and Israeli intensive care unit nurses and physicians. JAMA 2011;306:2694–703.
2. Lawrence RE, Curlin FA. Physicians' beliefs about conscience in medicine: a national survey. Acad Med 2009;84:1276–82.
3. Roe v. Wade (1973). Legal Information Institute. Available at: https://www.law.cornell.edu/wex/roe_v_wade_%281973%29 Accessed October 5, 2023.
4. Sawaki NN. The conscience defense to malpractice. Loyola University Chicago, School of law. LAW eCommons. 2020. Available at: https://lawecommons.luc.edu/cgi/viewcontent.cgi?article=1680&context=facpubs Accessed October 5, 2023.

5. Morrison SD, Nolan IT, Santosa K, et al. Conscientious objection to gender-affirming surgery: institutional experience and recommendations. Plast Reconstr Surg 2023;152:217–20.

6. Ejiogu NI. Conscientious objection, intersex surgeries, and a call for perioperative justice. Anesth Anag 2020;131:1626–8.

7. Wicclair MR. Conscientious objection in health care: an ethical Analysis. Cambridge UK: Cambridge University Press; 2011.

8. Rhodes R. Conscience, conscientious objections and medicine. Theor Med Bioeth 2019;40:487–506.

9. Symons X. Two conceptions of conscience and the problem of conscientious objection. J Med Ethics 2017;43:245–7.

10. Giubilini A. Objection to conscience: an argument against conscience exemptions in healthcare. Bioethics 2017;31:400–8.

11. Sulmasy DP. What is conscience and why is respect for it so important? Theoret Med Bioethics 2008;29:135–49.

12. Eberl JT. Protecting reasonable conscientious refusals in health care. Theoret Med Bioethics 2019;40:565–81.

13. Rousseau J-J. Emile, or on Education. New York, NY: Basic Books; 1979. Translated by Allan Bloom.

14. Card RF. Reasons, reasonability and establishing conscientious objector status in medicine. J Med Ethics 2017;43:222–5.

15. Card, Zolf B. No conscientious objection without normative justification: against conscientious objection in medicine. Bioethics 2019;33:146–53.

16. U.S. Supreme Court; Employment Division, Department of Human Resources of Oregon v. Smith. April 17, 1990. Available at: https://supreme.justia.com/cases/federal/us/494/872/#tab-opinion-1958252 Accessed March 27, 2023.

17. Maclure J, Durmont I. Selling conscience short: a response to Schuklenk and Smalling on conscientious objections by medical professionals. J Med Ethics 2017;43:241–4.

18. Verkade M, Karsten J, Koenraadt F, et al. Conscience as a regulatory function: an integrative theory put to the test. Int J Offender Ther Comp Criminol 2020;64:375–95.

19. Kochanska G, Aksan N. Children's conscience and self-regulation. J Pers 2006;74:1587–617.

20. Pies R. The ruined good boy. Am J Psychiatry 2011;168:1145–6.

21. Brown J, Goodridge D, Thorpe L, et al. Factors influencing practitioners who do not participate in ethically complex, legally available care: scoping review. BMC Med Ethics 2021;22:134.

22. Desmond Thomas Doss. The Congressional medal of Honor Society. Available at: https://www.cmohs.org/recipients/desmond-t-doss Accessed October 6, 2023.

23. Maddow R. Conscientious objectors to Trump border policy get free legal aid. MSNBC news. June 21, 2018 Available at: https://www.msnbc.com/rachel-maddow/watch/conscientious-objectors-to-trump-border-policy-get-free-legal-aid-1261516355689 Accessed October 6, 2023.

24. Williams A. Understanding conscientious objection and the acceptability of its practice in primary care. New Bioeth 2022;(Dec 14):1–25.

25. Wicclair MR. Conscientious objection in medicine. Bioethics 2000;14:205–27.

26. Wicclair MR. Preventing conscientious objection in medicine from running amok: a defense of reasonable accommodation. Theor Med Bioeth 2019;40:539–64.

27. Bayles MD. A problem of clean hands: refusal to provide professional services. Soc Theory Prac 1979;5:165–81.

28. Howard D. Civil disobedience, not merely conscientious objection, in medicine. HEC Forum 2021;33:215–32.
29. Combs MP, Anteil RM, Tilburt JC, et al. Conscientious refusals to refer: findings from a national physician survey. J Med Ethics 2011;37:397–401.
30. Lipora C, Goodin R. Assessing acts of complicity. In: On complicity and Compromise. Oxford UK: Oxford University Press; 2013. p. 97–129.
31. Emmerich N. Conscientious objection and the referral requirement a morally permissible moral mistakes. J Med Ethics 2023;49:189–95.
32. Stahl RY, Emanuel EJ. Physicians, not conscripts—conscientious objection in health care. N Eng J Med 2017;376:1380–5.
33. Savulescu J, Schuklenk U. Doctors have no right to refuse medical assistance in dying, abortion or contraception. Bioethics 2017;31:162–70.
34. Shuklenk U, Smalling R. Why medical professionals have no moral claim to conscientious objection accommodation in liberal democracies. J Med Ethics 2017; 43:234–40.
35. Carry your own load of responsibility. The Watchtower Announcing Jehovah's Kingdom. 1963 w63 2/15; pp121-5. Available at: https://wol.jw.org/en/wol/d/r1/lp-e/1963127 Accessed October 6, 2023.
36. American Society of Anesthesiologists. Guidelines for the Ethical Practice of Anesthesiology. American Society of Anesthesiologists, Park Ridge, Ill. 2020. Available at: https://www.asahq.org/standards-and-practice-parameters/guidelines-for-the-ethical-practice-of-anesthesiology Accessed October 5, 2023.
37. Davis JM, Haining CM, Keogh LA. A narrative literature review of the impact of conscientious objection by health professionals on women's access to abortion worldwide 2013-2021. Glob Public Health 2022;17:2190–220.
38. Kaye J, Amiri B, Melling L, Dalven J. Health care denied. American Civil Liberties Union. May 2016. Available at: https://www.aclu.org/issues/reproductive-freedom/religion-and-reproductive-rights/health-care-denied Accessed October 6, 2023.
39. Meyer H. Hospital merger in Washington state stokes fears about Catholic limits on care. KFF Health News. August 3, 2020. Available at: https://kffhealthnews.org/news/hospital-merger-in-washington-state-stokes-fears-about-catholic-limits-on-care/#:~:text=Already%2C%201%20in%206%20U.S.%20hospital%20beds%20are,systems%20to%20be%20released%20in%20September%20by%20Merger Watch. Accessed October 6, 2023.
40. Koksvik G. Practical and ethical complexities of MAiD: examples from Quebec. Wellcome Open Res. 2020; v5. Available at: https://www.ncbi.nlm.nih.gov/pmc/articles/PMC8063540/pdf/wellcomeopenres-5-18114.pdf Accessed October 5, 2023.
41. Little M, Lyerly AD. The limits of conscientious refusal: a duty to ensure access. AMA Virtual Mentor 2013;15:257–62.
42. Beauchamp TL, Childress JF. Principles of Biomedical ethics. 8th Edition. Oxford UK: Oxford University Press; 2019.
43. Lewis-Newby M, Wicclair M, Pope T, et al. An official American Thoracic Society policy statement: managing conscientious objections in intensive care medicine. Am J Respir Crit Care Med 2015;191:219–27.
44. Jackson S, Hunter J, Van Norman GA. Ethical Principles Do Not Support Mandatory Preanesthesia Pregnancy Screening Tests: A Narrative Review, . Anesth Analg. https://doi.org/10.1213/ANE.0000000000006669.
45. Harter TD. Towards accommodating physicians' conscientious objections: an argument for public disclosure. J Med Ethics 2015;41:224–8.

46. AMA Code of Medical Ethics, Opinion 1.1.7 Physician exercise of conscience. Available at: https://code-medical-ethics.ama-assn.org/ethics-opinions/physician-exercise-conscience Accessed October 5, 2023.
47. ASA Committee Ethics Committee's Statement on Ethical Guidelines for the Anesthesia Care of Patients with Do-Not-Resuscitate orders. Approved Oct 17, 2001; Reaffirmed Oct 17, 2018. Available at: https://www.asahq.org/standards-and-practice-parameters/statement-on-ethical-guidelines-for-the-anesthesia-care-of-patients-with-do-not-resuscitate-orders Accessed October 6, 2023.
48. Munthe C. Conscientious objection in healthcare: the Swedish solution. J Med Ethics 2017;43:257–9.
49. Glauser W. Canada and US going opposite directions on conscientious objection for doctors. CMAJ (Can Med Assoc J) 2018;190:e270–1.
50. White BP, Jeanneret R, Close E, et al. The impact on patients of objections by institutions to assisted dying: a qualitative study of family caregivers' perceptions. BMC Med Ethics 2023;24:22. https://doi.org/10.1186/s12910-023-00902-3. Accessed October 6, 2023.
51. Federal register. Protecting statutory conscience rights in health care; delegations of authority. A rule by the Health and Human Services Department on 05/21/2019. Available at: https://www.federalregister.gov/documents/2019/05/21/2019-09667/protecting-statutory-conscience-rights-in-health-care-delegations-of-authority Accessed Sept 23, 2023.
52. Informal rulemaking. Ballotpedia. Available at: https://ballotpedia.org/Informal_rulemaking Accessed September 23, 2023.
53. U.S. Government Office of Information and Regulatory Affairs. Reg Map. Available at: https://www.reginfo.gov/public/reginfo/Regmap/index.jsp Accessed September 23, 2023.
54. Federal register. Safeguarding the Rights of Conscience as Protected by Federal Statutes. Available at: https://www.federalregister.gov/documents/2023/01/05/2022-28505/safeguarding-the-rights-of-conscience-as-protected-by-federal-statutes Accessed Sept 23, 2023.
55. Callighan P, Brodsky J. HHS issues proposed rule to provide clarity on rights of conscience in healthcare. SheppardMullin In the Know. Jan 26, 2023 Available at: https://www.smintheknow.com/2023/01/hhs-issues-proposed-rule-to-provide-clarity-on-rights-of-conscience-in-healthcare/#more-85710.
56. First Amendment. Cornell Law School legal Information Institute .Available at: https://www.law.cornell.edu/constitution/first_amendment Accessed October 6, 2023.
57. James N. The Church amendment: in search of enforcement. Wash & Lee L Rev 2011;68:717–63.
58. Cornell Law School Legal Information Institute. 42 U.S. Code § 2000bb—Congressional findings and declaration of purposes. Available at: https://www.law.cornell.edu/uscode/text/42/2000bb Accessed October 6, 2023.
59. Cornell Law School Legal Information Institute. 42 U.S. code § 238n—abortion related discrimination in governmental activities regarding training and licensing of physicians. Available at: https://www.law.cornell.edu/uscode/text/42/238n Accessed October 6, 2023.
60. Cornell Law School Legal Information Institute. 42.U.S. code §18023(b)(4) Available at: https://www.law.cornell.edu/uscode/text/42/18023 Accessed October 6, 2023.
61. Sawaki NN. Protections from civil liability in state abortion conscience laws. JAMA 2019;322:1918–20.

62. Kogan R, Kraschel KL, Haupt CE. Which legal approaches help limit harms to patients from clinicians' conscience-based refusals? AMA J Ethics 2020;22: E209–16.
63. Rubin R. Government cites California for violating federal conscience laws. JAMA 2020;323:1123. https://doi.org/10.1001/jama.2020.301.
64. Fry-Bowers EK. A matter of conscience: examining the law and policy of conscientious objection in health care. Policy Polit Nurs Pract 2020;21:120–6.
65. FIGO Committee for the Ethical Aspects of Human Reproduction and Women's Health. FIGO Committee Report: Ethical guidelines on conscientious objection. Int J Gyn Obstet 2006;92:333–4.

Moving?

Make sure your subscription moves with you!

To notify us of your new address, find your **Clinics Account Number** (located on your mailing label above your name), and contact customer service at:

Email: journalscustomerservice-usa@elsevier.com

800-654-2452 (subscribers in the U.S. & Canada)
314-447-8871 (subscribers outside of the U.S. & Canada)

Fax number: 314-447-8029

Elsevier Health Sciences Division
Subscription Customer Service
3251 Riverport Lane
Maryland Heights, MO 63043

*To ensure uninterrupted delivery of your subscription, please notify us at least 4 weeks in advance of move.

Printed and bound by CPI Group (UK) Ltd, Croydon, CR0 4YY

08/05/2025

01864751-0001